D1195927

Memory, Brain, and Belief

Memory, Brain, and Belief

Edited by

Daniel L. Schacter
Elaine Scarry

Harvard University Press

Cambridge, Massachusetts
London, England / 2000

Copyright © 2000 by the President and Fellows of Harvard College
All rights reserved
Printed in the United States of America

Library of Congress Cataloging-in-Publication Data

Memory, brain, and belief / edited by Daniel L. Schacter and Elaine Scarry.
    p.   cm.
  Includes bibliographical references and index.
  ISBN 0-674-00061-7 (alk. paper)
  1. Memory Congresses. 2. Belief and doubt Congresses.
3. Cognitive neuroscience Congresses. I. Schacter, Daniel L.
[DNLM: 1. Memory Disorders—physiopathology Congresses. 2. Brain
Congresses. 3. Delusions Congresses. 4. Knowledge Congresses.
5. Memory—physiology Congresses. 6. Self Concept Congresses. WM
173.7 M53253   2000]
QP406.M44   2000
612.8'2—dc21
DNLM/DLC
for Library of Congress   99-40552

Acknowledgments

This volume is based on presentations at a three-day conference entitled "Memory and Belief" held at Harvard University May 16–18, 1997. The conference was sponsored by the Harvard Mind/Brain/Behavior Initiative, an interfaculty undertaking at the university dedicated to fostering new interdisciplinary approaches in research and teaching. We gratefully acknowledge the support of the initiative's leaders, Anne Harrington and Jerome Kagan, during the conception and planning of the conference. Ideas about the conference evolved in the context of a working group that met regularly to discuss memory and belief. We are thankful to members of the working group—Emery Brown, Joseph Coyle, Daniel Gilbert, Jerry Green, Jerome Kagan, and Robert Savoy—for intellectual stimulation and pragmatic advice that greatly improved the quality of the conference and of this volume.

Angela Healy provided extensive administrative support during all phases of conference planning and ensured that the meeting ran smoothly. Carrie Racine, an important member of the Schacter laboratory, has made invaluable contributions to the final preparation of the manuscript, carefully following up on and resolving all queries and inconsistencies. We are also extremely grateful to all the conference participants for their stimulating talks and chapters, which will no doubt enrich understanding of the relations among memory, brain, and belief.

D.L.S.

E.S.

Contents

Memory, Brain, and Belief

Introduction

Daniel L. Schacter
Elaine Scarry

Memory is central to mental functioning and plays a key role in numerous aspects of our everyday lives. Recollecting the concert we attended last week, recalling the plot of a favorite novel, acquiring the knowledge and skills to perform a new job—each of these and countless other cognitive feats depend on the effective operation of our memory systems. Without memory, our awareness would be confined to an eternal present and our lives would be virtually devoid of meaning.

In view of the pervasive role that memory plays in our everyday lives, it is perhaps not surprising that memory has been studied intensively by scientists and scholars in a variety of disciplines, ranging from cognitive psychology and neuroscience to psychoanalysis, history, and literary studies. Yet for the most part, studies of memory have proceeded within the boundaries of traditional scientific and scholarly disciplines, with relatively few attempts to bring together the insights of scientists and scholars who approach memory from the vantage points afforded by different disciplinary perspectives.

During the past several years, we have taken part in a small working group of scholars who have attempted to examine issues related to memory from a variety of disciplinary perspectives in both the sciences and the humanities, including cognitive psychology, social psychology, neurobiology, psychiatry, religious studies, economics, and literary analysis. Our memory working group has evolved within the context of Harvard University's Initiative in Mind/Brain/Behavior

1

(MBB)—an interdisciplinary undertaking that focuses on multilevel analyses of issues of mind, brain, and behavior. When the group was formed in 1993, we focused intensively on the nature of memory distortion: the ways in which, and mechanisms by which, the past may be sometimes remembered inaccurately. In May 1994 the working group organized a conference on memory distortion that brought together cognitive psychologists, neurobiologists, psychiatrists, historians, and sociologists. The conference sparked extensive discussion and debate concerning the bases of memory distortion at levels ranging from cells and synapses, to neural and mental systems, even to social groups (see Schacter, 1995, for the edited volume based on the conference that examines each of these levels of analysis).

In the aftermath of the memory distortion conference, the memory working group continued to meet and discuss pertinent issues, with discussion often focusing on the relations between cognitive and social expressions of memory on the one hand, and the brain bases of memory on the other. During these stimulating discussions of the relation between memory and brain, we often found ourselves confronting a seemingly inscrutable but undeniably important issue: the nature of belief and its role in memory. The problem was brought into focus most clearly by the large and ever-growing literature on so-called false memories, whereby people sometimes develop vivid and detailed recollections of events that never happened (Ceci, 1995; Conway, 1997; Loftus, 1997; Roediger, 1996; Schacter, 1999; Schacter, Norman, and Koutstaal, 1998). Perhaps the most striking feature of such inaccurate memories is that they are often expressed as powerful, seemingly unshakable beliefs about the past. Even though the events in question are sometimes highly unlikely or impossible—such as abductions by high-tech aliens or incidents from past lives—people nonetheless cling tenaciously to what Ceci (1995) has aptly referred to as "false beliefs."

Viewed from the perspective of what we ordinarily mean when we use the term "belief," observations of false beliefs about the past are perhaps not entirely surprising. For example, Webster's dictionary defines *belief* as "confidence in the truth or existence of something not immediately susceptible to a rigorous proof." To the extent that beliefs are defined by a subjective conviction about the truth of an assertion that cannot be proven, then memory could be viewed as a type of belief: it is often difficult to offer any "rigorous proof" of what did or did not happen in the past. And because memory is a fundamentally constructive process that is sometimes prone to error and distortion, it makes sense that such beliefs are occasionally misguided.

In addition to our construction of memory as a kind of belief about the past, discussions within the memory working group of pertinent literature quickly led us to see other possibly interesting relations between memory and belief. Studies concerned with the phenomenon of *retrospective bias* have revealed that one's memories of past experiences can be influenced by one's current beliefs. For example, various studies have shown that recollections of past political views can be distorted significantly by present political beliefs (Dawes, 1991; Levine, 1997). Similarly, exposure to material that influences one's beliefs about the value of such simple everyday activities as brushing one's teeth can likewise alter one's recollections of how often one carried out the activity (Ross, 1989). Retrospective biases of this kind have potentially significant implications for understanding how the stories we tell about our pasts—our autobiographical memories—are shaped by the beliefs we hold in the present (Conway and Rubin, 1993; Rubin, 1996; Schacter, 1996).

Just as memories are shaped by beliefs, so too are beliefs shaped by memories. In a phenomenon known as the *illusory truth effect,* for instance, mere repetition of a statement can lead to increases in the strength of one's belief that the statement is true (for an example see Begg, Anas, and Farinacci, 1992). Related research exploring nonconscious influences of past experience on current thought and behavior—known in cognitive psychology as implicit memory (Roediger, 1990; Schacter, 1987)—has shown that recent experiences can implicitly influence social judgments and beliefs (Greenwald and Banaji, 1995). Such phenomena suggest that our beliefs about the world may be more malleable than previously suspected.

Faced with these intriguing and seemingly rich points of intersection between memory and belief, and continuing to examine the way in which memory depends on brain activity, members of our working group concluded that the time was right to bring together scientists and scholars whose research and theorizing explores aspects of the relations among memory, brain, and belief. This volume is based on a

May 1997 conference at which all of the contributors presented and discussed their research.

Westbury and Dennett initiate the volume with a philosophical treatment of fundamental conceptions regarding memory and belief. As they note, both terms are susceptible to being used in multiple, sometimes confusing ways that can undermine any attempt to understand the nature of the relations between the two. These authors provide a useful historical overview of the ways in which philosophers have attempted to delineate the boundary conditions of both memory and belief, and they describe remaining—and still vexing—terminological and theoretical obstacles to exploring their relations. Although experimental scientists are familiar with issues related to the definition of "memory," and manage to use the term productively in their day-to-day research, the term "belief" is considerably less familiar and perhaps more problematic. Following Westbury and Dennett's lead, a number of the contributors who explicitly examine the nature of belief attempt to come to grips with defining the term. As will become apparent to the reader progressing through the volume, we are still some distance from an adequate working definition of belief that is shared across scientists and scholars. We are hopeful that the present volume will stimulate discussion and analysis that will ultimately lead to a shared definition of belief that will facilitate investigation of its relation to memory and brain.

The chapters in Part I offer cognitive, neurological, and pathological perspectives on relations among memory, brain, and belief. Each of the chapters provides striking illustrations of various aberrations of memory and belief, presents preliminary evidence illuminating how such disruptions in cognition depend on underlying brain processes, and considers theoretical ideas that are beginning to elucidate these fascinating phenomena. Johnson and Raye focus on cognitive and neural aspects of false memories and beliefs. They outline a conceptual model, known as the source monitoring framework, that emphasizes the constructive nature of remembering and believing and delineates the component processes on which they are based. These authors describe conditions in which inaccurate or false memories may be heightened, such as following damage to certain sectors of the frontal lobes, and also examine delusional beliefs in schizophrenic patients. They dissect these conditions from the perspective of the source monitoring framework, and describe converging evidence from studies of brain activity in healthy individuals that provide beginning insights into the neural processes that mediate remembering and believing.

Ramachandran describes an array of intriguing—and often bizarre—aberrations of memory and belief, and elucidates the nature of these conditions with cleverly conceived clinical experiments. Stroke patients with frank paralysis who nonetheless believe they can move their limbs, or who believe that familiar loved ones are impostor duplicates of the missing real person, are shocking to us because of the sheer magnitude of the cognitive distortions that the patients exhibit. Ramachandran enlists such cases in an emerging experimental epistemology that seeks to illuminate the mechanisms that produce these strange departures from normal memory and belief.

Frith and Dolan focus primarily on elucidating the nature of delusional perceptions and beliefs in schizophrenia and related conditions. They examine a variety of issues concerning both psychological and neurobiological aspects of the phenomena, including whether false perceptions are sufficient to explain false beliefs; the role of central monitoring processes in delusions; the relation between delusions and memory loss, as seen in the condition known as psychogenic amnesia; and the nature of memory distortion, as seen in confabulations of brain-damaged patients and false memories in healthy individuals. In addition, Frith and Dolan enrich their analysis with cutting edge data from studies using new neuroimaging techniques such as positron emission tomography (PET) and functional magnetic resonance imaging (fMRI) to illuminate the brain systems involved in remembering and believing. They focus in particular on the integrative role of the right prefrontal cortex and its possible function in the delusions and confabulations considered elsewhere in the chapter.

Part II of the volume examines the relation between conscious and nonconscious aspects of memory and belief and their relation to underlying brain mechanisms. Prior to the past decade or two, analyses of memory tended to focus on intentional, conscious recollections of past experiences. But beginning in the 1980s and continuing to the present, a growing number of studies have examined nonconscious influences of past experiences on subsequent performance and behavior—a type of memory most commonly referred to as implicit memory (Schacter, 1987). Numerous experiments have documented the existence of implicit memory in simple laboratory paradigms involving the study and testing of lists of words, pictures, and other materials (for reviews see Roediger and McDermott, 1993; Schacter and Buckner, 1998). More recently, research on implicit memory has been extended into the domain of social cognition, where new experimental paradigms are beginning to uncover fascinating and potentially important implicit influences on social beliefs and judgments. Banaji and Bhaskar review their own experimental evidence and that of others for the operation of such influences, describing experiments that use implicit testing techniques to reveal the operation of gender and racial stereotyping. They couch their theoretical discussion in the context of what they call the "humbling view" that behavior is not classically rational but rather boundedly rational—subject to limitations imposed by cognitive and memory abilities that result in various kinds of biases and other deviations from so-called optimal behavior. Banaji and Bhaskar consider the import of their data and theory on the operation of implicit social beliefs in real-world contexts.

Research on memory has benefited greatly from the development of animal models that allow researchers to unravel the complex web of brain structures and neurochemical influences underlying different forms of memory. A number of researchers have developed animal models that allow the separation of implicit memory (sometimes referred to as nondeclarative or procedural memory) from explicit memory (sometimes referred to as declarative memory; see for example Eichenbaum, 1994; Squire, 1994). However, one would be hard pressed to find any treatment of issues pertaining to belief in nonhuman animals. Eichenbaum and Bodkin take on the somewhat daunting task of extending work and thinking concerning animal memory into the domain of belief. They adopt the position that belief and knowledge can be viewed as distinct forms of memory. Whereas we ordinarily think of beliefs as propositions, often expressed in a verbal manner, Eichenbaum and Bodkin conceptualize belief as "a disposition to behave in a manner that is resistant to correction by experience." By contrast, they construe knowledge as "a disposition to behave that is constantly subject to corrective modification and updating by experience." Armed with these general definitions, Eichenbaum and Bodkin attempt to relate belief and knowledge to the performance of experimental animals on tests that are sensitive to different types of memory. They provide striking illustrations of how damage to the hippocampal formation can produce highly inflexible types of behavior that reflect, from their perspective, the operation of fixed beliefs. They also consider the relation between these phenomena and examples of implicit memory in humans, touching on the implications of their views for understanding pathological conditions such as psychosis, obsessive-compulsive disorder, and hysterical disorders.

Tulving and Lepage focus on the nature of awareness in memory for past events. They draw a sharp distinction between *consciousness,* a general capability of the brain that does not require an object (that is, one can be in a general state of consciousness), and *awareness,* a particular expression of the capability for consciousness that always has an object (one is always aware of something). They examine different forms of awareness of past events, drawing special attention to an "autonoetic" awareness that involves the ability to reexperience past events and imagine future ones. The crucial importance of this trait is illustrated by the case of an amnesic patient characterized by a selective and total loss of the capacity for autonoetic awareness. Turning to recent neuroimaging research, Tulving and Lepage summarize recent studies from their laboratory using positron emission tomography and event-related potentials to examine the nature of various forms of awareness for past events. Like Frith and Dolan, they are particularly concerned with the role of the frontal lobes in retrieval of past episodes.

The four chapters that constitute Part III of the volume consider memory and belief in autobiographical narratives from the perspective of psychologists who study autobiographical memory experimentally (Ross and Wilson, Nelson), or from the perspective of literary scholars who analyze the nature of autobiographies (Eakin, Bok). Ross and Wilson describe a pervasive phenomenon of human memory: current beliefs can shape and sometimes distort recollections of past events (see Schacter, 1999). They summarize studies that illustrate the numerous and varied manifestations of such retrospective biases, and propose a theoretical framework that attempts to account for how present beliefs influence appraisals of past selves, focusing in particular on the documented tendency of people to derogate past selves.

Nelson explores the developmental roots of autobiographical memory and belief. She is especially concerned with the roles of social interaction and language development in shaping the gradual emergence of coherent autobiographical narratives in young children. She also discusses the related issue of how memory for past experiences is sometimes changed or distorted by "reactivating" or "rehearsing" aspects of the experience. Examining autobiographical memory development in the broad context of related cognitive changes, Nelson also considers the development of belief, discussing the implications of the young child's seeming inability to grasp the occurrence or nature of mental states in others that involve holding false beliefs. Tying together the various strands, she points out commonalities among the various memory and cognitive abilities that develop between two and five years of age, emphasizing a major role for language in allowing the developing child to move from a "single-mind" representation of reality to a "multilevel" representational scheme.

Eakin, in his analysis of memory and belief in autobiography, explicitly builds on insights derived from developmental analyses of autobiographical memory and related cognitive perspectives that emphasize the constructive nature of remembering. Using as an example Christa Wolf's *Patterns of Childhood,* in which Wolf speaks of certain portions of her past in the first person and others in the second and third person, Eakin explores the role of memory in making possible the most fundamental beliefs about self and identity—the concept of a single, extended self that spans the different periods of one's life. From Eakin's perspective, the extended self is "a fiction of memory" that follows from accounts of memory described by cognitive and developmental psychologists.

Bok examines the nature and function of autobiography in a broad historical context. Examining what she calls "bitterly contested memories," Bok focuses on cases in which different autobiographers—the five children of Sofya and Lev Tolstoy, the French Enlightenment friends-turned-opponents Jean-Jacques Rousseau and Madame Louise d'Epinay—tell fundamentally different and sometimes conflicting stories about the past. To what extent do these accounts reflect the kinds of memory biases discussed by psychologists such as Ross and Wilson, where recollections of the past are altered in line with current beliefs? How can research concerning memory and belief inform our understanding of contested autobiographical recollections? These and related questions arise naturally from Bok's nuanced analysis of battles over the content and meaning of the past.

In his concluding comments, Damasio synthesizes themes developed in the preceding chapters by exploring definitional, conceptual, neurobiological, and pathological aspects of belief in relation to memory and other cognitive and affective phenomena. He suggests a number of ways to bring the analysis of belief into the mainstream of contemporary cognitive neuroscience. It is our hope that this volume will serve to stimulate such a development, and to build bridges between the various disciplines that can enrich our understanding of the relations among memory, brain, and belief.

References

Begg, I. M., Anas, A., and Farinacci, S. (1992). Dissociation of processes in belief: Source recollection, statement familiarity, and the illusion of truth. *Journal of Experimental Psychology: General, 121,* 446–458.

Ceci, S. J. (1995). False beliefs: Some developmental and clinical considerations. In D. L. Schacter (Ed.), *Memory distortion* (pp. 91–128). Cambridge, MA: Harvard University Press.

Conway, M. A. (Ed.). (1997). *Recovered memories and false memories.* Oxford: Oxford University Press.

Conway, M. A., and Rubin, D. C. (1993). The structure of autobiographical memory. In A. F. Collins, S. E. Gathercole, M. A. Conway, and P. E. Morris (Eds.), *Theories of memory* (pp. 103–137). Hillsdale, NJ: Lawrence Erlbaum.

Dawes, R. M. (1991). Biases of retrospection. *Issues in Child Abuse Accusations, 1,* 25–28.

Eichenbaum, H. (1994). The hippocampal system and declarative memory in humans and animals: Experimental analysis and historical origins. In D. L. Schacter and E. Tulving (Eds.), *Memory systems, 1994* (pp. 147–202). Cambridge, MA: MIT Press.

Greenwald, A. G., and Banaji, M. R. (1995). Implicit social cognition: Attitudes, self-esteem, and stereotypes. *Psychological Review, 102,* 4–27.

Levine, L. J. (1997). Reconstructing memory for emotions. *Journal of Experimental Psychology: General, 126*(2), 165–177.

Loftus, E. F. (1997). Memory for a past that never was. *Current Directions in Psychological Science, 6*(3), 60–64.

Roediger, H. L. III. (1990). Implicit memory: A commentary. *Bulletin of the Psychonomic Society, 28,* 373–380.

Roediger, H. L. III. (1996). Memory illusions. *Journal of Memory and Language, 35,* 76–100.

Roediger, H. L. III, and McDermott, K. B. (1993). Implicit memory in normal human subjects. In H. Spinnler and F. Boller (Eds.), *Handbook of neuropsychology,* Vol. 8 (pp. 63–131). Amsterdam: Elsevier.

Ross, M. (1989). Relation of implicit theories to the construction of personal histories. *Psychological Review, 96,* 341–357.

Rubin, D. C. (1995). *Memory in oral traditions: The cognitive psychology of epic, ballads, and counting-out rhymes.* New York: Oxford University Press.

Rubin, D. C. (Ed.). (1996). *Remembering our past: Studies in autobiographical memory.* Cambridge: Cambridge University Press.

Schacter, D. L. (1987). Implicit memory: History and current status. *Journal of Experimental Psychology: Learning, Memory, and Cognition, 13,* 501–518.

Schacter, D. L. (Ed.). (1995). *Memory distortion: How minds, brains, and societies reconstruct the past.* Cambridge, MA: Harvard University Press.

Schacter, D. L. (1996). *Searching for memory: The brain, the mind, and the past.* New York: Basic Books.

Schacter, D. L. (1999). The seven sins of memory. *American Psychologist, 54,* 182–203.

Schacter, D. L., and Buckner, R. L. (1998). Priming and the brain. *Neuron, 20,* 185–195.

Schacter, D. L., Norman, K. A., and Koutstaal, W. (1998). The cognitive neuroscience of constructive memory. *Annual Review of Psychology, 49,* 289–318.

Squire, L. R. (1994). Declarative and nondeclarative memory: Multiple brain systems supporting learning and memory. In D. L. Schacter and E. Tulving (Eds.), *Memory systems, 1994.* Cambridge, MA: MIT Press.

Mining the Past to Construct the Future: Memory and Belief as Forms of Knowledge

1

Chris Westbury
Daniel C. Dennett

The analogy between memory and a repository, and
between remembering and retaining, is obvious and is to
be found in all languages; it being natural to express the
operations of the mind by images taken from things
material. But in philosophy we ought to draw aside the
veil of imagery, and to view them naked.

Thomas Reid,
Essays on the Intellectual Powers of Man *(1815)*

Jacques Monod (1974) observed that "ever since its birth in the Ionian islands almost three thousand years ago, Western philosophy has been divided between two seemingly opposed attitudes. According to one of them the true and ultimate reality of the universe can reside only in perfectly immutable forms, unvarying by essence. According to the other, the only real truth resides in flux and evolution" (p. 98). Three thousand years of argument has so far failed to find a clear resolution to this ancient opposition. There are still two committed camps of "Neats" and "Scruffies," who fall on either side of the fundamental debate identified by Monod. Some of the most exciting points of intersection between the interests of philosophers and scientists today are those at which the apparent incompatibility between the two camps demands to be resolved—those points at which it becomes clear that the stable, neat objects of scientific inquiry are attaining their objective status by managing to separate themselves (often using scruffy means) from an underlying scruffy flux of dynamic phenomena. When we try to understand such objects, questions of science merge unavoidably with questions of epistemology. The questions that interest us about memory and belief exist at this intersection. We will briefly consider each of these phenomena in turn. In

11

doing so, we will try to point out some conceptual confusions that spring from the way we use their names in informal discourse, and emphasize a strong underlying similarity in the ways that memory and belief relate to knowledge.

Memory

Every event in the world has effects, and the chain of effects that spreads from any event continues essentially forever; but only some events leave long-lasting traces. We single out the best cases of this for special notice: footprints, scars, and various sorts of records. Of all the dinosaur footprints that ever pressed into mud, only a tiny fraction are discernible today; of all the clay tablets ever impressed with hieroglyphics, only a select few survive—but like the dinosaur footprints, they permit us to read the past in a way that the other long-lived effects of the same causes do not. Fifty light-years from Earth, a sphere of 1947 Jack Benny broadcasts is expanding into the galaxy, almost certainly unreconstructible by any technology. If those programs were not recorded here on Earth, they would be gone forever. Events that leave no salient long-term traces can be called inert historical facts; they happened, but the difference they made no longer makes a discernible difference. There is no fixed best way to count facts, but by almost any usable method we would have to say that most historical facts are inert. One of the following is a fact: (a) some of the gold in Dennett's teeth once belonged to Julius Caesar; (b) none of the gold in Dennett's teeth ever belonged to Julius Caesar. Although one of these statements is true, it is almost certainly beyond all powers of investigation to determine which.

The past consists of all historical facts, inert or recoverable. The whole point of brains, of nervous systems and sense organs, is to produce future, to permit organisms to develop, in real time, anticipations of what is likely to happen next, the better to deal with it. The only way—the only nonmagical way—organisms can do this is by prospecting and then mining the present for the precious ore of historical facts, the raw materials that are then refined into anticipations of the future. As Norbert Wiener (1948) pointed out long ago, the fundamental method is trajectory sampling or tracking: gathering data about the pattern of change in something of interest, then extrapolating the curve into the future. Whether an organism tracks temperature, or salinity, or the sun, or a prey, or a mate, or the Dow-Jones industrial average, the fundamental problem is the same: preventing selected historical facts from going inert, at least long enough to extract their portent for the future.

In his recent book *On the Origin of Objects,* Brian Smith (1996) avails himself of a similar idea of tracking to develop a metaphysical thesis about how the world came to split itself into the experiencer and the experienced, into organism and object. In discussing memory, he writes, "In order to make a memory more durable than a shadow, a . . . subject must first allow or arrange for an appropriate impression to be formed by the event in question, but must then take responsibility for storing it *in such a way as to ensure that it will continue to be effective* after the event it records has dissipated" (p. 221, emphasis added; see also Plotkin, 1994, pp. 149–152). Only organisms that can retrieve stored information in order to increase the likelihood of achieving some adaptive end will gain any advantage from memory. Memory must be rooted in use.

What is the simplest kind of use to which a rudimentary protomemory might be put? Consider the visual perception of motion or change. An organism's visual system could not tell the difference between something moving from left to right and something moving from right to left unless it had *some* way of getting the data from two moments of time into a single comparison process. Similarly, in order to tell that it is getting warmer, not colder, an organism has to have some way of "remembering" the temperature in the recent past. We put "remembering" in scare-quotes, because although this is the most fundamental form of memory, the basis for all others, it need not be much like conscious recollection. Protozoan memory, or the memory in a tree that reminds it to start pushing out buds in the spring, is not like recalling your first-grade teacher. Yet in one fundamental way, such functional use of stored information *is* like memory—that is why we call it memory, however scare-quoted. Memory in the fundamental sense is the ability to store useful information and to retrieve it in precisely those circumstances and that form which allow it to be useful.

Computer memory is memory in this fundamental sense—and only in this fundamental sense, obviously. The process of changing the electromagnetic properties of tiny areas on chips or disks may create many long-lasting local effects, but only those count as being stored in memory that can later be retrieved by the hardware in the ways intended when they were laid down. Any other changes wrought, however salient, long-lasting, or effective in altering the system's behavior, count as blemishes or scars, not memories. Scars are not memories. A dog whose body shows scars inflicted by some encounter but who exhibits no heightened caution, no discrimination of the harbingers of further scars—in short, who has learned nothing from the encounter—has no useful memory of the encounter, even if we others can read a lot about it in our examination of the scars. *We* can extract information from the traces left by the event; the dog, apparently, cannot.

Where do we draw the line? If one of the effects of the earlier encounter is that the dog now limps, and if this limp usefully avoids pain and further injury to the limb, does this count as memory? We need not answer each such question, but it is important to note that a long-lasting and salient trace is not enough, and that what more must be added—utility—comes in different grades and amounts. At one extreme, we find the paradigmatic cases of memory: conscious, reflective beliefs about the past, made manifest in episodes of articulate recollection: "Share your memories of the war with us, Grandpa." "I'd be delighted to: On April 22, 1943—I can see it as if it were this morning—I woke to the sound of mortar fire. . . . " At the other extreme, we find a slight tendency to crouch when a passing car backfires—all that remains of a past, once-useful response.

This twofold requirement—a trace and its utility—raises a quandary that has bedeviled philosophers and psychologists for several millennia. In its starkest form, it was articulated in Plato's *Meno*. In that early dialogue, the wealthy Meno challenges Socrates with an apparently paradoxical question: How is that we can ever discover anything new, given that we must either know what we are looking for (and therefore have no need to look for it) or not know what we are looking for (in which case we will have no way of recognizing it when we find it)? Socrates' answer is the doctrine that all knowledge is *anamnesis:* the recollection of innate knowledge, obtained from previous lives. It is hardly satisfactory. How, Meno might well have gone on to ask, do we tell veridical recollection from sheer fantasy? Reminiscence is problematical in the same way as knowledge: to recall something, we must already know what it is we are trying to recall (and therefore have no reason to recall it) or else not know it (and so have no ability to recall it).

In the *Theaetetus* Plato introduces two metaphors for memory, comparing it to an image inscribed on a wax tablet, which may be more or less smooth, muddy, and soft, and to a bird in an aviary:

> SOCRATES: Now consider whether knowledge is a thing you can possess in that way without having it about you, like a man who has caught some wild birds—pigeons or what not—and keeps them in an aviary for them at home. In a sense, of course, we might say that he "has" them all the time inasmuch as he possesses them, mightn't we?
>
> THEAETETUS: Yes.
>
> SOCRATES: But in another sense he "has" none of them, though he has got control of them, now that he has made them captive in an enclosure of his own; he can take and have hold of them whenever he likes by catching any bird he chooses, and let them go again; and it is open to him to do that as often as he pleases.

Neither metaphor provides a satisfactory answer to the question raised by Meno. If memory is an image carved in a wax tablet, we must somehow know where to look on the wax tablet, or at which wax tablet to look. If it is a bird in an aviary, we must not only be able to call it, but know which one to call and know that it will come when we call. Hotspur retorts to Glendower when he claims (in Shakespeare's *1 Henry IV*) that he "can call spirits from the vasty deep": "Why, so can I, or so can any man; But will they come when you do call for them?" Meno's problem of needing to know what you need to remember in order to remember it still presents a problem for modern theories of memory.

Plato's student Aristotle devoted a short treatise to the problem of memory (Aristotle, c. 350 B.C./1941), in which he proposed that memory was a picture *(eikon)* of the past thing remembered. This picture was causally related to a past object of perception, which was imprinted into a sense organ that was capable of perceiving it. Aristotle's proposal that the object of memory is an accurate picture of a perception, which can simply be consulted as if it were an object of perception, largely reduces the problem of memory to the problem of perception. In remembering *x,* we know that it is *x* for the same reason (whatever that might be!) that we were able to recognize *x* when we first sensed it, because a memory is simply another "viewing" of that same sensory impression. This viewpoint defines what was to become the standard representative theory of memory. Memory came to be seen as what John Locke (1700) called a "Store-house of our Ideas" (p. 150).[1]

There are numerous problems with the representative theory of memory, most of them echoes of Meno's question. A major difficulty is explaining how we can distinguish between imagination and memory. Aristotle's solution was to introduce the capacity of recognizing elapsed time, which allows one to connect the present memory image to an earlier act of perception. His conception of how this might work rested on a visual analogy, that of seeing objects at different distances (Aristotle, c. 350 B.C./1941, p. 615). Earlier memories have receded farther into the distance, and so are smaller and less distinct, than more recent memories.

David Hume (1739) suggested a way of differentiating memories from images that was similar to Aristotle's suggestion. According to Hume, what differentiated memory ideas from imaginative ideas was not a time stamp but the fact that the ideas of imagination are "fainter and more obscure" than the ideas of memory, which strike one with "superior force and vivacity" (p. 85). Thomas Reid (1815) was critical of Hume's view of memory, arguing that if Hume believed (as he claimed to) that ideas had only a contingent, rather than a necessary, relationship, then there could be no deductive argument that depended on the recognition of a relationship between one idea and another (that is, between a sense idea and a memory idea). Hume had himself recognized the difficulty and tried, in an appendix to his book, to replace the idea of "vivacity" with the idea of "apprehending the idea more strongly or taking a firmer hold of it" (Hume, 1739, p. 624). On this attempt, Reid commented dryly, "There is nothing more meritorious in a philosopher than to retract an error upon conviction, but in this instance I humbly apprehend Mr. Hume claims that merit upon too slight a ground" (Reid, 1815, p. 380). Reid's typically commonsensical solution to the problem begged the question by simply accepting that memory, like sense data, was a form of immediate and noninferential knowledge. (How do I tell a memory from a fantasy, Meno? I just do.)

John Stuart Mill (1869) proposed another mechanism for recognizing a memory as a memory. He suggested that in accessing a memory we run very quickly over all sense impressions since the remembered event, and use our understanding of the total number of events to locate the idea in its temporal location.

> In . . . recollection there is, first of all, the ideas or simple conceptions of the object and acts; and along with those ideas, and so closely combined as not to be separable, the idea of my formerly having had those same ideas. And this idea of my formerly having had those ideas is a very complicated idea, including the idea of myself at the present moment remembering, and that of myself of the past moment conceiving; and the whole series of the states of consciousness, which intervened between myself remembering, and myself conceiving. (pp. 330–331)

Many more recent philosophers have followed Thomas Reid in choosing to leave the difficult idea of "pastness" as an unanalyzed primitive. For example, William James wrote simply that memories were referred back in time by "a general feeling of the past direction of time" (James, 1890, p. 650). Similarly, Bertrand Russell (who ultimately remained skeptical of any necessary connection between memory and belief) suggested that a feeling of pastness and a feeling of familiarity gave rise to a feeling of belief, and that all three were essential constituents of memory (1921, pp. 161–163). (For further discussion of how philosophers subscribing to the representative theory have tried to explain the differentiation of memories from imagination, see Holland, 1954.)

Ironically, it is Plato's theory, rejected by Aristotle more than two thousand years ago, which is perhaps closest in spirit to modern theories of memory. Plato's theory of anamnesis is not to be scoffed at, even if we have to reinterpret his central metaphor in order to make any use of the idea. The main point he was making has been rediscovered again and again: there can be no learning—and so no knowledge—from the base of a tabula rasa. It follows that a memory cannot just be an isolated atomic fact, complete unto itself. James (1890) made this point explicitly, noting that

> what we began calling the "image," or "copy," of the fact in the mind, is really not there at all in that simple shape, as a separate idea. Or at least, if it be there as a separate idea, no memory will go with it. What memory goes with is, on the contrary, a very complex representation, that of the fact to be recalled *plus* its associates, the whole forming one "object" . . . and demanding probably a vastly more intricate brain-process than that on which any simple sensorial image depends. (p. 651; emphasis in original)

F. C. Bartlett (1932) would later reemphasize this same point in his criticisms of Ebbinghaus' early attempts to study memory with "meaningless" stimuli. He too recognized that for a memory to be *recognized,* there has to be *independent knowledge* against which it can be compared—how else? Even Skinnerians appreciated the need for an innate basis for distinguishing reinforcers, positive and negative. It was a failure to deal adequately with this necessity for independent knowledge that caused so many problems for the representationalists—they could find nothing to which their memory image might be compared, in order to recognize it *as* a memory. To compare it to another memory image would hardly do, since that would lead to an infinite regress.

Meno's question about how we can recognize our memories has been recast in its original form, as a question about how to recognize our own knowledge. It is a mistake, as everyone acknowledges, to assume that interpretation of recalled knowledge happens only at the preloading, perceptual stage—to assume that once knowledge "enters memory" (through the front door), it is happily stored away, to be "retrieved" intact at later times of "recollection." Though everyone recognizes this as a bad view, it still haunts discussions subliminally.

The importance of interpretation in accessing memory has of course been known for a long time. Starting with Bartlett's (1932) famous experiments examining the recollection of stories, which led him to conclude that organisms have an "effort after meaning," it has been repeatedly demonstrated that our ability to recall is inextricably linked to our assumptions about how the world is, and is subject to "top-down" schematization dictated by those assumptions (see Goldman, 1986, for a review and analysis of empirical evidence for this claim). What we recall is not what we actually experienced, but rather a reconstruction of what we experienced that is consistent with our current goals and our knowledge of the world. As Bartlett put it: "Remembering is not the re-excitation of innumerable fixed, lifeless, and fragmentary forms. It is an imaginative reconstruction, or construction, built out of the relation of our attitude towards a whole active mass of organized past reactions or experience, and to a little outstanding detail which commonly appears in image or in language form" (1932, p. 213, cited in Zechmeister and Nyberg, 1982, p. 301).

The assessment of what constitutes an acceptable reconstruction of the past must be dynamically computed by an organism under the constraints imposed by its built-in biological biases and the history of the interaction of those biases with the environment in which the organism has lived. The apparently stable objects of memory—the representations of the things being recalled—are not retrieved from some Store-house of Ideas where they have been waiting intact, but rather are constructed on the fly by a computational process. As H. R. Maturana (1970) wrote, "Memory as an allusion to a representation in the learning animal of its past experiences is also a description by the observer of his ordered interactions with the observed animal [which may be the observer himself]; memory as a storage of representations of the environment to be used on different occasions in recall does not exist as a neurophysiological function" (p. 37). What we call recollection can never be more than the most plausible story we come up with (or, perhaps, only a story which is plausible enough) within the context of the constraints imposed by biology and history.

Belief

The word "belief" is difficult to define, in part because it is used in different ways in different contexts. In his closing statements at the conference from which the chapters in this volume have been drawn,

Antonio Damasio pointed out that a person who talked about his beliefs about everyday things—about the shape or purpose of doorknobs, pencils, telephones, and irons—would be taken for either a comic or a lunatic (or, as one of us added, a philosopher!). Damasio was trying to capture a commonly held intuition: that beliefs cannot be about just anything at all; they must be about important or notably uncertain things. In ordinary usage, the term "belief" is reserved for referring only to linguistically encoded convictions and doctrines, not to the mass of unexpressed and widely held background knowledge that we all implicitly use to navigate through our world.

We would not normally be willing to say that a person who makes himself a cup of coffee is thereby expressing his beliefs about the physical characteristics of electrical outlets, coffee machines, ceramic containers, hot liquids, and organic compounds such as coffee beans, sugar, and milk, or even that he is expressing a belief about the desirability of coffee. He is simply making a cup of coffee. However, within the cognitive science and philosophy of mind communities, the word "belief" is often used much more generally, to refer to any implicit or explicit information that guides an agent's voluntary actions. One benefit of this way of thinking is that it allows us to speak of the beliefs of nonhuman agents (see Dennett, 1987a, 1995, 1996). By widening the meaning of the word, we lose certainty about exactly when it applies. Does the duckling who follows Konrad Lorenz truly believe that the large bearded man is its mother? Does the ant following a pheromone trail or the amoeba swimming up a chemical gradient really believe that following those signals will lead to a food supply? When we see a cow in a field, do we believe simultaneously that our eyes are not fooling us, that an object that looks like a cow is a cow, that our memory for names of animals is functioning properly, that we are not dreaming, and so on for the thousands of other propositions that must all be true in order for us to believe that the cow in the field is indeed precisely that? Are we to accept that any cognitive state must encode all the implicit beliefs which must be held in order for that state to be interpreted properly?

We will consider two possible recent approaches to these kinds of questions: the "language of thought" approach and the "intentional stance" approach.

The Language of Thought

The tradition in cognitive science and philosophy of mind that we characterize as the language of thought tradition shares some philosophical roots with the representative theory of memory. This language of thought tradition has considered beliefs to be individual data structures to be found somewhere in the brain (in the Golden Age of Neurocryptology, presumably). To those who hold this strange view, this has seemed to follow from the fact that beliefs are, in philosophical parlance, "propositional attitudes," instances of the formula

$$x \text{ believes that } p,$$

where p is replaced by some sentence expressing the proposition believed. But we need not, and indeed should not, jump so blithely to the conclusion that the beliefs about which we want to have theories in cognitive science are anything like that. To see why not, consider the following experiment, with yourself as subject:[2]

> Here is a joke. See if you get it. (Newfies are people from Newfoundland; they are the Poles of Canada—or the Irish of Canada, if you're British.)
>
> A man went to visit his friend the Newfie and found him with both ears bandaged. "What happened?" he asked, and the Newfie replied, "I was ironing my shirt, you know, and the telephone rang." "That explains one ear, but what about the other?" "Well, you know, I had to call the doctor!"

The experiment yields a positive result if you get the joke. Most people do, but not all. If we were to pause, in the fashion of Eugene Charniak, whose story-understanding AI (artificial intelligence) program (Charniak, 1974) first explored this phenomenon, and ask what one has to believe in order to get the joke, we would generate a very long list of different propositions. We would need to include propositions about the shape of an iron and the shape of a telephone; about the supposed fact that when people are stupid they often cannot simultaneously do different things with the left hand and the right hand; about the fact that the heft of a telephone receiver and an iron are approximately the same; about the fact that when telephones ring, people generally answer them; and many, many more.

What makes the brief narrative a joke and not just a boring story is that it is radically enthymematic; it leaves out a lot of facts and counts on the listener's filling them in, which the listener is able to do only if she believes all those propositions. Now here is a daft theory about how you got the joke—and it is probably not quite fair to Jerry Fodor and other language-of-thought fans, but they haven't offered any alternatives: In come some sentences (exactly the sentences written above), through the eyes of those who read the joke and the ears of those who hear it. Their arrival provokes a mechanism that goes hunting for all the relevant sentences—all those on our list—and soon brings them into a common workspace, where a resolution theorem prover takes over, filling in all the gaps by logical inference.

Some such sententialist theory of cognitive processing is the direction in which Fodor has gestured, but nobody has produced a plausible version. No one believes the theory sketch just given, we trust, but even if it and all its near kin (the other sententialist/inference engine theories) are rejected as theories about how you got the joke, our list of propositions is not for that reason otiose or foolish or spurious. It actually does describe cognitive conditions (very abstractly considered) that do have to be met by anyone who gets the joke.

We can easily imagine running the experiments that would prove this. Strike off one belief on that list and see what happens. That is, find some people who lack that belief (but have all the others) and tell them the joke. They will not get it. They *cannot* get it, because each of the beliefs is necessary for comprehension of the story. In other words, we have counterfactual-supporting generalizations of the following form: If you don't believe (have forgotten) that *p*, then you won't get the joke.

Here is an empirical prediction that relies on the scientific probity of talking about this list of beliefs, even though the items on that list do not refer to anything *salient* in the head, but are mere *abstracta*: This joke will soon be extinct, rendered too obsolete to provoke a laugh in a generation or two. Why? Because in this age of wash-and-wear clothing, young people are growing up without ever having seen anybody iron. Some do not know what an iron looks and feels like, and their numbers are growing. For that matter, telephones are changing shape and heft all the time too, so the essential belief in the similarity of shape and heft of telephone receiver and iron is also going to vanish. That belief is not going to be reliably in the belief pool of normal audiences, so they would not get the joke. You would have to explain it to them—"Well, back in the olden days, irons sorta looked and felt like . . . "—and then of course it would no longer be a joke. This example could be multiplied many times over, showing that the power of folk psychology or the intentional stance as a calculus of abstracta is not in the least threatened by the prospect that no version of Fodor's "language of thought" model of belief is sustained by cognitive neuroscience.

Note that introspection leaves open the question of what cognitive mechanisms are involved in getting the joke. Some people may report having had quite detailed imagery while listening to the joke. Others may say they "got it" with only the faintest traces of imagery. In either case, the list of beliefs on which their amusement depended would be surprisingly long. No one has the experience of consciously entertaining such a lengthy set of propositions, even though it must be true that the information expressed by those propositions is somehow in their possession, and has aptly and swiftly enabled them to see the point.

We should not be fooled by the apparent immediacy of the reaction to the joke—or by the absence of any discernible steps between hearing the joke and getting it, or by the impossibility of listing all the propositions required to get the joke—into thinking that those who get the joke must therefore have made a mental jump that did not require any cognitive representation of the intermediate computational steps. Such a viewpoint simply reflects a "fossil trace" of the Cartesian sententialist metaphor, as if propositions must necessarily be processed in their sentential form simply because it is possible and seems natural to us to state them in that form. The neural processes that allow us to get a joke are, by definition, cognitive processes, however nonsentential, emotionally mediated, parallel, and widely distributed in the brain they may be. The problem facing neuroscientists who wish to understand belief is not to discover *how* "belief propositions" are processed by the brain, but rather to discover *if* beliefs are processed in propositional form at all, and if not, to discover what those neural processes which admit of high-level descriptions in terms of propositional processing are actually computing.[3]

We consider it extremely unlikely that beliefs are represented in the brain as sentence-like data structures. Beliefs are ubiquitous guides and influences on our every action and waking reaction, but they are not the familiar items of daily phenomenology. We are unaware of our beliefs, for the most part. We just act on them. Are such "sub-propositional" beliefs "memories"? In the fundamental sense defined earlier, yes—for they involve the ability to encode useful information and to decode it in precisely those circumstances where it can be useful. In the stronger, more common sense of the word, however, they are not memories. Any use of the brain's plasticity to store information can be counted as memory in the most basic sense, but we must be careful not to conflate this sense of the word with the everyday concept of memory.

The Intentional Stance

Because we do not want to explain beliefs by first assuming their existence, in the manner of the sententialist theories that assume the existence of proposition-like data structures in the brain, we suggest that the most useful way to think of a belief is as an explanatory tool, rather than as an object in need of explaining. Instead of continuing the attempt to define a belief as an entity that an organism might have or not have (in the concrete, binary-valued way that a library can have a particular book or a poem can have a particular line), a belief must be defined in terms of the circumstance under which a belief could be justifiably *attributed* to that organism. What is meant when it is asserted that an organism has a belief, we propose, is that its behavior can be reliably predicted by ascribing that belief to it—an act of ascription we call taking the intentional stance.

The suggestion is not simply that the adoption of such a definition might be a heuristic for sidestepping the question of what a belief "really" is, but the stronger suggestion that all there is to having a belief that p is a system that is efficiently (and, in the strongest cases, most efficiently) predictable under the assumption that it believes that p.

This suggestion is intended to carry ontological, rather than simply methodological, weight.

We do not propose to justify this claim in detail here, as much space has already been devoted to that end elsewhere (see Dennett, 1987a, 1988, 1991). Rather, we want to emphasize only that this definition means that we must define a (propositional) belief in the same way that we have defined a memory, as a particular kind of useful knowledge. To say that x believes that p is to assert that x's behavior (verbal and otherwise) demonstrates a particular kind of regularity; namely, just that kind of regularity which justifies the "projection" (the subjective assumption by the observer) of x's intentionality about p. Although there might be many different ways in which (and mechanisms by which) x can behave so as to allow for the ascription of intentionality about p, we can be sure that the following must be true of all such x's:

1. x must "know how" (in a loose sense that includes "be structured so as") to act in order to produce a regularity that allows for the ascription of p (and, trivially, must either be able to produce it or be unable to produce it for purely mechanical or external, rather than epistemological, reasons);
2. x must be self-motivated (in a loose sense that includes "be structured so as") to produce the regularity described above) (because simply knowing how to state or act in accordance with a belief—or being forced at gunpoint to state or act in accordance with a belief—does not entail believing);
3. the observer (which may be x himself) who is making the attribution to x of a belief that p must be (implicitly or explicitly) satisfied that he is able to discern (independently of whether he actually is able to discern) the regularity that x's behavior demonstrates. In other words, in order to attribute a belief that p, an organism must simultaneously attribute to himself (that is, act in a way that seems to him to accord with) the belief "I know what it means to believe that p." In order to adopt the intentional stance toward others, one must also adopt it toward oneself.

The third requirement is of particular interest, for a couple of reasons.

The first reason is that the requirement that an organism must be satisfied that it is able to discern the intentionality-defining regularity, is recursively dependent on the very requirements to which it belongs. To be able to discern a regularity in x's behavior is to hold a belief about what it means for x to believe that p. It is therefore necessary that the attributor fulfill the three conditions outlined above for attributing a belief (in this case, toward himself): he must know how to act consistently with his belief that x believes that p, must be self-motivated to do so, and must be satisfied that he is able to do so. The recursion is grounded (that is, infinite recursion on the third requirement is avoided) by the fact that the attributor will, by definition, certainly be satisfied that he is able to recognize just those regularities which he himself must be satisfied that he is able to recognize. This is not to say that we must know everything that we believe, which is not necessarily true, but only that, in order to satisfy the above three requirements for believing any proposition p, we must also satisfy those requirements for believing another proposition: namely, the proposition that we know what it means to believe that p.

The second reason that the third requirement is of particular interest is because it states that the intentional stance can be grounded in an organism's own satisfaction with its ability to detect a relevant regularity, rather than its actual (objectively measurable) ability to detect any such regularity. The existence of an implicit or explicit subjective satisfaction that an organism can detect an appropriate regularity with respect to a proposition p (the existence of a belief that it knows what it means to believe that p) in the absence of any empirical supporting evidence is not a rare or unlikely event: jealous lovers who unjustly accuse their mates of infidelity, sports fans who treat their home team as if it had a consistent personality across changes in its membership, and people who believe political campaign promises, among many others in our world, all exhibit signs that they have projected belief onto a system that can be demonstrated to be undeserving of the honor. In a less forgiving world than the one we humans have managed to create for ourselves, such errors would be little tolerated. Natural selection would act as the quick and final judge of which systems for recognizing intentional patterns had sufficient practical utility. In our human world, however, it is possible to mix in a great many idio-syncratically grounded intentional projection systems with the few that are required by us all—hence the great variance in the beliefs that human beings are willing to agree they hold.

Note that the claim that beliefs depend on an organism's ability to self-assess its own beliefs should not be interpreted as supporting a radical epistemological relativism, since it is evident that the most important means by which human beings assess their satisfaction with their beliefs is by being satisfied that they hold the beliefs that society taught them how be satisfied that they held.[4] Children raised to believe that *p* are much more likely to grow up believing that *p* than children raised to believe that not-*p*, a fact which has been the source of considerable distress in the course of recorded human history among the more adamant proponents of not-*p*.

Many of the objections raised against the view of belief offered by the intentional stance spring from a desire once identified by Ludwig Wittgenstein as a "need": the desire to maintain a folk psychological category of belief, which views belief as some sort of mysterious essence inherent in the entity to which the belief is attributed. Wittgenstein (1983) wrote: "If you talk about essence—you are merely noting a convention. But here one would like to retort: there is no greater difference than that between a proposition about the depth of the essence and one about—a mere convention. But what if I reply: to the depth that we see in the essence there corresponds the deep need for a convention" (p. 65).

Acceptance of the view of belief offered by the intentional stance means that a wide variety of objectively different phenomena (including those that may demonstrably be modulated by different brain regions within a single species) may justifiably be called belief. The demand for a definition which defines belief in terms that are independent of situational contingencies is ill founded, in the same way that the demand for a detailed but context-free definition of evolutionary fitness is unfounded. In both cases, the only definitions that can be provided must either be so general as to be unhelpful as an explanatory device in any specific situation (for instance, "an organism is fit because it is well suited for living in its environment") or so specific that no wide generalization of it will be possible (we should not expect to learn much about why swallows have survived as a species from a detailed understanding of the eating and mating habits of a species of jellyfish).

We would like to discourage the demand for a context-independent definition of belief, and encourage the idea that the definition of a belief in any particular circumstance is equivalent to the identification of the contingencies which allow that belief to be attributable. (Language, of course, allows us to produce behaviors that make it very easy to attribute beliefs to ourselves and to each other.) In just the same way that the biologist who wishes to discuss "fitness" must identify the relevant constraints in both the species under discussion and the environment in which its members are competing for the chance to reproduce, we suggest that the psychologist who wishes to discuss "belief" with scientific precision must identify both the environment in which the belief under discussion is attributed (that is, the relevant rules of interpretation under which the attribution is made) and the actions of the organism that fall under those rules of interpretation.[5]

It might be further clarifying to compare the current status of beliefs in scientific terminology with the status of genes prior to Crick and Watson's identification of DNA as the vehicle of genetic transmission. At that point in time, genes had already been identified by their functional roles as characterized in the (over-) simplifications of transmission genetics. They were "whatever they are" that could play those relatively well-defined roles. The attempt to fit old-style gene talk into the realities of molecular biology required some large adjustments in the understanding of what a gene might be, to the point that serious controversy exists about whether it is right to talk about genes at all.

Although the situation with beliefs is much less sanguine, the dimly imagined hope that beliefs may turn out to be like what genes were once thought to be—salient structures, identifiable (with minimal procrustean adjustments) as the vehicles of previously well-defined content elements—presupposes what is simply not true: that there is a relatively rigorous, precise, predictive science of beliefs and their functional interactions. This is the myth of "East Pole" Cognitive Science (see Dennett, 1987b, 1998) and the "physical symbol system" hypothesis, which has not yet been borne out at all. We can keep this fond hope in mind without succumbing to the imperative that urges us to consider it an inevitable development.

Conclusion

In terms of Monod's dialectical view of the history of philosophy, we have offered definitions of memory and belief that fall rather closer to the side of the Scruffies than that of the Neats. Although it may be dismaying or frustrating to some, the history of the concepts clearly demonstrates that neater definitions are likely to be philosophically problematical. The complex network of implicit and explicit knowledge that underlies the categories of both "belief" and "memory" rests on the ability of that network to both define and recognize its own coherence. Belief and memory thus fall under the definition of knowledge that the Italian anti-Cartesian philosopher Giambattista Vico (1710/1988) gave nearly three centuries ago: the process of making the objects of the mind (or, as we might say today, the apparent objects of the mind) correspond to each other in shapely proportion.[6] Because organisms may have developed numerous different methods for making the apparent objects of the mind correspond to one another in shapely proportion—and because the methods by which such shapeliness may be detected are informed by many different kinds of learning—we must be wary of any definition that treats memory and belief as if they could be simple primitives existing only inside the brain. They are rather summary descriptions, imposed from the top down, of a set of diverse and complex mechanisms that are all attempting to achieve a single common end: to keep the useful facts of history from going immediately inert.

References

Aristotle. (c. 350 B.C./1941). On memory and reminiscence. In *The basic works of Aristotle* (J. I. Beare, Trans.). New York: Random House.

Bartlett, F. C. (1932). *Remembering*. Cambridge: Cambridge University Press.

Broad, C. D. (1925/1962). *The mind and its place in nature*. London: Routledge and Kegan Paul.

Charniak, E. (1974). Toward a model of children's story comprehension. Unpublished. MIT lab report 266.

Dennett, D. (1987a). *The intentional stance*. Cambridge, MA: MIT Press.

Dennett, D. (1987b). The logical geography of computational approaches: A view from the East Pole. In M. Brand and M. Harnish (Eds.), *Problems in the representation of knowledge*. Tucson: University of Arizona Press.

Dennett, D. (1988). Précis of *The intentional stance. Behavioral and Brain Sciences, 11*, 495–546.

Dennett, D. (1991). Real patterns. *Journal of Philosophy, 87*, 27–51.

Dennett, D. (1995). Do animals have beliefs? In H. L. Roitblat and J-A Meyer (Eds.), *Comparative approaches to cognitive science*. Cambridge, MA: MIT Press.

Dennett, D. (1996). *Kinds of minds*. New York: Basic Books.

Dennett, D. (1998). *Brainchildren: Essays on designing minds*. Cambridge, MA: MIT Press.

Efran, J., Lukens, M., and Lukens, R. (1990). *Language, structure, and change*. New York: W. W. Norton.

Goldman, A. I. (1986). *Epistemology and cognition*. Cambridge, MA: Harvard University Press.

Holland, R. F. (1954). The empiricist theory of memory. *Mind, 63*, 464–468.

Hume, D. (1739/1896). *Treatise of human nature* (L. A. Selby-Bigge, Ed.). Oxford: Clarendon Press.

James, W. (1890/1950). *Principles of psychology*, Vol. 1. New York: Dover.

Locke, J. (1700/1979). *An essay concerning human understanding*, (P. N. Nidditch, Ed.). Oxford: Clarendon Press.

Malcolm, N. (1963). *Knowledge and certainty: Essays and lectures*. Englewood Cliffs, NJ: Prentice-Hall.

Marr, D. (1982). *Vision*. New York: Freeman.

Maturana, H. R. (1970). Biology of cognition. In H. R. Maturana and F. J. Varela. (1980). *Autopoesis and cognition: The realization of the living* (pp. 1–58). Dordrecht, The Netherlands: D. Reidel.

Mill, J. (1869). *Analysis of phenomena of the human mind*, Vol. 1. London: Long, Green, Reader, and Dyer.

Monod, J. (1974). *Chance and necessity* London: Fontana.

Plato (347 B.C./1928). *The works of Plato* (I. Edman, Ed.). New York: Tudor.

Plotkin, H. (1994). *Darwin machines and the nature of knowledge*. Cambridge, MA: Harvard University Press.

Reid, T. (1815/1969). *Essays on the intellectual powers of man*. Cambridge, MA: MIT Press.

Russell, B. (1921). *The analysis of mind.* London: Allen and Unwin.

Ryle, G. (1949). *The concept of mind.* London: Penguin Books.

Smith, B. C. (1996). *On the origin of objects.* Cambridge, MA: MIT Press.

Vico, G. (1710/1988). *On the most ancient wisdom of the Italians unearthed from the origins of the Latin language* (L. M. Palmer, Trans.). Ithaca: Cornell University Press.

Wiener, N. (1948/1991). *Cybernetics.* Cambridge, MA: MIT Press.

Wittgenstein, L. (1958). *Philosophical investigations.* Oxford: Blackwell.

Wittgenstein, L. (1983). *Remarks on the foundations of mathematics.* Cambridge, MA: MIT Press.

Zechmeister, E. B., and Nyberg, S. E. (1982). *Human memory: An introduction to research and theory.* Monterey, CA: Brooks/Cole.

Notes

1. Notwithstanding his common association with the representative theorists, Locke's view of memory was actually more subtle than this metaphor suggests. He goes on to note that "our Ideas being nothing, but actual Perceptions in the Mind, which cease to be anything, when there is no perception of them, this laying up of our Ideas in the Repository of Memory, signifies no more but this, that the Mind has a Power, in many cases, to revive Perceptions, which it has once had . . . And in this Sense it is, that our Ideas are said to be in our Memories, when indeed, they are actually no where, but only there is an ability in the Mind, when it will, to revive them again" (p. 150). This passage suggests that Locke did not think of the memory simply as a static storehouse of images, but rather as a dynamic ability to evoke or reconstruct an image, a metaphor more closely in keeping with modern scientific views of memory, which is close to the view of memory we champion here.

2. This example is drawn from Dennett, 1987, pp. 76–77.

3. David Marr (1982) made a relevant distinction between what he (rather misleadingly) called the computational level and a lower level he referred to as the algorithmic level. We might prefer to call his computational level the functional level, concerned as it is with what function, in an abstract and idealized sense, the system under consideration is intended to compute: that is, concerned as it is with competence rather than performance. The lower algorithmic level is concerned with the abstract details of how that function is actually implemented by the system. (A third, lowest level—the hardware level—is concerned with the concrete engineering details of the implementation of that particular algorithm.) Marr's point was that mistakes at the highest (computational) level made it difficult or im-

possible to adequately address questions at the lower levels, because errors at the computational level made it difficult or impossible to distinguish between informative fact and artifact at the lower levels. Looking for propositions in the brain might be very much like looking for perfect earth-centered circles in the orbits of the heavenly bodies. The high-level requirements of the theory mislead one into blurring a distinction we decidedly do not wish to blur: the one between noise (theoretically neutral facts relating to performance) and data (theoretically important facts relating to competence).

4. As Efran, Lukens, and Lukens (1990, p. 111) put it in discussing the closely related phenomena of meaning: "Although we understand (and agree with) the notion that meanings are social constructions, that does not imply that they can or should be modified at will. Participating in a culture is a commitment to abide by established language conventions. Capricious renaming of actions for short-term gain may entail unexpected, hidden, long-term risks. If you cheapen the verbal coin of the realm now, it is hard to escape the inflationary effects later."

5. In actual practice, of course, the rules of interpretation that seem to be commonly accepted in the company in which the attribution of beliefs takes place, can often be simply assumed by the attributor to be accepted by the intended audience of his intentional attribution. If they are not, he is communicating with the wrong audience.

6. This view is reflected in the etymology of "belief." According to the Oxford English Dictionary, the word derives from a degraded form of the original Teutonic "galaubian," which means "to hold estimable or pleasing; to be satisfied with," intensified by the addition of the prefix "be." Thus, etymologically, a belief is something with which one is thoroughly satisfied or much pleased.

Cognitive, Neurological, and Pathological Perspectives

Cognitive and Brain Mechanisms
of False Memories and Beliefs

2

Marcia K. Johnson
Carol L. Raye

This chapter describes some of the cognitive processes that give rise to false memories and beliefs and discusses possible underlying brain mechanisms. Cognitive studies of normal individuals, in combination with observations from neuropsychology and psychopathology, and with evidence from newer brain imaging techniques, permit a reasonably rich characterization of how distortion may come about. Such distortions include both everyday errors and the more profound constructions and fabrications categorized as confabulations and delusions.

Despite some differences in terminology, theoretical ideas about normal distortions of memory and belief (for example, Bartlett, 1932; Bransford and Johnson, 1973; Ceci and Bruck, 1993; Hasher, Goldstein, and Toppino, 1977; Johnson and Raye, 1981; Loftus, 1979; Roediger, 1996; Ross, 1989; Schacter, 1995; Zaragoza, Lane, Ackil, and Chambers, 1997) and about delusions and confabulation (Baddeley, Thornton, Chua, and McKenna, 1996; Burgess and Shallice, 1996; Conway, 1992; Dalla Barba, 1995; Frith, 1992; Johnson, 1988, 1991; Kopelman, 1987; Maher, 1974; Moscovitch, 1989, 1995; Norman and Schacter, 1996; Stuss, Alexander, Lieberman, and Levine, 1978), converge on a common set of themes—for example, the constructive and reconstructive nature of memory, the importance of retrieval cues, and the need for monitoring mechanisms. Our discussion is organized around the source monitoring framework (SMF) (Johnson, 1988, 1991; Johnson and Raye, 1981, 1998), an integrative approach that incorporates these central themes and also provides a developed description of the evaluation or monitoring functions that most theorists agree are critical to understanding confabulations and delusions.

False Memories and Beliefs

The phenomena in which we are interested include everyday distortions of memory (remembering that a conversation took place in a restaurant when it actually took place in a car) and erroneous beliefs (most people on welfare are black), as well as clinically significant phenomena such as confabulations (remembering a trip on a spacecraft) and delusions (believing that someone is controlling your thoughts). For present purposes, we will not make a sharp distinction between memory and belief in discussing normal cognition, or between confabulation and delusion in talking about abnormal cognition. We believe the cognitive processes described in this paper apply to both (see also Kopelman, Guinan, and Lewis, 1995). However, it should be emphasized that what people *call* memories and beliefs reflects the outcomes of these source monitoring processes. People tend to use the word "memory" when a mental experience or report of a mental experience is detailed, including information indicating that one experienced the event oneself, and they tend to use the word "belief" when it does not have contextual details and for a broad range of mental experiences or reports that seem to assert present or past general states of affairs which may or may not involve personally experienced events (including the events from which the belief was derived, such as reading the newspaper). Nevertheless, where veridicality is concerned, it is difficult to draw a sharp distinction between the concepts of memory and belief. Memories are beliefs about what happened, and beliefs are constructed from, and reinforced by, memories.

In the neuropsychological and clinical literatures, the term "confabulation" is often used to refer to a false memory and "delusion" to a false belief, but the usage is not consistent. It is equally likely to be driven by etiology: distortions of memory and belief that are associated with known or presumed *brain damage* tend to be called confabulations, and distortions of memory and belief associated with *psy-*

chopathology tend to be called delusions. As evidence accumulates that patients with psychotic delusions may have brain pathology in some of the same or related brain areas as do confabulating organic brain-damaged patients or abnormalities in one or more neurotransmitter systems (Frith, 1992; Gray, 1995), an etiology-based distinction between delusions and confabulations becomes questionable.

The Source Monitoring Framework (SMF)

Two earlier papers outlined an approach to understanding delusions (Johnson, 1988) and confabulations (Johnson, 1991) based on theoretical ideas derived from cognitive studies of reality monitoring and source monitoring. According to this view, false perceptions, false memories, and false beliefs can all be understood within a common source monitoring framework.

> The characteristics of mental experience that provide it with the quality of reality are similar for perception, event memories, and beliefs: sensory detail; embeddedness in spatial and temporal context; embeddedness in supporting memories, knowledge, and beliefs; and the absence of consciousness of or memory for the cognitive operations producing the event or belief. Reality testing of ongoing perception and reality monitoring of memories and beliefs are complex judgment processes that are subject to error and more difficult in some situations than others. (Johnson, 1988, p. 57)

A characterization of those judgment processes provided the background for suggestions about the various ways that distortions in memories and beliefs could come about through pathological operation of normal processes (such as rehearsal and embellishment) or disruption of normal processes as a consequence of brain damage (retrieval deficits or failure to access cognitive operations). Because much of the relevant evidence has been described elsewhere (Johnson, 1997a; Johnson, Hashtroudi, and Lindsay, 1993; Mitchell and Johnson, 2000), here we will highlight certain central ideas and further consider the brain mechanisms that are implicated (see also Johnson, 1997b).

The SMF assumes that memories consist of distributed features, more or less well bound together, that are a result of perceptual processing (identifying objects, locations and colors, and the like) and reflective processing (imagining a conversation, planning a meeting, ruminating on the past).[1] Errors can be introduced when a memory is first acquired and anytime thereafter when it is activated and when it is evaluated. That is, memories are initially constructed from perceptions, thoughts, beliefs, and goals active together at the time. Subsequently they are reconstructed, often differently, in the context of different goals and different activated information, with the result that they may be reactivated incompletely with different features active at different times, conflated with similar memories from other events, and embellished or otherwise changed by additional perceptual or reflective processing. Because of this indeterminacy about the origin of various aspects of mental experience, we need inferential processes to evaluate the veridicality or source of an activated "memory." The SMF proposes that we evaluate activated information and infer, from its phenomenal properties and/or its relation to other memories, beliefs, and knowledge, that it is veridical or make other source attributions about it—for example, whether we did X or only thought about doing it, who said or did Y, where, and so on. Evaluation processes vary from relatively automatic (heuristic) to more deliberate or reflectively complex (systematic). The parameters of these evaluation (monitoring) processes—such as how different types of information are weighted in the decision, and whether we rely on a quick heuristic decision or engage systematic processes—vary as a function of the consequences of an error, social factors, and the like.

Distortions Arise from Normal Cognition

Knowing the source of information is an important element in judging the accuracy or veridicality of that information—it matters if we have seen something with our own eyes or heard it third hand, or dreamed it or fantasized it, or if we saw it on the nightly news or in a movie. But the source of information typically is not something stored as a propositional tag along with our memories, beliefs, and knowledge. Rather, we infer source. We use heuristic source monitoring processes to attribute a source to information based on an evaluation of various features of the information. If activated information from the memory being evaluated has qualities that we expect memories from a certain source to have, we attribute the information to that source (see Figure 2.1).

We are not always conscious of these processes. Heuristic source attributions take place constantly without notice, and are relatively automatic or effortless. In contrast, the systematic processes engaged in source monitoring (for example, extended retrieval and reasoning) require more of the reflective processes (Johnson and Hirst, 1993) that are likely to give rise to a sense of effort (Hasher and Zacks, 1979) or control (Posner and Snyder, 1975; Shallice, 1988).

As noted above, we believe aspects of an activated memory are evaluated with respect to our expectations or beliefs about the distinguishing qualities of different sources of memories, for example, how familiar we expect them to be or the kind of perceptual detail we expect them to have. Depending on the circumstances of the moment— our objectives, how important it is to be accurate, the particular subset of features of the target memory that is currently activated—we may be more or less specific in the information we use to evaluate the source, and therefore the accuracy, of a reactivated memory.

For example, suppose an advertisement for a movie triggers a vague memory that someone told us recently that they had seen a good movie. We may be very cursory in our *heuristic source evaluation*. We may decide that the movie in the ad is the movie someone told us about simply because its name seems familiar, as if someone might have mentioned it recently; that is, we may use very undifferentiated information. (And we may be wrong if we stop there, because we may have seen the movie title in another context or its title may be similar to that of another movie we have heard about.)

If veridicality is somewhat more important, we will likely require more specific (differentiated) information to make a particular source attribution. We may focus on (increase our weightings of) other features of the activated information. For example, if the activated information, although sketchy, includes a sense of a hallway conversation, we may conclude it is an accurate memory because it has some small degree of the detail that we would expect from a recent, possibly brief, casual event. If we have time to see only one movie this month, we

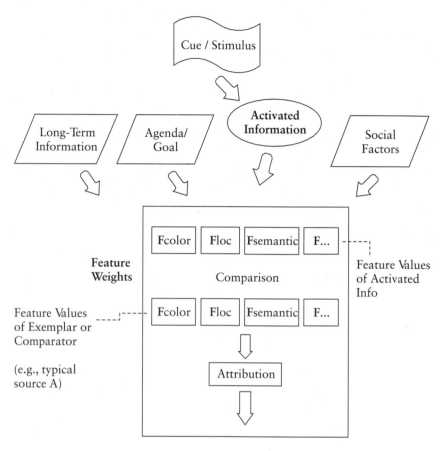

Figure 2.1   SMF heuristic processes.

may require yet more specific information and use systematic processes to retrieve additional candidate memories of recent social occasions until we find one that seems an appropriate match. It could be a recent dinner at a particular restaurant with two friends at which we talked about films—a highly detailed memory, which may in fact be accurate or inaccurate, but which we infer to be accurate based on its perceptual, temporal, semantic, and other features. Thus, depending on our motives, the types of information we expect or require to make a source decision will vary, whether we are engaging a heuristic process or systematic processes or both.

Qualitative Characteristics of Mental Experience

As we have described, heuristic source decision processes often are based on the phenomenal characteristics of activated information. Several lines of evidence support the idea that qualitative cues to source are evaluated in source attribution processes.

1. Source monitoring accuracy is influenced by manipulations that are specifically designed to vary the qualitative features of memories, such as perceptual detail, cognitive operations, and semantic information (Durso and Johnson, 1980; Lindsay, Johnson, and Kwon, 1991; Markham and Hynes, 1993). For example, if people imagine in another person's voice as opposed to their own voice, they are likely to claim later that that person said those words (Johnson, Foley, and Leach, 1988); and the more times people imagine an item, the more times they later think they saw it (Johnson, Raye, Wang, and Taylor, 1979). Visual imagery during reading leads people to say they saw in a picture what they only read about in text (Belli, Lindsay, Gales, and McCarthy, 1994; Intraub and Hoffman, 1992; Zaragoza et al., 1997), and hearing the sound an object makes (for instance, a barking dog) leads people to err and say they saw a picture of a dog (Henkel, Franklin, and Johnson, in press). And increasing the *semantic* similarity between two speakers increases source errors (Lindsay, 1991).

2. People often offer specific details of a target memory as evidence that the remembered event really happened: "I can remember what the dentist's office looked like" or "I can remember how long it took" (Johnson, Foley, Suengas, and Raye, 1988).

3. When subjects rate the qualitative characteristics of their memories using, for example, a Memory Characteristics Questionnaire (MCQ), ratings typically are higher for perceived than for imagined events, and for correct than for incorrect source attributions (Henkel, Johnson, and De Leonardis, 1998; Johnson, Foley, Suengas, and Raye, 1988; Mather, Henkel, and Johnson, 1997; Norman and Schacter, 1997; see also Brewer, 1992; Conway and Dewhurst, 1995; Conway, Collins, Gathercole, and Anderson, 1996).

4. Confidence in source judgments tends to be associated with level of rated detail (Hashtroudi, Johnson, and Chrosniak, 1990) and confidence in autobiographical recall is related to amount of visual information recalled (Brewer, 1988).

5. The more differentiated the information required to make a source attribution, the more vulnerable the decision is to disruption from distraction or speeded responding (Johnson, Kounios, and Reeder, 1994; Jacoby, Woloshyn, and Kelley, 1989; see also Zaragoza et al., 1997).

Accessing and Weighting Information

According to the SMF, schemas and other prior knowledge (for example, about a particular person or about newsprint versus television as a news source) and categories constructed for the task (Barsalou, 1985; see also retrieval task processing in Burgess and Shallice, 1996) help define source-typical exemplars in heuristic source evaluation processes and in systematic evaluation of consistency and plausibility. Which features are weighted most heavily can be determined by long-term experience or by more immediate situational conditions (see Figure 2.1).

The MCQ rating procedure can be used to help identify what information is available for source discrimination and, together with performance data, to what extent that information is being used. For example, subjects who have heard sets of words in which all items within a set are related to a "theme" word that was not presented (*thread, sharp, haystack* are all related to *needle*) are very likely to falsely recall the theme word or recognize the theme word *(needle)* when it is presented as a lure (Deese, 1959; Roediger and McDermott, 1995). Using the MCQ, Mather, Henkel, and Johnson (1997) found that correctly recognized words had more perceptual detail than falsely recognized lure words, but did not have more associative information (see also Norman and Schacter, 1997). The high level of false memories typically found in this paradigm suggests that the weight given to perceptual information in this situation is less than that given to semantic, associative information or to familiarity.

People can flexibly access features or assign different weights to different features, as indicated by the fact that source accuracy varies with test conditions (Dodson and Johnson, 1993; Hasher and Griffin 1978; Raye, Johnson, and Taylor, 1980). For example, subjects are less likely to misattribute information suggested in a description to a previously seen picture if they are asked to indicate which of the possible sources the information came from (picture, description, both, neither) than if they are asked only to indicate whether it came from the picture or was new (Lindsay and Johnson, 1989; Zaragoza and Koshmider, 1989). One interpretation is that the source identification instructions induce subjects to more completely or more carefully assess the various qualitative characteristics of their memories in light of possible sources; thus, they are less likely to say "picture" if the item is simply familiar or exceeds some minimal threshold for perceptual detail. In the SMF, familiarity is treated as a phenomenal quality of memories that can serve as input to heuristic and systematic judgment processes. Even when subjects are making source judgments heuristically based on familiarity, as often occurs in old-new recognition, they adjust their criteria depending on expectations about the probability that an item is familiar and what familiarity signals (Dodson and Johnson, 1994; Skurnik, 1998).

The weight given to certain characteristics may also change as we grow older. Hashtroudi et al. (1990, reported in Johnson and Multhaup, 1992) found that although older and younger adults showed similar correlations between clarity (a factor derived from MCQ ratings) and confidence in the accuracy of a memory, older adults showed significantly higher correlations between emotion and confidence in accuracy. Johnson and Multhaup suggested that, compared to young adults, older individuals may give more weight to emotional aspects of memories in evaluating their veridicality.

In general, mental experiences are assessed according to certain expectations—that is, in light of the weights assigned to various types of information and the threshold amount or pattern (criteria) required for any particular attribution.[2] Both the qualitative and quantitative standards used to evaluate memories and beliefs may be adjusted in short-term, situational ways, as when test conditions induce subjects to look more carefully or to look at information they might have previously ignored (Lindsay and Johnson, 1989; Mather et al., 1997) or when subjects adjust to the relative proportions of types of items in a test set (Dodson and Johnson, 1996). Long-term changes may also occur in the habitual or default requirements. For example, older adults may come to require less perceptual information in order to attribute something to memory if they generally have less perceptual detail encoded, or come to weight emotional detail more heavily because they find the emotional aspects of events more interesting.

Feature Binding

Features that are poorly bound to other features of an event during initial encoding or not consolidated afterward will be poor cues for those other features later (Johnson, 1992; Johnson and Chalfonte, 1994). Features of episodes may be poorly bound for any of a number of reasons, including distraction during encoding (Craik and Byrd, 1982; Jacoby, Woloshyn, and Kelley, 1989) or failure to think about the event subsequently (Suengas and Johnson, 1988).

Emotion is a particularly interesting factor that can affect the extent to which other features are bound together during encoding or during subsequent thinking or talking about events. Suengas and Johnson (1988) reported evidence that thinking about emotional aspects of prior events decreased the availability of perceptual information. Hashtroudi, Johnson, Vnek, and Ferguson (1994) had subjects act in a short play and then manipulated whether subjects thought about either the factual aspects of the play or their emotional reactions. Compared to young adults, older adults were less able to identify the origin (themselves or another person) of statements from the play when they had thought about emotional aspects, but did not differ significantly from young adults when they had thought about factual aspects. Johnson, Nolde, and De Leonardis (1996) had young adults listen to two speakers making various statements (such as "I support the death penalty"; "Interracial relations do not bother me") while subjects thought about either how they felt or how the speakers felt. Later, subjects were poorer at identifying the source of various statements if they had focused on how they themselves felt.

These studies suggest that when subjects are thinking about their feelings, they are less likely to be engaged in processes that bind perceptual detail with content than are subjects whose attention is focused on the factual aspects (Hashtroudi et al., 1994) or more external features of a situation (including other people's apparent emotion). Later these weakly bound features, if they are reactivated at all, are less likely to be sufficient for correctly identifying the source of statements. That is, a test probe statement is likely to reactivate only remembered emotion as a feature of the original event and not reactivate perceptual features of the speaker. Interestingly, Johnson, Nolde, and De Leonardis (1996) found that when subjects thought about how they felt, their old-new recognition was better than when they thought about how the speakers felt. Their reactivated emotional response was a cue for distinguishing experimental sentences from new sentences (which is a less specific, more general source decision) but not for distinguishing which speaker said an old item (which is a more specific source decision). Thus, emotional self-focus can yield memories that are "strong" but lack the features needed for some source decisions.

Effects of Thinking about Events

A fundamental premise of the SMF is that cognition is constructive; memories and beliefs are the joint product of perceptual inputs and the assumptions, knowledge, and motives we bring to them (Alba and Hasher, 1983; Bartlett, 1932; Bransford and Johnson, 1973; Johnson and Sherman, 1990; Ross, 1997). Such constructive processes import elements in the very acts of comprehension and remembering (Johnson, Bransford, and Solomon, 1973), elements that may later be attributed to the wrong source through the normal operation of imperfect source monitoring mechanisms (Johnson and Raye, 1981). For example, in simply understanding the sentence "John pounded the nail," one might infer a hammer and later claim to have heard it (Johnson et al., 1973) or in understanding the word "candy," concepts such as "sweet" might be activated and later falsely recognized (Deese, 1959; Underwood, 1965). Similarly, such constructive intrusions can happen during remembering, as associative and inferential processes fill in around incomplete memorial information.

An important dynamic in constructive memory is that we not only are able to think while we are experiencing events, but we also are able to think back on them (ruminate) after the fact. Suengas and Johnson (1988) showed that thinking about events maintains the vividness of memories, and that thinking about imagined events can have the same impact on vividness ratings as thinking about perceived events. They suggested that if one were to selectively rehearse imagined events, the vividness of these memories would begin to approximate that of memories of perceived events.

Suggestibility effects are a major case of thinking about events in which new information is introduced via a description or questions referring to a prior event, and the new information is later misattributed to the original event—for example, on the basis of perceptual or other details that were imagined when the suggestion was processed (Belli and Loftus, 1994; Hyman and Pentland, 1996; Loftus, 1979; Zaragoza and Lane, 1994). Furthermore, repeating suggestions increases the likelihood of false memory for the suggested events (Mitchell and Zaragoza, 1996).

Conflating Information

As discussed above, heuristic source attributions may rely on specific feature evidence (for example, auditory information if we are trying to decide if we heard something) or on less specific, more global assessments (perceptual information in general if we are deciding whether we imagined or whether we perceived something). For example, *hearing* something (say, a dog barking) increases the chances subjects will claim to have *seen* something (a *dog*) they only imagined (Henkel, Franklin, and Johnson, in press). Also important is that normal memory distortion can arise through the combination of elements that have no obvious semantic or referential relation to each other. For example, Henkel and Franklin (1998) showed that seeing one object (for instance, a magnifying glass) increased the chances subjects claimed to have seen a perceptually similar item they had only imagined (a lollipop). Such false conjunctions of features (the semantic detail associated with a lollipop along with perceptual information about a round object) may be a consequence of poor binding as described above (see also Reinitz, Lammers, and Cochran, 1992).

More Systematic Processes

A number of investigators have noted that remembering can be an extended process involving systematic (or strategic) retrieval using self-presented cues, problem-solving strategies, and reasoning (Baddeley, 1982; Burgess and Shallice, 1996; Conway, 1992; Johnson and Raye, 1981; Reiser, 1986; Williams and Hollan, 1981). Source attributions are often made on the basis of evaluating an activated "memory" in relation to other knowledge, beliefs, and supporting memories related to the target. This additional information used to assess the veridicality of a memory is sometimes activated by cues that are self-generated. Such reflective (effortful, intentional) use of a retrieval strategy from a repertoire of strategic possibilities that help elaborate or constrain retrieval cues (as going through one's day to remember where one left some object) is a process that we include in the category of systematic source monitoring processes. It should be noted that we view the actual activation of memories and knowledge as an associative process that is directed by current goals or agendas; the existing associative relations among memories, knowledge, and beliefs; and active retrieval cues including self-generated cues and external cues (stimuli). Either or both systematic and heuristic evaluation processes may operate, in different ways, on the activated (retrieved) information.

In addition to the self-generation of retrieval cues, a second important function of systematic source monitoring processes is another type of source evaluation process. We have sometimes referred to the systematic evaluation of additional source information as extended reasoning because, compared to heuristic processes, it often relies on a broader range of abstract relational knowledge as well as on event information and more complex comparisons of the two: noting the internal consistency or inconsistency in a memory, or between it and related memories; noting the reliability or unreliability in recall of an event at different times, noting the degree of consensus with other people's memories; or evaluating the plausibility of a memory based on general knowledge or beliefs (Johnson, 1988; Johnson and Raye, 1981) (see Table 2.1). For example, people may decide that a social event happened because they remember noting it on their calendar beforehand or talking about it later to others. Or they may decide that a dream about a scientific discovery did not happen because it is not consistent with what they know to be possible (Johnson et al., 1988). These more effortful or systematic processes are more likely to be observed in studies of autobiographical recall than in studies using simple laboratory materials because of the greater complexity of the memories and the longer retention intervals involved.

As with heuristic source processes, systematic processes may rely on less-differentiated information (for example, simply the fact that additional information is or is not retrieved; or the amount of infor-

Table 2.1   Systematic processes used in making source monitoring judgments

While heuristic source monitoring processes rely on a relatively nondeliberative comparison of phenomenal characteristics of an activated target memory to a set of expected or prototypic characteristics, systematic processes are responsible for a more reflective retrieval of additional knowledge, beliefs, and memories, and more deliberative reasoning about the target memory with respect to the additional information.

Examples of Systematic Processes

Reflective generation of retrieval cues—use of knowledge to generate retrieval cues to gain additional information relevant to the particular source question at hand, for instance:

- in trying to remember who told you a work-related fact, you might generate retrieval cues based on members of your department or recent phone calls and e-mails;
- to remember the source of a news item, you generate news sources, TV, radio, and so on.

Retrieving supporting memories—retrieving other memories related to the target, and the inability to retrieve additional information related to the target memory, for example:

- remembering a conversation about the event which took place soon before or after the event;
- "I know I said X because I remember my train of thought at the time";
- you decide you must be wrong in thinking that person X told you a particular fact a little while ago because you cannot recall any recent occasion when the two of you met or spoke.

Noting consistency or inconsistency in remembering from one time to another time (reliability), in remembering from person to person (consensus), or among the attributes of a specific memory (internal coherence), for instance:

- if in recounting a dinner party you realize that you recall Sam was there but recalled Phil was there the last time you described the party, you conclude you do not remember the event well;
- when your account and another's differ, you know one of you must be wrong;
- when you realize that some perceptual details in the memory reveal a perspective that you could not have, given other components of the memory (you did not go backstage at the play, yet you have vivid perceptual details of the dressing room).

Evaluating plausibility or likelihood of the target memory, given what is generally known or believed, for example:

- "It's not the kind of thing I would say, therefore I could not have said it";
- you remember seeing a politician give a speech at a park when you were young, but then you realize that you were not yet born at the time of the speech.

mation retrieved) or may require a more critical evaluation of specific information for coherence, plausibility, or consensus (Johnson, 1988; Ross, 1997). A new senator recently described his emotional response to a political speech that he had heard as a child in the park where it was given. If he had been more cautious and used a higher criterion to judge the veridicality of whatever he was about to say to the press, he might have invoked more systematic evaluation processes and realized, before the press pointed it out, that he was not born at the time of the speech.

Binding deficits operating when memories are encoded will, like strategic retrieval deficits, affect the success of retrieval cues and will affect the quality of related memories that are available to be retrieved. Like heuristic evaluation, systematic evaluation (plausibility and consistency checks) will suffer from polluted input, caused for example by rumination. *How* memories are thought about later will of course determine if veridicality is strengthened or weakened. As noted above, some types of emotional focus during or after an event potentially decrease the likelihood that perceptual features are bound together. In addition, emotional focus may produce memory deficits by increasing the chances that elaborations, interpretations, or constructions take place, thus increasing the chances for later source confusions. For example, Hashtroudi et al. (1994) found that both younger and older adults were more likely to include elaborations in their recall of a short play in which they had participated if they had thought about their affective reactions than if they had thought about factual details. Consistent with these findings, data recently collected by Mather (1998) suggest that subjects who focus on how they feel while reading a story are later more likely to show recall protocols that distort the story in ways that make it more consistent with their expectations than are subjects who focus on the factual aspects of the story. Again, both heuristic and systematic source attributions would be expected to be negatively affected by rumination that distorts the content of memories.

By capitalizing on the potential effects of rumination in creating the conditions for source monitoring errors (for example, increasing relative vividness of some features; elaboration and embedding in other memories and beliefs), some subjects can be induced to report constructed or fabricated complex autobiographical memories (Ceci,

Crotteau Huffman, Smith, and Loftus, 1994; Ceci, Loftus, Leichtman, and Bruck, 1994; Hyman, Husband, and Billings, 1995). In these studies people are asked to think about long-past events, including some that they did not actually experience (going to the hospital with an ear infection or getting lost at a shopping mall). These tend to be events for which there is reasonably rich schematic or script knowledge (what hospitals and malls are like), which should make it relatively easy for subjects to imagine specific details of the situation. In a particularly compelling demonstration, Ceci and colleagues showed that with repeated tellings, some children came to produce vivid and coherent accounts of fictional events, and that clinicians and researchers who viewed videotapes of children describing events could not discriminate above chance between accounts of real and fictional events.

Interaction of Processes

Heuristic and systematic source monitoring processes often interact. Memories and other information may be revived via relatively effortless associative processes or via cues generated through the reflectively controlled use of systematic retrieval strategies. As shown schematically in Figure 2.2, the activated information may then be subject to heuristic evaluation, or may be more systematically evaluated for coherence or plausibility.

Figure 2.2 also illustrates that heuristic and systematic processes serve as checks on each other (Johnson, 1991; cf. Burgess and Shallice, 1996, and Norman and Bobrow, 1979). For example, the inappropriate heuristic use of familiarity can be countered by more systematic processing (Jacoby, 1991). If a memory has much detail, it may pass a heuristic check but fail a more systematic check for plausibility. Conversely, if a memory seems very plausible but has no specific detail, one might question whether it is, in fact, a veridical memory. A related point is that source information is not only useful when it appears to specify source unambiguously; when source monitoring processes are working normally, ambiguities and vagueness in mental experiences provide meaningful information as well. The lack of clear detail or of coherence signals "caution, this might not be an accurate memory of an actual event or defensible belief." If a memory or belief has inconsequential implications, it can be ignored or treated as a cu-

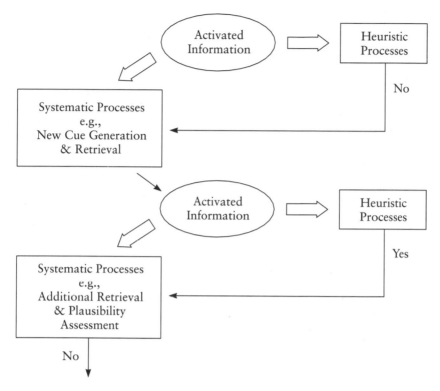

Figure 2.2   Interaction between systematic and SMF heuristic processes.

riosity. If it is important, additional efforts can be made to gather more information through further retrieval efforts, consulting records, documents, other people's memories and beliefs, and so forth. Without such confirming evidence, it may be better not to "act" on such a memory or belief.

One way that cognitive monitoring mechanisms could be disrupted is if such cautionary signals were ignored or misread. For example, it probably would be a mistake to assume that vague memories signal that something significant has been forgotten or repressed. Even supposing that one were especially likely to forget highly salient but unpleasant experiences, the quality of ambiguity or vagueness would not be a particularly reliable cue that a memory is meaningful. This is not to say that there are no important life events for which memories are dim or unavailable, only that there are a great many dim or unavailable memories that are not particularly important or accurate.

Both heuristic and systematic monitoring processes are embedded in an interindividual social context and a broader cultural context that influence the nature of the events we experience initially. They also affect how we interpret those events, what we subsequently think about them (including how we embellish memories), and the criteria we use (both what we focus on and the amount of evidence required) later in making attributions about their origin. For example, the impact that the social interaction between therapists and patients can have on the source monitoring of patients is at the heart of recent controversy over the recovery of repressed memories. Lindsay and Read (1994) draw on the SMF to discuss the potential for inducing false memories in a therapeutic situation.

Brain Mechanisms

Insofar as binding processes are crucial for creating event memories, and retrieval and evaluation processes are vital for monitoring them, it seems reasonable to suppose that those areas of the brain that have been identified as important for feature binding (medial-temporal structures—Cohen and Eichenbaum, 1993; Johnson and Chalfonte, 1994; Kroll, Knight, Metcalfe, Wolf, and Tulving, 1996; Squire and Knowlton, 1995) and strategic or executive functions (frontal areas—Daigneault, Braun, and Whitaker, 1992; Shallice, 1988; Stuss and Benson, 1986) are critical for veridical memories and beliefs (see Baddeley and Wilson, 1986; Johnson, 1991, 1997a, 1997b; Moscovitch, 1995). Indeed, confabulations and delusions have been associated with neuropathology in these regions (Baddeley and Wilson, 1986; Stuss, Alexander, Lieberman, and Levine, 1978).

Frontal Patients

Disrupted Processes. Brain damage from head injuries, tumors, aneurysm of the anterior communicating artery (ACoA), and other diseases and traumas affecting frontal and adjacent subcortical brain regions have wide-ranging effects on cognition (Shimamura, 1995; Stuss, Eskes, and Foster, 1994). Of particular interest are those effects that would be expected to reduce the veridicality of memories and beliefs by affecting processes critical for source monitoring.

Frontal damage can result in various source memory deficits: remembering modality, visual versus auditory (Shoqeirat, 1989, cited in DeLuca and Diamond, 1995), speaker identification (Johnson, O'Connor, and Cantor, 1997), temporal judgments (Milner, 1971; Shimamura, Janowsky, and Squire, 1990), and identifying whether facts were learned in an experiment or known preexperimentally (Janowsky, Shimamura, and Squire, 1989; Schacter, Harbluk, and McLachlan, 1984). There is also evidence that systematic encoding and retrieval processes are likely to be disrupted. For example, Parkin, Leng, Stanhope, and Smith (1988) reported an ACoA patient, JB, who performed very poorly on a paired-associate learning task but improved dramatically when instructed to use imagery. This result suggests that frontal patients may fail to engage more systematic encoding processes that might be effective if they were engaged. And certainly some of the above judgments, especially temporal discriminations among autobiographical or historical events, may depend on systematic retrieval and extended reasoning processes.

Systematic retrieval deficits of frontal patients are especially apparent in their generally poor recall of autobiographical events (Baddeley and Wilson, 1986). For example, Johnson, O'Connor, and Cantor (1997) compared three patients with left frontal damage and three age-matched controls on autobiographical recall of preexperimental events (a vacation) and recall of complex experimental "minievents" (hammering a nail, imagining cutting out a paper snowflake). Relative to the controls, the frontal patients showed typically impoverished memories (they were less likely to recall an event and events, when recalled, had fewer details) and they tended to profit from additional cues.

Johnson and colleagues also found that although the amount of detail reported by the frontal patients was much lower than that reported by the normal controls, the distribution of characteristics (relative frequency of mention of actions, perceptual details, affect, spatial information) was about the same as for the normal controls. These results suggest that in these patients retrieval was not selectively disrupted for one or another type of information; rather, it was generally disrupted because the deficits were distributed across scoring categories. Such an unselective deficit argues for dysfunction of the processes that initiate and guide strategic retrieval, not of access to any particular type of information. Because additional cues did help autobiographical recall, at least some of the deficits appear to be related to poor self-initiated cueing (Baddeley and Wilson, 1986; Moscovitch, 1995; Norman and Schacter, 1996).

In future work with larger patient groups, a systematic comparison of the qualitative characteristics of autobiographical recall of right, left, and bilateral frontal patients would be quite interesting, to see if this unselective deficit pattern is general or is specific to left frontal patients.

In addition to their disrupted contextual and temporal memory, and strategic encoding and retrieval deficits, some frontal patients may use inappropriate feature weights and/or lax criteria in evaluating memories. Schacter, Curran, Galluccio, Milberg, and Bates (1996) reported a patient, BG, who had an infarction of the right frontal lobe and who showed an unusually high false recognition rate on old-new tests involving words, sounds, pronounceable nonwords, or pictures. When the distractors were drawn from a different semantic category than the studied items, this patient had a normal false recognition rate. It was as if he remembered that he had seen items of a given type, and then said "old" to any items of that type on the recognition test.

With the usual recognition test in which distractors are drawn from the same class(es) as studied items, this simple heuristic evaluation would lead to a high false recognition rate. If BG had only categorical information (as a consequence of poor feature binding or selective, schematic encoding), then the best heuristic he could adopt would be to give the greatest (or only) weight to categorical information. On the other hand, if he had additional potentially discriminating information, then category information would have been weighted inappropriately highly.

Given these various deficits in information or processes that have been shown to be important for normal source memory, it is not surprising that frontal patients may become confused about the origin of information, conflate elements from various sources (including, very likely, their own imaginations, television programs, dreams, and the like) and may produce quite bizarre and fantastic confabulations and delusions (Baddeley and Wilson, 1986; Damasio, Graff-Radford, Eslinger, Damasio, and Kassell, 1985; Luria, 1976; Moscovitch, 1995; Stuss, Alexander, Lieberman, and Levine, 1978).

Nevertheless, only some frontal patients confabulate, not all. The three frontal patients in Johnson, O'Connor, and Cantor (1997) illustrate that severe source deficits (including poor temporal information) and autobiographical recall deficits do not necessarily produce confabulation. Similarly, in spite of the high false recognition rate, the Schacter group's patient BG did not confabulate. However, the absence of confabulation in such patients is not difficult to understand from the perspective of the SMF.

According to the SMF, various mechanisms together constrain the extent to which memories and beliefs can get out of control or become distorted. Avoiding confabulations and delusions is not the specific responsibility of any one of these mechanisms. If, for example, certain pieces of temporal or spatial contextual information are missing, one might retrieve other related information that would allow the correct source to be identified based on plausibility. Or without retrieving additional related confirming or disconfirming information, one might remember some particular striking detail that would suggest the memory was veridical. If sufficient detail and supporting or disconfirming information are not available, an appropriate set of weights and criteria might indicate that one should remain in doubt. Recognition that one has poor memory or judgment processes (or feedback about this problem from others) might even cause one to adjust weights and tighten criteria in order to avoid mistakes. Thus, deficits in systematic retrieval alone, for example, would not necessarily produce confabulation.

Of course, the more of these "reality constraints" that break down, the more likely one should be to show confabulations and delusions. Consistent with this hypothesis, Fischer, Alexander, D'Esposito, and Otto (1995) found that clinical judgment of severity of confabulation was correlated with *extent* of lesion in ACoA patients. If we assume that various reality monitoring processes (such as assessing specific feature qualities, retrieving additional information, maintaining appropriate criteria) are mediated by different frontal regions (presumably in combination with more posterior projection areas), increased likelihood of confabulation with disruption of more frontal regions would be expected (see Johnson, Hayes, D'Esposito, and Raye, forthcoming).

The Johnson, O'Connor, and Cantor (1997) study included a fourth ACoA patient, GS, who had bilateral frontal damage and who confabulated. Like the nonconfabulating unilateral frontal patients, GS showed deficits on speaker identification. In addition, he showed a greater deficit than the other frontal patients on autobiographical recall—his ability to report specific autobiographical details was extremely impoverished. Bilateral damage may be especially disruptive to recursive retrieval or retrieval and evaluation processes; interhemispheric cooperation may be necessary to keep information refreshed while new cues are generated, new information is retrieved, or retrieved information is evaluated.

One finding suggests that GS had particular difficulty self-generating retrieval cues or sustaining a recursive retrieval strategy: when specific memories were cued, he did much better. In fact, he produced somewhat more detailed reports of the minievents than did the other frontal patients. In addition, when asked to recall a specific anniversary party several months earlier, his recall was quite detailed (but also included some confabulated elements). Another factor that may have been critical is that his reports of memories of events he had been asked to *imagine* in the lab (cutting out a paper snowflake) were more detailed than those of other frontal patients (cf. David and Howard, 1994). Thus, the combination of poor contextual memory, disrupted ability to self-initiate retrieval processes, and a propensity to vivid imagination may have combined to produce confabulations in this patient.

Qualitative Characteristics of Confabulations and Delusions. In addition to comparing confabulators to nonconfabulating control patients, we can also try to compare the qualitative characteristics of a confabulating patient's veridical and nonveridical recall. Questions of interest include: Do confabulations have the same phenomenal characteristics as real memories, and hence seem real to the patient? Do they have the same coherence and embeddedness in supporting knowledge and beliefs as real memories? What is the relative importance of vividness and embeddedness in creating the sense of reality for a patient? (Johnson, 1988, 1991). A few studies provide preliminary evidence regarding such issues.

Dalla Barba (1995) tested whether a confabulating patient's real memories and confabulations differed in the phenomenal experience of "remembering" versus "knowing," or R/K (Tulving, 1985). In this technique, when a memory is recalled, individuals are typically asked to judge its qualities and answer "Remember" if they recollect specific characteristics of the event and "Know" if the memory is familiar but they cannot recall specific details (Gardiner and Java, 1993; Rajaram and Roediger, 1997). Dalla Barba emphasized "remembering" as the conscious experience of a particular episode of one's life (rather than recollecting detail) and found that a confabulating patient, MB, was as likely to indicate that he "remembered" a confabulated event as an actual event.

From our point of view, R/K judgments are based on an evaluation of features similar to source judgments, albeit perhaps with a different, lower criterion (see also Conway et al., 1996). If a confabulation is reasonably detailed and does not have strong cognitive-operations information associated with generating it, then it would be judged either "real" in a source monitoring judgment or R in an R/K judgment—and neither judgment alone might be sensitive enough to show qualitative differences between real and confabulated memories (see Mather et al., 1997). That is, it could be that confabulated memories have characteristically different details (features) but about the same number of details, or they may have less detail than true memories but still enough to qualify for a "remember" (or "perceived") response rather than a "know" response.

Johnson, O'Connor, and Cantor (1997) compared confabulated and real memory by asking two independent raters to use an MCQ to evaluate the qualitative characteristics of GS's confabulated memory for the circumstances of his aneurysm, and his real memory for a party he had attended that same week. The confabulated memory had a level of qualitative detail similar to that of the veridical memory. But this is just one case. It might be useful to see if confabulating patients could rate their own confabulations and real memories using an MCQ and compare subjective with objective MCQ ratings.

Damage in Other Brain Regions.   Right hemisphere damage in non-frontal cortical regions appears to lead to perceptual and attentional deficits that can, especially in combination with frontal damage, produce confabulations and delusions of recognizable types. For example, quite bizarre or illogical confabulations and delusions sometimes center around misidentifications of place (right posterior temporoparietal lesions associated with reduplicative paramnesia), misidentification of persons (right inferior temporal lesions associated with Capgras syndrome), or somatic distortions (anterior right parietal lesions associated with infestation or somatic delusions) (Malloy and Duffy, 1994, p. 212); or they are associated with neglect (right inferior parietal lesions associated with anosognosia for hemiparalysis—Heilman, 1991; Ramachandran, 1995) and may represent responses to disrupted perceptual-attentional information (Maher, 1974).

These syndromes are generally consistent with a model such as the SMF in which (a) source attributions are made on the basis of qualitative features of experience and (b) either the input into, or the functioning of, evaluation/monitoring processes can be selectively disrupted for different types of information. Inasmuch as we assume the evaluation/monitoring processes to involve frontal systems, the neuropsychological findings suggest that disruption can occur in the information received by frontal regions from other cortical regions, or in the ability of frontal regions to either access or assess the information from various other regions, or both—thus resulting in a variety of confabulatory or delusional syndromes.

In summary, there is general consensus that confabulations and delusions shown by frontal patients involve disruptions in encoding, retrieval, and evaluation or monitoring processes (Baddeley and Wilson, 1986; Burgess and Shallice, 1996; Dalla Barba, 1993; Frith, 1992; Johnson, 1991; Moscovitch, 1989; Norman and Schacter, 1996; Stuss, Eskes, and Foster, 1994). Furthermore, neuropsychological studies of frontal patients find disruptions in various processes central for source monitoring (see also Schacter, Norman, and Koutstaal, 1998). Because of the multiple constraints arising from the multiple source monitoring factors outlined in the SMF, the kinds of severe confabulations and delusions seen in some patients may require a breakdown in more than one type of information or process. For example, poor contextual memory (especially, perhaps, poor temporal memory) in combination with other factors—such as strategic retrieval deficits, evaluation deficits (inappropriate feature weights or criteria), and a propensity for vivid imagery in some individuals— could contribute to false memories and beliefs through their effects on source monitoring attributions. The specific regions most frequently implicated in confabulation include the ventromedial frontal area, basal forebrain, and anterior cingulate (DeLuca, 1993; DeLuca and Diamond, 1995; Johnson, 1991; Johnson, Hayes, D'Esposito, and Raye, forthcoming; Moscovitch, 1995). These would be the most likely candidates or "regions of interest" in future attempts to sort out which brain systems are associated with which processes in the SMF.

Schizophrenic Patients

Neuropathological, neuropharmacological, neuroimaging, and neuropsychological approaches to determining the brain correlates of schizophrenia have not produced a consensus (see, for example, Andreasen, 1997; David and Cutting, 1994; Frith, 1996; Weinberger, 1988). Nevertheless, the brain areas that tend to be implicated (frontal and temporal cortex, hippocampal formation, basal ganglia, and other basal forebrain structures) overlap with areas of brain damage associated with confabulation and delusions in cases of documented brain damage. Furthermore, damage in more posterior brain regions, especially in combination with frontal dysfunction, can produce a range of exotic delusions such as reduplicative paramnesia and Capgras syndrome. Such disruptions in experience could provide the grain of sand around which more complex delusional syndromes form (Maher, 1974), perhaps through selective rumination (Johnson, 1988). For example, the fact that Capgras syndrome is common in schizophrenia (Cutting, 1994) implicates underlying brain pathology in at least some cases of schizophrenia (Ellis and De Pauw, 1994; Fleminger, 1994). Insofar as perceptions of (and memory for) qualitative characteristics of experience provide the inputs for evaluation and source attribution, distorted inputs may lead to false perceptions, memories, and beliefs.

The most prevalent hypotheses today relative to a neural basis for schizophrenia focus on possible defects in neurotransmitter (dopamine) systems (Andreasen, 1997; Fibiger, 1997; Gray, 1995). So-called positive and negative symptoms of schizophrenia respond to different drug therapies and differ by other assessments of brain correlates as well. For example, negative symptoms (apathy, lack of initiative) seem more likely to be associated with neuropsychological tests of frontal function (Frith, 1996). Positive symptoms of schizophrenia (hallucinations, delusions) do not show strong associations with neuropsychological tests of frontal function, nor with neuroimaging evidence of frontal pathology. However, positive symptoms appear to respond to neuroleptics that block dopamine, especially in the lateral septal nucleus and nucleus accumbens (Fibiger, 1997). Notably, these two structures are in the basal forebrain area, which is also generally implicated in confabulation resulting from brain damage (DeLuca and Diamond, 1995).

Positive symptoms of schizophrenia, like the confabulations and delusions of frontal patients, can be viewed as a product of normal source monitoring processes applied to unusual input (for example, vivid perceptual or strong affective features from imaginations) or dysfunctional processes applied to usual input (for example, lower criteria) or both. According to the SMF, source monitoring processes not only assess information about visual, auditory, semantic, affective, and other features, they also assess information about cognitive operations associated, for example, with imagery in various modalities, inference, or reflective initiation and manipulation of images and thoughts (Johnson and Raye, 1981).

Cognitive operations (self-generated or reflective processes) are important for identifying oneself as the origin of thoughts or actions (see also Johnson and Reeder, 1997). Disruptions in either the quality of the cognitive operations information available, or in the ability to evaluate it, lead to self-generated experiences that one would not have the sense of having initiated or controlled. For example, the disruption of brain regions associated with either the cognitive control of or the initial phenomenal experience of cognitive operations, or with the evaluation of cognitive operations features associated with a mental experience, could lead to a variety of psychotic experiences such as hallucinations, beliefs about thought insertion, and delusions of external control.

Consistent with this idea, Bentall, Baker and Havers (1991) proposed a reality monitoring deficit specific to cognitive operations to account for hallucination in schizophrenia patients. They found that hallucinating patients, compared to psychiatric controls and normals, were more likely to attribute self-generated items to the experimenter. This effect was especially noticeable on items that required more effort to generate and that should have had the most cognitive operations information, suggesting that the hallucinators did not store or were less able to access information about cognitive operations in making source attributions.

Frith's (1992) suggestion that first-rank symptoms of schizophrenia result from disorders of self-monitoring of willed intentions is similar to the SMF idea that deficits can occur selectively in monitoring cognitive operations (Bentall et al., 1991; Johnson, 1988, 1991). This theme is also present in Gray's (1995) proposal that positive symptoms may result from a limbic-basal ganglia-based system that compares expected and actual outcomes, and in which a disruption could make self-initiated events appear novel or unexpected.

Based on the SMF, deficits can occur in different ways in monitoring cognitive operations. One possibility is that little or no cognitive operations information may be associated with hallucinatory or delusional phenomenal experiences. Of course, normally, some thoughts seem to occur spontaneously, without conscious effort or intention, much as dreams do or as images may arise while reading a novel. Nevertheless, in most waking thought, the modulating influence of goals and agendas typically restrict conscious cognitive activity to relevant information (Shallice, 1988).

Spontaneous thoughts may occur more frequently in schizophrenia for several reasons. For example, reduced inhibition of weak or unintentional mental experiences (Hasher and Zacks, 1988) or a reduced ability to maintain the task-relevant context, and thus less goal-directed modulation of cognitive activity (Cohen and Servan-Schreiber, 1992), could render conscious that which ordinarily would not be conscious. Thus source evaluation processes may be presented with many more candidates than normally that have no cognitive operations features and hence are more likely to be attributed to other agents or sources—for example, aliens or a radio transmitter implanted in the head. If these ordinarily inhibited ideas were to include vivid perceptual or affective detail as well, they might seem especially compelling. An increase in the frequency of spontaneous mental experiences would not necessarily be accompanied by a decrease in the cognitive operations information associated with deliberate goal-directed thoughts. Thus, schizophrenic patients may show greater deficits in identifying themselves as the origin of unintentional thoughts than as the origin of intentional thoughts.

Another possibility is that information about the cognitive operations that produced a delusion or hallucination is present but is unavailable to or not used in reality-monitoring evaluation processes. For example, Johnson (1991) proposed that two reflective subsystems (R-1 and R-2) ordinarily cooperate (monitor each other), but their ability to communicate could be disrupted, thereby reducing access of one subsystem to the cognitive operations information from the other.

Insofar as initiating and later reactivating reflective operations such as those involved in agenda-controlled thoughts and actions are frontally based (Shallice, 1988), and monitoring (evaluation) processes also are frontally based, an inability to access or use cognitive operations information might be expected to result from disruption of frontal functioning, particularly if two or more cooperative processes or systems underlie these functions. If R-1 and R-2 processes are disproportionately represented in the right and left hemispheres respectively (Johnson, 1997), deficits in the interaction of the two systems would be consistent with characterizations of schizophrenia that emphasize some kind of hemispheric imbalance or disconnection (Cutting, 1990). Alternatively, systematic R-2 processes important for source monitoring may require interhemispheric cooperation (Nolde, Johnson, and Raye, 1998).

Although a reality-monitoring deficit specific to cognitive operations information could lead to experiences of sensory hallucinations and delusions of external control, more complex delusions, such as delusions of persecution, are likely to involve additional factors. Especially important, we believe, in more complex delusions and other psychotic syndromes is the role of repetition and rumination. Thinking about events (both real and fantasized) can make them more vivid, make them come to mind more readily, and embed them in related thoughts and beliefs that will then be taken as evidence of their veridicality (Johnson, 1988).

David and Howard (1994) addressed such issues in a study of the phenomenal experiences of four patients with delusional memories (three late paraphrenia cases and one person diagnosed with schizoaffective psychosis). These researchers compared patients' MCQ ratings for their delusional memories with their ratings for nondelusional memories from the same period. Delusional memories had higher ratings on aspects such as clarity, contextual information, and feelings. High ratings on these attributes were correlated with ratings of frequency of rehearsal, and patients indicated that they had rehearsed the delusional memories more frequently than the real memories. Of course, delusional ideas may be rehearsed because they are vivid rather than the reverse, but David and Howard's findings are at least consistent with laboratory findings on the effects of rehearsal (Suengas and Johnson, 1988).

One's worldviews, schemas, and chronic anxieties are likely to influence one's rumination, as well as the way various features of experience, including memories, are likely to be weighted in any monitoring process. Thus a number of cognitive, social, and motivational mechanisms exist by which clinically significant confabulations and delusions can occur in the absence of or in combination with specific brain damage (Kopelman, Guinan, and Lewis, 1995; O'Connor, Walbridge, Sandson, and Alexander, 1996).

Aging and Memory Distortion

Because normal aging is likely to be accompanied by neuropathology in medial temporal and frontal regions, studies of older adults provide one way of investigating the brain mechanisms underlying disruption of source monitoring processes. There are many more people older than age sixty-five than there are amnesics, frontal patients, or schizophrenics. Furthermore, healthy older individuals can engage in a wider range of tasks, so they constitute a promising population for studying the processes involved in true and false memories and beliefs.

Numerous studies show that older adults have deficits in source memory. For example, older adults are less likely to accurately remember contextual features of events such as the speaker (Bayen and Murnane, 1996; Ferguson, Hashtroudi, and Johnson, 1992), the color or font of the stimuli (Kausler and Puckett, 1980; Park and Puglisi, 1985), the location of items (Light and Zelinski, 1983; Pezdek, 1983), the origin of trivia facts (Craik, Morris, Morris, and Loewen, 1990), whether something was seen in a video or a photograph (Schacter, Koustaal, Johnson, Gross, and Angell, 1997), and the orienting task performed (De Leonardis and Johnson, 1997).

Chalfonte and Johnson (1996) found that even when older and younger adults had apparently equivalent information about individual features (item and color), the older adults were less likely to bind those features to each other. Chalfonte and Johnson suggested that such binding deficits might be related to neuropathology in the medial-temporal regions associated with aging (Ivy, MacLeod, Petit, and Markus, 1992), but their study provided no direct evidence for such a link.

Henkel, Johnson, and De Leonardis (1998) explored the potential link between source memory and age-related deficits in medial-temporal and frontal-lobe function. The subjects in their study viewed some pictures and imagined others, and then were given a source monitoring test (older adults were tested after a fifteen-minute retention interval and younger adults after a two-day interval, to equate groups on old-new recognition). Whereas older adults were no more likely than young adults to claim to have seen imagined items that were unrelated to any other items, they were much more likely to claim to have seen imagined items (for example, *lollipop* or *banana*) that were perceptually (or conceptually) related to perceived items (for example, *magnifying glass* or *apple*). Thus, older adults were not simply more confused in general, but suffered in particular from similarity among features of candidate memories. Henkel and colleagues suggested that such memory distortions arise because certain memory records of features (for example, round shape) are not tightly bound to the context of their occurrence, which can affect judgment about the source of another memory. As would be expected based on the likelihood of age-related neuropathology in medial-temporal regions, source memory scores of older adults were correlated with their scores on a neuropsychological battery of tests often used to assess medial-temporal function (Glisky, Polster, and Routhieaux, 1995).

A second group of older adults were tested after a two-day delay. In addition to a correlation between source accuracy and medial-temporal scores, a correlation was found between source accuracy and scores on a neuropsychological battery of tests often used to assess frontal function (Glisky et al., 1995). Henkel, Johnson, and De Leonardis suggested that this correlation reflects the greater importance of systematic retrieval and evaluation processes after a delay, and is consistent with evidence for age-related neuroanatomic and neurochemical changes in frontal-lobe regions (Kemper, 1984; West, 1996) and with other observations of correlations between source memory and frontal measures in older adults (Craik, Morris, Morris, and Loewen, 1990; see also Mather, Johnson, and De Leonardis, 1999).

These results are consistent with the idea that medial-temporal and frontal regions play somewhat different roles in source memory, with medial-temporal regions more important for binding features into complex memories and frontal regions more important for evaluation and systematic retrieval (Johnson et al., 1993; Moscovitch, 1995). Of course, this is an oversimplification because frontal and medial-temporal regions typically work together. Thus frontal damage can interfere with binding processes by disrupting the agendas that affect binding—for instance, reflectively controlled agendas that promote rehearsal and elaborative encoding. Similarly, medial-temporal damage can decrease the effectiveness of elaborative frontal processes at encoding and self-cuing at retrieval because fewer features are bound together.

In any event, the combination of medial-temporal and frontal damage should be particularly devastating because of the combined effects of poor binding of features and disrupted reflective processes that maintain agendas and retrieve and evaluate information. In fact, some of the most severe cases of confabulation come from patients with both medial-temporal and frontal damage (Baddeley and Wilson, 1986; DeLuca and Diamond, 1995).

Brain Activity and Source Memory Processes
Techniques for recording metabolic (positron emission tomography or PET; and functional magnetic resonance imaging, or fMRI) and elec-

trical (event-related potentials, or ERPs) brain activity offer an opportunity to bridge the gap between evidence and theoretical ideas derived from the study of normal individuals in cognitive tasks, and those derived from the neuropsychological study of brain-damaged patients and from clinical studies of psychiatric patients (for reviews of brain imaging research see Buckner and Tulving, 1995; McCarthy, 1995; Nolde, Johnson, and Raye, 1998; Rugg, 1995; Ungerleider, 1995). Evidence suggests that these techniques will be useful in exploring the heuristic and systematic processes that go into the construction and reconstruction of memories and beliefs, including the agenda-driven selective probing for and weighting of memory features and their evaluation in light of task goals.

Selective Access and Weighting. Johnson, Kounios, and Nolde (1996) reported a study in which subjects saw pictures (line drawings) and words under one of two orienting tasks. Subjects in the Function task rated the number of functions they could think of for each item on a scale from 1 to 3 or more, and subjects in the Artist task rated how difficult a picture would be to draw (for picture items), or they imagined a picture (for word items) and rated how difficult that would be to draw on a scale from 1 (easy) to 3 (difficult). Subsequently, ERPs were recorded while subjects were shown words and for each one indicated whether it corresponded to an item previously presented as a picture, previously presented as a word, or was new.

Johnson and colleagues found marked negativities at about 400 milliseconds following the onset of the test stimulus that appeared at occipital sites in the Function group and at frontal sites in the Artist group. They suggested that this different topographical pattern was consistent with the idea that different attributes of memory are distributed in different regions of the neocortex (Damasio, 1989; see also Martin et al., 1995), and that the two groups differentially probed or weighted different types of information in their judgments. It appears that Function subjects were making picture/word judgments largely on the basis of the amount of visual detail evoked by the stimulus, hence the large occipital negativity. In contrast, although Artist subjects presumably encoded as much (and probably more) visual detail about the stimuli, the amount of remembered visual detail was not a particularly diagnostic cue for source because the test subjects generated visual details (imaged line drawings) for objects represented by word stimuli as well. Artist subjects were thus more likely to probe for information about the cognitive operations engaged at encoding rather than the visual detail stored as a result of that encoding, hence the frontal negativity.

A subsequent study by Nolde (1997) supported this interpretation that the observed negativities reflected selective access and/or weighting of different attributes. Subjects at acquisition engaged in the Function task for some items and the Artist task for other items, then were given the same source monitoring task as in the previous study. If our interpretation of the earlier study is accurate, the ERP data in the Nolde study should not show a difference in information probed as a function of acquisition task, since in that study it was not possible for subjects to adopt a selective strategy at test (any individual test item might have been in the Function or the Artist condition). Our prediction was correct: test trial ERPs for Artist and Function items did not differ in topographical distribution of activation. For both Artist and Function items, both occipital and frontal negativities occurred, suggesting that subjects were using the two types of information. Also, response latencies were slower in this more complex decision situation, as would be expected if subjects were considering both types of information. Taken together, the two studies suggest that people adjust the information that they probe or evaluate to fit the particular conditions of the source discrimination task (see also Johnson, Nolde, Mather, et al., 1997).

Retrieval versus Evaluation. Recent brain imaging studies have yielded hemispheric asymmetries, with the right frontal areas more active than the left in episodic memory tasks (Buckner, 1996). Such asymmetries have led to the suggestion that retrieval is a right frontal function (Shallice, Fletcher, Frith, Grasby, et al., 1994; Tulving, Kapur, Markowitsch, Craik, Habib, and Houle, 1994). One possibility is that this right lateralized activity represents a "retrieval mode" that is engaged during the test stage of episodic tasks (Nyberg, Cabeza, and Tulving, 1996). Or the right frontal activity may represent the amount of retrieval effort required by a task (Schacter, Alpert,

Savage, et al., 1996). Still a third possibility is that the right frontal activity represents not retrieval processes per se, but evaluation or monitoring of the output of activation and retrieval processes (Shallice et al., 1994). Sorting out these possibilities is a challenge because every episodic memory study is a source monitoring study, just as every episodic memory study is a retrieval study; that is, every memory that is attributed to some particular past event is so ascribed on the basis of source attribution processes.

The ERP study by Johnson, Kounios, and Nolde (1996) provides some evidence that the right lateralized activity seen in PET and fMRI studies may not reflect either a retrieval mode or retrieval per se, but perhaps some component(s) of postretrieval evaluation of the activated information. In addition to the subjects who made source monitoring judgments at test, other subjects had the same acquisition conditions (Function or Artist task) and then received an old-new recognition test. In that test, all old items (pictures and words) and new items were presented as words, and subjects were asked to identify items as "old" (from the previous list) or "new."

Collapsed across subjects who were given old-new and those given source identification tests, test-trial ERPs showed a frontal, right-lateralized asymmetry. However, this frontal asymmetry was greater in the later interval of individual trials, suggesting it did not reflect an overall retrieval mode adopted for the task. Also, the asymmetry was larger starting at a point past where critical access probes for specific information evidently took place (around 400 milliseconds, as discussed above). Further, the degree of hemispheric asymmetry did not interact with whether subjects were making old-new judgments or more specific source judgments (picture, word, new). Because this lateralized activity did not vary between test tasks, we believe it may represent commonalities in the evaluation processes of old-new recognition and source identification. Nevertheless, despite commonalities, these processes are not necessarily identical (Johnson and Raye, 1981; Raye, 1976). Is there further evidence that reflects differences in old-new and source decision processes?

Although the frontal, right-lateralized effect was not different for old-new and source monitoring conditions, Johnson, Kounios, and Nolde (1996) did find a marked difference in ERP waves (superimposed on the right-lateralized effect mentioned above) between old-new recognition and source identification groups that was frontally, but bilaterally, distributed (see also Senkfor and Van Petten, 1998). Source identification typically is a more difficult source monitoring task than is old-new recognition—that is, it requires more differentiated information, or a closer inspection of the nature of the activated information, or the attempted retrieval of additional information (Johnson et al., 1994). Thus, this late frontal, bilateral difference between recognition and source identification suggests that difficult source monitoring tasks require the activation and perhaps cooperation of both hemispheres (for relevant evidence see Nolde, Johnson, and D'Esposito, 1998; Nolde, Johnson, and Raye, 1998).

In short, these ERP studies are consistent with the behavioral evidence suggesting that not all information in memory is equally accessed or weighted during remembering (Lindsay and Johnson, 1989; Hashtroudi et al., cited in Johnson and Multhaup, 1992; Mather et al., 1997). Brain imaging in combination with ERPs can provide converging evidence about where in the brain and when in the processing (during memory access, during evaluation) agendas are having their impact.

We speculate that the right-frontal effect in episodic memory tests seen with brain imaging may index a common component of heuristic evaluation processes that operates on activated information in light of whatever task agenda has been set. For example, a target representation in perceptual cortical sites (say P-2 in MEM; Johnson, 1992) might be evaluated by frontal heuristic reflective processes (R-1 in MEM) for familiarity in old-new recognition, or for amount of perceptual detail in source identification. (In fact, there is some evidence that the right hemisphere may be better than the left in discriminating at test between old items and similar items—Metcalfe, Funnell, and Gazzaniga, 1995; Phelps and Gazzaniga, 1992.)

We further speculate that the bilateral frontal effect we observed represents interhemispheric cooperation or coordination. We would expect more systematic R-2 type processing (or processing that requires coordination between R-1 and R-2 subsystems) to be necessary more often in source identification than in old-new recognition tasks. This expectation is not specific to source monitoring, of course. Other reflectively demanding tasks, such as recall, should require interaction between hemispheres as well (see Phelps, Hirst, and Gazzaniga, 1991).

The example of heuristic processing above illustrates "metaprocessing" in MEM, whereby one representation (in this case a P-2 target) is taken as the object of another (in this case a reflective R-1 agenda) (Johnson and Reeder, 1997; cf. Nelson and Narens, 1990). (Similar ideas are Jacoby and Kelley's 1987 notion of memory as "object," and Frith's 1992 concept of "metarepresentation.")

Our example of bilateral systematic processing also illustrates metaprocessing. Again assume that a target representation is activated in a P-2 representation system. If a decision cannot be made quickly (heuristically), the activated information will need to be kept refreshed while, perhaps, other recent items are systematically retrieved in order to make a judgment that is consistent with other recent judgments. One hemisphere may be needed to keep the activated information refreshed while the other is retrieving additional information. Or one hemisphere may represent and keep refreshed information (such as perceptual detail) while the other hemisphere retrieves other information (perhaps semantic interpretations or elaborations; see Metcalfe et al., 1995). According to the SMF, information represented in or retrieved by the two hemispheres would be weighted and evaluated in order to yield a source attribution.

We further speculate that certain types of reasoning, problem solving, or cyclical retrieval (that is, activities involving subgoals) involved in autobiographical recall and in evaluating memories for plausibility or coherence with other memories would also involve cooperation between hemispheres. Thus, we expect that these complex (reflective R-2) retrieval and evaluation processes are more likely to require interhemispheric cooperation. They should therefore be particularly likely to be disrupted by bilateral frontal damage (as in the case of GS described above, Johnson, O'Connor, and Cantor, 1997) or by disruption in the communication between the two hemispheres as in split-brain patients (Metcalfe et al., 1995). That is, if interhemispheric cooperation is central to more difficult source judgments, or those that depend on the retrieval and integration of various sources of information, that fact would explain why bilateral frontal damage can produce severe confabulation. Hemispheric imbalance and disrupted communication have also been proposed as basic deficits in schizo-phrenia (Cutting, 1994).

SMF Functions and Brain Regions. The broad outlines of a model relating brain mechanisms to the cognitive processes involved in re-membering can be described and would have reasonable consensus (see Table 2.2). Memories result from a complex balance between me-dial-temporal and frontal brain regions, in interaction with other cor-tical and subcortical regions that encode information about visual, au-ditory, spatial, affective, and other features of events. The accuracy of memories and beliefs is determined by feature-binding processes medi-ated by medial-temporal regions, often in the service of frontally mediated agendas, and by frontally mediated strategic retrieval and evaluation processes, themselves dependent on medial-temporal reac-tivation of bound features. Thus this delicate system can be disturbed by the disruption of brain regions supporting any of these processes or perceptual processing or their interaction, as indicated by studies of aging and of brain-damaged patients. Confabulations and delusions seem particularly likely when damage to more than one part occurs, especially when damage includes the basal forebrain region and in-creases in frontal regions. Similarly, drugs that target neurotransmitter systems critical to these regions, especially dopamine circuits, have therapeutic effects on positive symptoms of schizophrenia.

We can also begin to propose some more specific aspects of a cog-nitive model of these processes (Figures 2.1 and 2.2) and of their neural mapping. Processes mediated by frontal systems adjust weights for possible types of evidence—for features such as visual or auditory detail, location, and so forth. Confidence in the accuracy of a memory is especially related to the amount of evidence in the most heavily weighted features. Decision criteria determine how discrete judgments or attributions are mapped onto the weighted evidence. Consistent with these ideas, ERP studies show differential brain activation related to the presumably differential weighting of features in memory source decisions (Johnson, Kounios, and Nolde, 1996; Johnson, Nolde, Mather, et al., 1997).

Among the various types of information available during perceiv-ing, remembering, and thinking, we have suggested that evidence from

Table 2.2   Brain regions and cognitive functions important in evaluating veridicality

Brain area	Cognitive functions	Evidence cited
Cerebral cortex (various cortical areas)	Feature perception	Clinical syndromes caused by brain damage (e.g., Capgras, neglect)
	Distributed feature representation in memory	Brain damage, PET, ERP studies
Medial-temporal area (e.g., hippocampal formation)	Feature binding, reactivation (nondeliberative)	Brain damage (amnesia patients), aging
Frontal regions	Reflective processing (e.g., self-generated cognition)	Brain damage (Korsakoff, frontal patients), aging, schizophrenia (positive symptoms)
Right frontal cortex	Heuristic evaluation processes (e.g., heuristic source monitoring attributions)	ERP, PET studies, brain damage
Bilateral frontal cortex ·	Systematic processes (e.g., cue generation, strategic retrieval, evaluating consistency or plausibility)	ERP, PET, fMRI studies, brain damage

reflective cognitive operations is especially important in distinguishing real from imagined events, memories, and beliefs (Johnson, 1992; Johnson and Raye, 1981). Disruptions in the deliberative control of mental operations or in the ability to evaluate this information as evidence of source of an experience or memory could produce hallucinations, delusions, or confabulations. ERP data showed frontal brain activation when individuals attempted to use information about past cognitive operations to make source decisions, and activation in posterior brain regions when decisions could be based on remembered visual information (Johnson et al., 1996). These data could indicate that stored cognitive operations are represented frontally.

Frontally maintained agendas not only modulate feature weights and criteria, they initiate further processing if the task goals are not met. The further processing that might be needed—for example, strategic retrieval or comparing the relative amounts of evidence contained in mental experiences on the current trial with those from past trials—also requires a frontally maintained agenda. Processing is said to be heuristic when a relatively simple agenda or a single reflective subsystem is sufficient for the task. Processing is said to be systematic when two or more synchronously interacting agendas or reflective subsystems are required. ERP, fMRI, and PET data suggest that right prefrontal regions are disproportionately involved in heuristic processing during source monitoring and other memory tasks, and that left and right prefrontal regions coordinate when more complex or systematic processing is required (Nolde, Johnson, and D'Esposito, 1998; Nolde, Johnson, and Raye, 1998).

Conclusion

A common set of themes has arisen from neuropsychological and clinical studies of confabulations and delusions. A number of these are similar to ideas that have arisen in the study of normal cognition and have been proposed as mechanisms by which false memories and beliefs come about. The source monitoring framework provides a way of integrating these two traditions. The SMF points to the importance of encoding and consolidation processes, cognitive events and experiences that happen after events (such as rumination), and cue conditions and agendas (schemas, plans, and the like) that are active at both encoding and test. These factors determine which information will receive selective processing, how much additional strategic processing takes place, and how elements of mental experiences are evaluated. Normal distortions in perceptions, memories, and beliefs arise because these processes are not perfect and because they are subject to the influence of cognitive contexts and motivational and social factors. Clinically significant confabulations and delusions arise when these imperfect processes are further disrupted by brain damage and functional abnormalities. Such clinical findings have provided valuable information identifying general brain regions implicated in remembering and believing.

As additional data become available from brain imaging and ERP studies designed to isolate various components of critical cognitive processes underlying memories and beliefs, the exact nature and location of the transactions or brain circuits required for binding, reactivating, retrieving, and evaluating information of various types should become more apparent. We will then come closer to characterizing the brain activity associated with the phenomenal experiences of remembering and believing.

References

Alba, J. W., and Hasher, L. (1983). Is memory schematic? *Psychological Bulletin, 93,* 203–231.

Andreasen, N. C. (1997). Linking mind and brain in the study of mental illnesses: A project for a scientific psychopathology. *Science, 275,* 1586–93.

Baddeley, A. (1986). *Working memory,* Vol. 2. New York: Oxford University Press.

Baddeley, A., Thornton, A., Chua, S. E., and McKenna, P. (1996). Schizophrenic delusions and the construction of autobiographical memory. In D. C. Rubin (Ed.), *Remembering our past: Studies in autobiographical memory* (pp. 384–428). New York: Cambridge University Press.

Baddeley, A. D., and Wilson, B. (1986). Amnesia, autobiographical memory and confabulation. In D. C. Rubin (Ed.), *Autobiographical memory* (pp. 225–252). New York: Cambridge University Press.

Barsalou, L. W. (1985). Ideals, central tendency, and frequency of instantiation as determinants of graded structure in categories. *Journal of Experimental Psychology: Learning, Memory, and Cognition, 11,* 629–654.

Bartlett, F. C. (1932). *Remembering: A study in experimental and social psychology.* Cambridge: Cambridge University Press.

Bayen, U. J., and Murnane, K. (1996). Aging and the use of perceptual and temporal information in source memory tasks. *Psychology and Aging, 11,* 293–303.

Belli, R. F., Lindsay, D. S., Gales, M. S., and McCarthy, T. T. (1994). Memory impairment and source misattribution in postevent misinformation experiments with short retention intervals. *Memory and Cognition, 22,* 40–54.

Belli, R., and Loftus, E. (1994). Recovered memories of childhood abuse: A source monitoring perspective. In S. J. Lynn and J. W. Rhue (Eds.), *Dissociation: Clinical and theoretical perspectives* (pp. 415–433). New York: Guilford Press.

Bentall, R. P., Baker, G. A., and Havers, S. (1991). Reality monitoring and psychotic hallucinations. *British Journal of Clinical Psychology, 30,* 213–222.

Bransford, J. D., and Johnson, M. K. (1973). Considerations of some problems of comprehension. In W. Chase (Ed.), *Visual information processing* (pp. 383–438). New York: Academic Press.

Brewer, W. F. (1988). Memory for randomly sampled autobiographical events. In U. Neisser and E. Winograd (Eds.), *Remembering reconsidered: Ecological and traditional approaches to the study of memory. Emory symposia in cognition,* Vol. 2 (pp. 21–90). New York: Cambridge University Press.

Brewer, W. F. (1992). Phenomenal experience in laboratory and autobiographical memory tasks. In M. A. Conway, D. C. Rubin, H. Spinnler, and W. A. Wagenaar (Eds.), *Theoretical perspectives on autobiographical memory* (pp. 31–51). Boston: Kluwer Academic Publishers.

Buckner, R. L. (1996). Beyond HERA: Contributions of specific prefrontal brain areas to long-term memory retrieval. *Psychonomic Bulletin and Review, 3,* 149–158.

Buckner, R. L., and Tulving, E. (1995). Neuroimaging studies of memory: Theory and recent PET results. In F. Boller and J. Grafman (Eds.), *Handbook of neuropsychology,* Vol. 10 (pp. 439–46). New York: Elsevier.

Burgess, P. W., and Shallice, T. (1996). Bizarre responses, rule detection and frontal lobe lesions. *Cortex, 32*(2), 241–259.

Ceci, S. J., and Bruck, M. (1993). Suggestibility of the child witness: A historical review and synthesis. *Psychological Bulletin, 113,* 403–439.

Ceci, S. J., Crotteau Huffman, M. L., Smith, E., and Loftus, E. F. (1994). Repeatedly thinking about a non-event: Source misattributions among preschoolers. *Consciousness and Cognition, 3*(3/4), 388–407.

Ceci, S. J., Loftus, E., Leichtman, M., and Bruck, M. (1994). The possible role of source misattributions in the creation of false beliefs among preschoolers. *International Journal of Clinical and Experimental Hypnosis, 42*(4), 304–320.

Chalfonte, B. L., and Johnson, M. K. (1996). Feature memory and binding in young and older adults. *Memory and Cognition, 24*(4), 403–416.

Cohen, J. D., and Servan-Schreiber, D. (1992). Context, cortex, and dopamine: A connectionist approach to behavior and biology in schizophrenia. *Psychological Review, 99,* 45–77.

Cohen, N. J., and Eichenbaum, H. (1993). *Memory, amnesia, and the hippocampal system.* Cambridge, MA: MIT Press.

Conway, M. A. (1992). A structural model of autobiographical memory. In M. A. Conway, D. C. Rubin, H. Spinnler, and W. Wagenaar (Eds.), *Theoretical perspectives on autobiographical memory* (pp. 167–193). Boston: Kluwer Academic Publishers.

Conway, M. A. (1996). Autobiographical knowledge and autobiographical memories. In D. C. Rubin (Ed.), *Remembering our past: Studies in autobiographical memory* (pp. 67–93). New York: Cambridge University Press.

Conway, M. A., Collins, A. F., Gathercole, S. E., and Anderson, S. J. (1996). Recollections of true and false autobiographical memories. *Journal of Experimental Psychology: General, 125,* 69–95.

Conway, M. A., and Dewhurst, S. A. (1995). Remembering, familiarity, and source monitoring. *Quarterly Journal of Experimental Psychology, 48A*(1), 125–140.

Craik, F. I. M., and Byrd, M. (1982). Aging and cognitive deficits: The role of attentional resources. In F. I. M. Craik and S. E. Treehub (Eds.), *Aging and cognitive processes* (pp. 191–211). New York: Plenum Press.

Craik, F. I. M., Morris, L. W., Morris, R. G., and Loewen, E. R. (1990). Relations between source amnesia and frontal lobe functioning in older adults. *Psychology and Aging, 5,* 148–151.

Cutting, J. (1990). *The right cerebral hemisphere and psychiatric disorders.* Oxford: Oxford University Press.

Cutting, J. C. (1994). Evidence for right hemisphere dysfunction in schizophrenia. In A. S. David and J. C. Cutting (Eds.), *The neuropsychology of schizophrenia* (pp. 231–242). Hove, England: Lawrence Erlbaum.

Daigneault, S., Braun, C. M. J., and Whitaker, H. A. (1992). An empirical test of two opposing theoretical models of prefrontal function. *Brain and Cognition, 19,* 48–71.

Dalla Barba, G. (1993). Confabulation: Knowledge and recollective experience. *Cognitive Neuropsychology, 10,* 1–20.

Dalla Barba, G. (1995). Consciousness and confabulation: Remembering "another" past. In R. Campbell and M. A. Conway (Eds.), *Broken memories: Case studies in memory impairment* (pp. 101–114). Oxford: Blackwell.

Damasio, A. R. (1989). Time-locked multiregional retroactivation: A systems-level proposal for the neural substrates of recall and recognition. *Cognition, 33,* 25–62.

Damasio, A. R., Graff-Radford, N. R., Eslinger, P. J., Damasio, H., and Kassell, N. (1985). Amnesia following basal forebrain lesions. *Archives of Neurology, 42,* 263–271.

David, A. S., and Cutting, J. C. (1994). The neuropsychology of schizophrenia—introduction and overview. In A. S. David and J. C. Cutting (Eds.), *The neuropsychology of schizophrenia* (pp. 231–242). Hove, England: Lawrence Erlbaum.

David, A. S., and Howard, R. (1994). An experimental phenomenological approach to delusional memory in schizophrenia and late paraphrenia. *Psychological Medicine, 24,* 515–524.

Deese, J. (1959). On the prediction of occurrence of particular verbal intrusions in immediate recall. *Journal of Experimental Psychology, 58,* 17–22.

De Leonardis, D. M., and Johnson, M. K. (1997). *Aging and source monitoring: The relation between cognitive operations and perceptual information.* Manuscript.

DeLuca, J. (1993). Predicting neurobehavioral patterns following anterior communicating artery aneurysm. *Cortex, 29,* 639–647.

DeLuca, J., and Diamond, B. J. (1995). Aneurysm of the anterior communicating artery: A review of neuroanatomical and neuropsychological sequelae. *Journal of Clinical and Experimental Neuropsychology, 17*(1), 100–121.

Dodson, C. S., and Johnson, M. K. (1993). Rate of false source attributions depends on how questions are asked. *American Journal of Psychology, 106*(4), 541–557.

Dodson, C. S., and Johnson, M. K. (1996). Some problems with the process dissociation approach to memory. *Journal of Experimental Psychology: General, 125*(2), 181–194.

Durso, F. T., and Johnson, M. K. (1980). The effects of orienting tasks on recognition, recall, and modality confusion of pictures and words. *Journal of Verbal Learning and Verbal Behavior, 19*, 416–429.

Ellis, H. D., and de Pauw, K. W. (1994). The cognitive neuropsychiatric origins of the Capgras delusion. In A. S. David and J. C. Cutting (Eds.), *The neuropsychology of schizophrenia* (pp. 317–335). Hove, England: Lawrence Erlbaum.

Ferguson, S., Hashtroudi, S., and Johnson, M. K. (1992). Age differences in using source-relevant cues. *Psychology and Aging, 7*, 443–452.

Fibiger, H. C. (1997). Anti-psychotic drugs: Insights provided by immediate early genes. Paper presented at the Langfeld Conference on Current Issues in Comparative and Developmental Psychobiology, Princeton.

Fischer, R. S., Alexander, M. P., D'Esposito, M., and Otto, R. (1995). Neuropsychological and neuroanatomical correlates of confabulation. *Journal of Clinical and Experimental Neuropsychology, 17*(1), 20–28.

Fleminger, S. (1994). Delusional misidentification: An exemplary symptom illustrating an interaction between organic brain disease and psychological processes. First International Conference on Delusional Misidentification Syndromes (1993), Paris. *Psychopathology, 27*(3–5), 161–167.

Frith, C. D. (1992). *The cognitive neuropsychology of schizophrenia.* Hove, England: Lawrence Erlbaum.

Frith, C. D. (1996). Neuropsychology of schizophrenia: What are the implications of intellectual and experiential abnormalities for the neurobiology of schizophrenia? *British Medical Bulletin, 52*(3), 618–626.

Gardiner, J. M., and Java, R. I. (1993). Recognising and remembering. In A. E. Collins, S. E. Gathercole, M. A. Conway, and P. E. Morris (Eds.), *Theories of memory* (pp. 163–188). Hove, England: Lawrence Erlbaum.

Glisky, E. L., Polster, M. R., and Routhieaux, B. C. (1995). Double dissociation between item and source memory. *Neuropsychology, 9*(2), 229–235.

Gray, J. A. (1995). A model of the limbic system and basal ganglia: Applications to anxiety and schizophrenia. In M. S. Gazzaniga (Ed.), *The cognitive neurosciences* (pp. 1165–76). Cambridge, MA: MIT Press.

Hasher, L., Goldstein, D., and Toppino, T. (1977). Frequency and the conference of referential validity. *Journal of Verbal Learning and Verbal Behavior, 16*(1), 107–112.

Hasher, L., and Griffin, M. (1978). Reconstructive and reproductive processes in memory. *Journal of Experimental Psychology: Human Learning and Memory, 4,* 318–330.

Hasher, L., and Zacks, R. T. (1979). Automatic and effortful processes in memory. *Journal of Experimental Psychology: General, 108,* 356–388.

Hasher, L., and Zacks, R. T. (1988). Working memory, comprehension, and aging: A review and a new view. *Psychology of Learning and Motivation, 22,* 193–225.

Hashtroudi, S., Johnson, M. K., and Chrosniak, L. D. (1990). Aging and qualitative characteristics of memories for perceived and imagined complex events. *Psychology and Aging, 5,* 119–126.

Hashtroudi, S., Johnson, M. K., Vnek, N., and Ferguson, S. A. (1994). Aging and the effects of affective and factual focus on source monitoring and recall. *Psychology and Aging, 9*(1), 160–170.

Heilman, K. M. (1991). Anosognosia: Possible neuropsychological mechanisms. In G. P. Prigatano and D. L. Schacter (Eds.), *Awareness of deficit after brain injury: Clinical and theoretical issues* (pp. 53–62). New York: Oxford University Press.

Henkel, L., and Franklin, N. (1998). Reality monitoring of physically similar and conceptually related objects. *Memory and Cognition, 26,* 659–673.

Henkel, L. A., Franklin, N., and Johnson, M. K. (1998). Cross-modal source monitoring confusions between perceived and imagined events. Manuscript.

Henkel, L. A., Johnson, M. K., and De Leonardis, D. M. (1998). Aging and source monitoring: Cognitive processes and neuropsychological correlates. *Journal of Experimental Psychology: General, 127,* 251–268.

Hyman, I. E., Jr., Husband, T. H., and Billings, F. J. (1995). False memories of childhood experiences. *Applied Cognitive Psychology, 9,* 181–197.

Hyman, I. E., and Pentland, J. (1996). The role of mental imagery in the creation of false childhood memories. *Journal of Memory and Language, 35,* 101–117.

Intraub, H., and Hoffman, J. E. (1992). Reading and visual memory: Remembering scenes that were never seen. *American Journal of Psychology, 105,* 101–114.

Ivy, G. O., MacLeod, C. M., Petit, T. L., and Markus, E. J. (1992). A physiological framework for perceptual and cognitive changes in aging. In F. I. M. Craik and T. A. Salthouse (Eds.), *The handbook of aging and cognition* (pp. 273–314). Hillsdale, NJ: Lawrence Erlbaum.

Jacoby, L. L. (1991). A process dissociation framework: Separating automatic from intentional uses of memory. *Journal of Memory and Language, 30,* 513–541.

Jacoby, L. L., and Dallas, M. (1981). On the relationship between autobiographical memory and perceptual learning. *Journal of Experimental Psychology: General, 110*(3), 306–340.

Jacoby, L. L., and Kelley, C. M. (1987). Unconscious influences of memory for a prior event. *Personality and Social Psychology Bulletin, 13,* 314–336.

Jacoby, L. L., Woloshyn, V., and Kelley, C. M. (1989). Becoming famous without being recognized: Unconscious influences of memory produced by dividing attention. *Journal of Experimental Psychology: General, 118*(2), 115–125.

Janowsky, J. S., Shimamura, A. P., and Squire, L. R. (1989). Source memory impairment in patients with frontal lobe lesions. *Neuropsychologia, 27,* 1043–56.

Johnson, M. K. (1988). Discriminating the origin of information. In T. F. Oltmanns and B. A. Maher (Eds.), *Delusional beliefs* (pp. 34–65). New York: John Wiley.

Johnson, M. K. (1991). Reality monitoring: Evidence from confabulation in organic brain disease patients. In G. P. Prigatano and D. L. Schacter (Eds.), *Awareness of deficit after brain injury: Clinical and theoretical issues* (pp. 176–197). New York: Oxford University Press.

Johnson, M. K. (1992). MEM: Mechanisms of recollection. *Journal of Cognitive Neuroscience, 4*(3), 268–280.

Johnson, M. K. (1997a). Identifying the origin of mental experience. In M. S. Myslobodsky (Ed.), *The mythomanias: The nature of deception and self-deception* (pp. 133–180). Mahwah, NJ: Lawrence Erlbaum.

Johnson, M. K. (1997b). Source monitoring and memory distortion. *Philosophical Transactions of the Royal Society of London, 352,* 1733–45.

Johnson, M. K., Bransford, J. D., and Solomon, S. K. (1973). Memory for tacit implications of sentences. *Journal of Experimental Psychology, 98,* 203–205.

Johnson, M. K., and Chalfonte, B. L. (1994). Binding complex memories: The role of reactivation and the hippocampus. In D. L. Schacter and E. Tulving (Eds.), *Memory systems 1994* (pp. 311–350). Cambridge, MA: MIT Press.

Johnson, M. K., Foley, M. A., and Leach, K. (1988). The consequences for memory of imagining in another person's voice. *Memory and Cognition, 16,* 337–342.

Johnson, M. K., Foley, M. A., Suengas, A. G., and Raye, C. L. (1988). Phenomenal characteristics of memories for perceived and imagined autobiographical events. *Journal of Experimental Psychology: General, 117,* 371–376.

Johnson, M. K., Hashtroudi, S., and Lindsay, D. S. (1993). Source monitoring. *Psychological Bulletin, 114*(1), 3–28.

Johnson, M. K., Hayes, S. M., D'Esposito, M., and Raye, C. L. (Forthcoming). Confabulation. In F. Boller and J. Grafman (Eds.), *Handbook of Neuropsychology* (2nd ed.), Vol. 4. Amsterdam: Elsevier Science.

Johnson, M. K., and Hirst, W. (1993). MEM: Memory subsystems as processes. In A. F. Collins, S. E. Gathercole, M. A. Conway, and P. E. Morris (Eds.), *Theories of memory* (pp. 241–286). Hove, England: Lawrence Erlbaum.

Johnson, M. K., Kounios, J., and Nolde, S. F. (1996). Electrophysiological brain activity and memory source monitoring. *NeuroReport, 7,* 2929–32.

Johnson, M. K., Kounios, J., and Reeder, J. A. (1994). Time-course studies of reality monitoring and recognition. *Journal of Experimental Psychology: Learning, Memory, and Cognition, 20*(6), 1409–19.

Johnson, M. K., and Multhaup, K. S. (1992). Emotion and MEM. In S.-A. Christianson (Ed.), *The handbook of emotion and memory: Research and theory* (pp. 33–66). Hillsdale, NJ: Lawrence Erlbaum.

Johnson, M. K., Nolde, S. F., and De Leonardis, D. M. (1996). Emotional focus and source monitoring. *Journal of Memory and Language, 35*(2), 135–156.

Johnson, M. K., Nolde, S. F., Mather, M., Kounios, J., Schacter, D. L., and Curran, T. (1997). The similarity of brain activity associated with true and false recognition memory depends on test format. *Psychological Science, 8,* 250–257.

Johnson, M. K., O'Connor, M., and Cantor, J. (1997). Confabulation, memory deficits, and frontal dysfunction. *Brain and Cognition, 34,* 189–206.

Johnson, M. K., and Raye, C. L. (1981). Reality monitoring. *Psychological Review, 88,* 67–85.

Johnson, M. K., and Raye, C. L. (1998). False memories and confabulation. *Trends in Cognitive Science, 2,* 137–145.

Johnson, M. K., Raye, C. L., Wang, A. Y., and Taylor, T. H. (1979). Fact and fantasy: The roles of accuracy and variability in confusing imaginations with perceptual experiences. *Journal of Experimental Psychology: Human Learning and Memory, 5,* 229–240.

Johnson, M. K., and Reeder, J. A. (1997). Consciousness as meta-processing. In J. D. Cohen and J. W. Schooler (Eds.), *Scientific approaches to consciousness* (pp. 261–293). Mahwah, NJ: Lawrence Erlbaum.

Johnson, M. K., and Sherman, S. J. (1990). Constructing and reconstructing the past and the future in the present. In E. T. Higgins and R. M. Sorrentino (Eds.), *Handbook of motivation and cognition: Foundations of social behavior* (pp. 482–526). New York: Guilford Press.

Kausler, D. H., and Puckett, J. M. (1980). Adult age differences in recognition memory for a nonsemantic attribute. *Experimental Aging Research, 6,* 349–355.

Kemper, T. (1984). Neuroanatomical and neuropathological changes during aging and dementia. In M. L. Albert and Janice E. Knoefel (Eds.), *Clini-*

cal neurology of aging (2nd ed.) (pp. 3–67). New York: Oxford University Press.

Kopelman, M. D. (1987). Two types of confabulation. *Journal of Neurology, Neurosurgery, and Psychiatry, 50*(11), 1482–87.

Kopelman, M. D., Guinan, E. M., and Lewis, P. D. R. (1995). Delusional memory, confabulation, and frontal lobe dysfunction: A case study in De Clerambault's syndrome. *Neurocase, 1*, 71–77.

Kroll, N. E. A., Knight, R. T., Metcalfe, J., Wolf, E. S., and Tulving, E. (1996). Cohesion failure as a source of memory illusions. *Journal of Memory and Language, 35*(2), 176–196.

Light, L. L., and Zelinski, E. M. (1983). Memory for spatial information in young and old adults. *Developmental Psychology, 19*(6), 901–906.

Lindsay, D. S., and Johnson, M. K. (1989). The eyewitness suggestibility effect and memory for source. *Memory and Cognition, 17*(3), 349–358.

Lindsay, D. S., Johnson, M. K., and Kwon, P. (1991). Developmental changes in memory source monitoring. *Journal of Experimental Child Psychology, 52*(3), 297–318.

Lindsay, D. S., and Read, J. D. (1994). Psychotherapy and memories of childhood sexual abuse: A cognitive perspective. *Applied Cognitive Psychology, 8*(4), 281–338.

Loftus, E. F. (1979). *Eyewitness testimony.* Cambridge, MA: Harvard University Press.

Luria, A. R. (1976). *The neuropsychology of memory.* Washington, D.C.: V. H. Winston.

Maher, B. (1974). Delusional thinking and perceptual disorder. *Journal of Individual Psychology, 30*(1), 98–113.

Malloy, P., and Duffy, J. (1994). The frontal lobes in neuropsychiatric disorders. In F. Boller and J. Grafman, *Handbook of neuropsychology,* Vol. 9 (pp. 203–232). New York: Elsevier.

Markham, R., and Hynes, L. (1993). The effect of vividness of imagery on reality monitoring. *Journal of Mental Imagery, 17*(3–4), 159–170.

Martin, A., Haxby, J. V., Lalonde, F. M., Wiggs, C. L., and Ungerleider, L. G. (1995). Discrete cortical regions associated with knowledge of color and knowledge of action. *Science, 270*, 102–105.

Mather, M. (1998). Emotional review and memory distortion. Manuscript.

Mather, M., Henkel, L. A., and Johnson, M. K. (1997). Evaluating characteristics of false memories: Remember/know judgments and memory characteristics questionnaire compared. *Memory and Cognition, 25*, 826–837.

Mather, M., Johnson, M. K., and De Leonardis, D. (1999). Stereotype reliance in source monitoring: Age differences and neuropsychological test correlates. *Cognitive Neuropsychology, 16*, 437–458.

McCarthy, G. (1995). Functional neuroimaging of memory. *Neuroscientist, 1*, 155–163.

McKay, A. P., McKenna, P. J., and Baddeley, A. D. (1995). Memory pathology in schizophrenia. In R. Campbell and M. A. Conway, (Eds.), *Broken memories: Case studies in memory impairment* (pp. 124–136). Oxford: Blackwell.

Metcalfe, J., Funnell, M., and Gazzaniga, M. S. (1995). Right-hemisphere memory superiority: Studies of a split-brain patient. *Psychological Science, 6*(3), 157–164.

Milner, B. (1971). Interhemispheric difference in the localization of psychological processes in man. *British Medical Bulletin, 27,* 272–277.

Milner, B., Petrides, M., and Smith, M. L. (1985). Frontal lobes and the temporal organization of memory. *Human Neurobiology, 4,* 137–142.

Mitchell, K. J., and Johnson, M. K. (2000). Source monitoring: Attributing memories to sources. In E. Tulving and F. I. M. Craik (Eds.), *The Oxford Handbook of Memory* (pp. 179–195). New York: Oxford University Press.

Mitchell, K. J., and Zaragoza, M. S. (1996). Repeated exposure to suggestion and false memory: The role of contextual variability. *Journal of Memory and Language, 35*(2), 246–260.

Moscovitch, M. (1989). Confabulation and the frontal systems: Strategic versus associative retrieval in neuropsychological theories of memory. In H. L. Roediger and F. I. M. Craik (Eds.), *Varieties of memory and consciousness: Essays in honour of Endel Tulving* (pp. 133–160). Hillsdale, NJ: Lawrence Erlbaum.

Moscovitch, M. (1995). Confabulation. In D. L. Schacter (Ed.), *Memory distortions: How minds, brains, and societies reconstruct the past* (pp. 226–251). Cambridge, MA: Harvard University Press.

Nelson, T. O., and Narens, L. (1990). Metamemory: A theoretical framework and some new findings. In G. H. Bower (Ed.), *The psychology of learning and motivation,* Vol. 26 (pp. 125–173). New York: Academic Press.

Nolde, S. F. (1997). Event-related potentials: Studies of memory access during source monitoring and old/new recognition. Doctoral dissertation, Princeton University.

Nolde, S. F., Johnson, M. K., and D'Esposito, M. (1998). Left prefrontal activation during episodic remembering: An event-related fMRI study. *NeuroReport, 9,* 3509–14.

Nolde, S. F., Johnson, M. K., and Raye, C. L. (1998). The role of prefrontal cortex in episodic memory. *Trends in Cognitive Sciences, 2,* 399–406.

Norman, D. A., and Bobrow, D. G. (1979). Descriptions: An intermediate stage in memory retrieval. *Cognitive Psychology, 11*(1), 107–123.

Norman, D. A., and Schacter, D. L. (1996). Implicit memory, explicit memory, and false recollection: A cognitive neuroscience perspective. In L. M.

Reder (Ed.), *Implicit memory and metacognition.* Hillsdale, NJ: Lawrence Erlbaum.

Norman, K. A., and Schacter, D. L. (1997). False recognition in younger and older adults: Exploring the characteristics of illusory memories. *Memory and Cognition, 25*, 838–848.

Nyberg, L., Cabeza, R., and Tulving, E. (1996). PET studies of encoding and retrieval: The HERA model. *Psychonomic Bulletin and Review, 3*, 135–148.

O'Connor, M., Walbridge, M., Sandson, T., and Alexander, M. (1996). A neuropsychological analysis of Capgras syndrome. *Neuropsychiatry, Neuropsychology and Behavioral Neurology, 9*, 265–271.

Park, D. C., and Puglisi, J. T. (1985). Older adults' memory for the color of pictures and words. *Journal of Gerontology, 40*(2), 198–204.

Parkin, A. J., Leng, N. R., Stanhope, N., and Smith, A. P. (1988). Memory impairment following ruptured aneurysm of the interior communicating artery. *Brain and Cognition, 7*, 231–243.

Pezdek, K. (1983). Memory for items and their spatial locations by young and elderly adults. *Developmental Psychology, 19*, 895–900.

Phelps, E. A., and Gazzaniga, M. S. (1992). Hemispheric differences in mnemonic processing: The effects of left hemisphere interpretation. *Neuropsychologia, 30*(3), 293–297.

Phelps, E. A., Hirst, W., and Gazzaniga, M. S. (1991). Deficits in recall following partial and complete commissurotomy. *Cerebral Cortex, 1*(6), 492–498.

Posner, M. I., and Snyder, C. R. R. (1975). Attention and cognitive control. In R. L. Solso (Ed.), *Information processing and cognition: The Loyola symposium* (pp. 55–85). Hillsdale, NJ: Lawrence Erlbaum.

Rajaram, S., and Roediger, H. L. III. (1997). Remembering and knowing as states of consciousness during retrieval. In J. D. Cohen and J. W. Schooler (Eds.), *Scientific approaches to consciousness* (pp. 213–240). Mahwah, NJ: Lawrence Erlbaum.

Ramachandran, V. S. (1995). Anosognosia in parietal lobe syndrome. *Consciousness and Cognition, 4*(1), 22–51.

Raye, C. L. (1976). Recognition: Frequency or organization? *American Journal of Psychology, 89*, 645–658.

Raye, C. L., Johnson, M. K., and Taylor, T. H. (1980). Is there something special about memory for internally generated information? *Memory and Cognition, 8*(2), 141–148.

Reinitz, M., Lammers, W., and Cochran, B. (1992). Memory-conjunction errors: Miscombination of stored stimulus features can produce illusions of memory. *Memory and Cognition, 20*(1), 1–11.

Reiser, B. J. (1986). The encoding and retrieval of memories of real-world experiences. In J. A. Galambo, R. P. Abelson, and J. B. Black (Eds.), *Knowledge structures* (pp. 71–99). Hillsdale, NJ: Lawrence Erlbaum.

Roediger, H. (1996). Memory illusions. *Journal of Memory and Language,* 35(2), 76–100.

Roediger, H. L., and McDermott, K. B. (1995). Creating false memories: Remembering words not presented in lists. *Journal of Experimental Psychology: Learning, Memory, and Cognition,* 21(4), 803–814.

Ross, M. (1989). Relation of implicit theories to the construction of personal histories. *Psychological Review,* 96(2), 341–357.

Ross, M. (1997). Validating memories. In N. L. Stein, P. A. Ornstein, B. Tversky, and C. Brainerd (Eds.), *Memory for everyday and emotional events* (pp. 49–81). Hillsdale, NJ: Lawrence Erlbaum.

Rugg, M. D. (1995). Event-related potential studies of human memory. In M. S. Gazzaniga (Ed.), *The cognitive neurosciences* (pp. 789–801). Cambridge, MA: MIT Press.

Schacter, D. L. (1995). Memory distortion: History and current status. In D. L. Schacter (Ed.), *Memory distortion* (pp. 1–43). Cambridge, MA: Harvard University Press.

Schacter, D. L., Alpert, N. M., Savage, C. R., et al. (1996). Conscious recollection and the human hippocampal formation: Evidence from positron emission tomography, *Proceedings of the National Academy of Sciences of the United States of America,* 93, 321–325.

Schacter, D. L., Curran, T., Galluccio, L., Milberg, W. P., and Bates, J. F. (1996). False recognition and the right frontal lobe: A case study. *Neuropsychologia,* 34(8), 793–808.

Schacter, D. L., Harbluk, J. L., and McLachlan, D. R. (1984). Retrieval without recollection: An experimental analysis of source amnesia. *Journal of Verbal Learning and Verbal Behavior,* 23(5), 593–611.

Schacter, D. L., Koutstaal, W., Johnson, M. K., Gross, M. S., and Angell, K. E. (1997). False recollection induced via photographs: A comparison of older and younger adults. *Psychology and Aging, 12,* 203–215.

Schacter, D. L., Norman, K. A., Koutstaal, W. (1998). The cognitive neuroscience of constructive memory. *Annual Review of Psychology, 49,* 289–318.

Schacter, D. L., Reiman, E., Curran, T., Yun, L. S., Bandy, D., McDermott, K. B., and Roediger, H. L. III. (1996). Neuroanatomical correlates of veridical and illusory recognition memory: Evidence from positron emission tomography. *Neuron, 17,* 267–274.

Senkfor, A. J., and Van Petten, C. (1998). Who said what: An event-related potential investigation of source and item memory. *Journal of Experimental Psychology: Learning, Memory and Cognition, 24,* 1005–25.

Shallice, T. (1988). *From neuropsychology to mental structure.* New York: Cambridge University Press.

Shallice, T., Fletcher, P., Frith, C. D., Grasby, P., Frackowiak, R. S. J., and Dolan, R. J. (1994). Brain regions associated with acquisition and retrieval of verbal episodic memory. *Nature, 368,* 6472.

Shimamura, A. P. (1995). Memory and frontal lobe function. In M. S. Gazzaniga (Ed.), *The cognitive neurosciences* (pp. 803–813). Cambridge, MA: MIT Press.

Shimamura, A. P., Janowsky, J. S., and Squire, L. R. (1990). Memory for the temporal order of events in patients with frontal lobe lesions and amnesic patients. *Neuropsychologia, 28*(8), 803–813.

Skurnik, I. W. (1998). Metacognition and the illusion of truth. Doctoral dissertation, Princeton University.

Squire, L. R., and Knowlton, B. J. (1995). Memory, hippocampus, and brain systems. In M. S. Gazzaniga (Ed.), *The cognitive neurosciences* (pp. 825–837). Cambridge, MA: MIT Press.

Stuss, D. T., Alexander, M. P., Lieberman, A., and Levine, H. (1978). An extraordinary form of confabulation. *Neurology, 28*(1), 1166–72.

Stuss, D. T., and Benson, D. F. (1986). *The frontal lobes.* New York: Raven Press.

Stuss, D. T., Eskes, G. A., and Foster, J. K. (1994). Experimental neuropsychological studies of frontal lobe functions. In F. Boller and J. Grafman (Eds.), *Handbook of neuropsychology,* Vol. 9 (pp. 149–185). New York: Elsevier.

Suengas, A. G., and Johnson, M. K. (1988). Qualitative effects of rehearsal on memories for perceived and imagined complex events. *Journal of Experimental Psychology: General, 117*(4), 377–389.

Tulving, E. (1983). *Elements of episodic memory.* New York: Clarendon Press.

Tulving, E. (1985). Memory and consciousness. *Canadian Psychology, 26*(1), 1–12.

Tulving, E., Kapur, S., Markowitsch, H. J., Craik, F. I. M., Habib, R., and Houle, S. (1994). Neuroanatomical correlates of retrieval in episodic memory: Auditory sentence recognition. *Proceedings of the National Academy of Sciences of the United States of America, 91,* 2012–15.

Ungerleider, L. G. (1995). Functional brain imaging studies of cortical mechanisms for memory. *Science, 270,* (5237).

Underwood, B. J. (1965). False recognition produced by implicit verbal responses. *Journal of Experimental Psychology, 70,* 122–129.

Weinberger, D. R. (1988). Schizophrenia and the frontal lobe. *Trends in Neuroscience, 11*(8), 367–370.

West, R. L. (1996). An application of prefrontal cortex function theory to cognitive aging. *Psychological Bulletin, 120*(2), 272–292.

Williams, M. W., and Hollan, J. D. (1981). The process of retrieval from very long-term memory. *Cognitive Science, 5,* 87–119.

Zaragoza, M. S., and Koshmider, J. W. III. (1989). Misled subjects may know more than their performance implies. *Journal of Experimental Psychology: Learning, Memory, and Cognition, 15*(2), 246–255.

Zaragoza, M. S., and Lane, S. M. (1994). Source misattributions and the sug-
    gestibility of eyewitness memory. *Journal of Experimental Psychology:
    Learning, Memory, and Cognition, 20*(4), 934–945.
Zaragoza, M. S., Lane, S. M., Ackil, J. K., and Chambers, K. L. (1997). Con-
    fusing real and suggested memories: Source monitoring and eyewitness
    suggestibility. In N. L. Stein, P. A. Ornstein, B. Tversky, and C. Brainerd
    (Eds.), *Memory for everyday and emotional events* (pp. 401–425). Hills-
    dale, NJ: Lawrence Erlbaum.

Notes

1. We assume features of memories are distributed in those brain areas that
   originally processed the information (see for example Damasio, 1989).
   When we say that features must be "bound" together to form memories,
   we are not implying that a new single representation replaces these features. Rather, we mean that a process ("binding") relates the feature representations in such a way that they are more likely to be activated together
   later (Cohen and Eichenbaum, 1993).
2. We sometimes use the words "criterion" and "criteria" in an everyday
   sense to include what features are considered and how different features
   are weighted, as well as the threshold amount (or match of such information to a standard) that is required for a given source attribution. This
   usage may confuse some readers because the same terms are sometimes
   employed in the literature to refer to the decision threshold in a signal detection analysis of old-new recognition in which information is assumed to
   vary only along a single dimension (such as strength). In the SMF, both the
   qualitative and quantitative characteristics of mental experiences affect
   source attributions. Here we refer to "weights" when emphasizing flexibility in which qualities of mental experience are given the most focus or
   highest importance, and to "criteria" when we are emphasizing flexibility
   in the nature (amount or pattern) of information that is required for a particular source attribution. The two factors together are components of
   overall evaluative processes that make attributions about the nature of
   mental experiences.

Acknowledgments

This research was supported by NIA grant AG09253.

Memory and the Brain: New Lessons from Old Syndromes

V. S. Ramachandran

Canst thou not minister to a mind diseas'd,
Pluck from the memory a rooted sorrow,
Raze out the written troubles of the brain,
And with some sweet oblivious antidote
Cleanse the stuff'd bosom of that perilous stuff
Which weighs upon the heart?

William Shakespeare

During the last three decades, considerable progress has been made in understanding the neural basis of memory formation. Most of this research falls into two categories:

1. Investigation of the actual synaptic changes involved—studied elegantly in aplysia (Alkon et al., 1993; Bailey and Kandel, 1995) and in in-vitro hippocampal slices (Lynch, 1989; Stanton and Sejnowski, 1989);
2. Investigation of anterograde amnesia resulting from medial temporal lobe/hippocampal damage (Milner, Corkin, and Teuber, 1968; Mishkin, 1978; Schacter, 1996; Squire, 1987; Weiskrantz, 1987).

Surprisingly, the equally important narrative or "constructive" aspects of human memory (the mechanisms of retrieval, the creation of new categories, and a tacit taxonomy of these categories), the encoding of spatial and temporal context, and the binding of objects across successive episodic memories, have rarely been studied experimentally—although their importance was recognized long ago by Bartlett (1932). The vast psychological literature on this topic is largely uninformative; in particular, we have no idea of what the neural substrates of these elusive mechanisms might be.

87

In this chapter I will suggest that other neurological syndromes can help elucidate mnemonic mechanisms in the brain: anosognosia, phantom limbs, and Capgras syndrome. These syndromes may provide a valuable experimental opportunity for studying aspects of memory that have hitherto remained inaccessible to scientific scrutiny.

Anosognosia

This disturbance is observed in patients with left-sided paralysis caused by damage to the right hemisphere, usually the result of a stroke. Most patients with right hemisphere stroke acknowledge their paralysis, but a small proportion (approximately 5 percent) vehemently deny it. This syndrome was first described at the turn of the century by the French neurologist Joseph Babinski (1914). Since then, numerous fascinating clinical cases have been described, but the tendency has been to regard them as outlandish or bizarre. I have attempted to bring this syndrome into the domain of modern cognitive neuroscience, as it raises some fundamental questions concerning the organization of the human mind.

As an illustration of anosognosia, consider my conversation with an elderly woman, FD, who had had a right hemisphere stroke eight days previously, resulting in a complete left hemiplegia. She was unable to move without a wheelchair and had no use of her left arm.

VSR: Mrs. D, how are you feeling today?
FD: I've got a headache. I've had a stroke so they brought me to the hospital.
VSR: Mrs. D, can you walk?
FD: Yes. (She had been in a wheelchair for the past two weeks and could not walk.)
VSR: Mrs. D, hold out your hands. Can you move your hands?
FD: Yes.
VSR: Can you use your right hand?
FD: Yes.
VSR: Can you use your left hand?
FD: Yes.

VSR: Are both hands equally strong?
FD: Yes, of course they are.

These responses are quite typical of a person with anosognosia. I wondered what would happen if I pushed the patient further. I did so with some hesitation, for fear of precipitating what Goldstein (1940) called a catastrophic reaction—medical jargon for "the patient starts to cry because her defenses crumble."

VSR: Can you point to my nose with your right hand?
FD: (She pointed to my nose.)
VSR: Point to me with your left hand.
FD: (Her hand lay paralyzed in front of her.)
VSR: Are you pointing to my nose?
FD: Yes.
VSR: Can you clearly see it pointing?
FD: Yes, it is about two inches from your nose.

The woman had now produced a frank confabulation. She had no problems with her vision and could see her arm perfectly clearly, yet she experienced a delusion about her own body image. (I had verified previously that she had no left hemineglect, and also took the precaution of standing on her right side.)

VSR: Can you clap?
FD: Of course I can clap.
VSR: Will you clap for me?
FD: (She proceeded to make clapping movements with her right hand as if clapping with an imaginary hand near the midline.)
VSR: Are you clapping?
FD: Yes, I'm clapping.

Here at last we may have an answer to the Zen master's eternal riddle, What is the sound of one hand clapping? Mrs. D obviously knew the answer!

Mrs. D's responses are quite extreme. What is much more common in patients with anosognosia is a tendency to come up with assorted rationalizations to explain why the arm does not move; they do not usually say they can actually see the arm moving. Consider the following conversation with a more typical patient, LR. She too had sustained a right hemisphere stroke that had paralyzed the left side of her body.

VSR: Mrs. R, how are you doing?
LR: I'm fine.
VSR: Can you walk?
LR: Yes.
VSR: Can you use your arms?
LR: Yes.
VSR: Can you use your right arm?
LR: Yes.
VSR: Can you use your left arm?
LR: Yes, I can use my left arm.
VSR: Can you point to me with your right hand?
LR: (She pointed to me with her right hand.)
VSR: Point to me with your left hand?
LR: (Her hand remained lying in front of her.)
VSR: Are you pointing?
LR: I have severe arthritis in my shoulder, you know that doctor. It hurts.

These patients often come up with ingenious excuses and poignantly comic euphemisms to evade the main thrust of the question.

VSR: How come you are not using your left arm?
LR: I've never been very ambidextrous.

There is a striking similarity between the strategies used by these patients and what Anna and Sigmund Freud called psychological defense mechanisms (A. Freud, 1946; S. Freud, 1996), employed when people are confronted with disturbing facts about themselves. Examples are rationalization, denial, repression of unpleasant memories, and reaction formation. Individuals suffering from anosognosia utilize these strategies but in grossly exaggerated form (Ramachandran, 1994, 1995). For example, a normal person who has peripheral nerve damage and is left with a paralyzed arm may play down the extent of the deficit ("Oh, I think I'll recover soon"), but he (or she) is unlikely to declare that the arm does not belong to him or that he sees it pointing about two inches from his physician's nose. Most people would not carry defense mechanisms to such limits.

One interpretation of anosognosia would be in psychodynamic terms: the patient is confronted with something unpleasant, paralysis, and plays it down or even denies it. This explanation is invalid for one simple reason—the disorder is rarely seen when the left hemisphere is damaged and right-sided paralysis results. That paralysis ought to be just as unpleasant, yet these patients rarely engage in denial. Such asymmetry suggests that anosognosia is a neurological rather than a psychological syndrome. Indeed, it is fascinating precisely because it straddles the borderline between neurology and psychiatry.

A more cognitive interpretation of the syndrome would be in terms of the hemineglect–hemi-inattention that often accompanies denial. That is, one could argue that the patient neglects her paralysis in much the same way that she neglects everything else on the left side. This hypothesis is probably at least partially correct, but it does not account for the persistence of the denial even when the patient's attention is drawn to the paralysis. Nor does it explain why she does not intellectually correct her misconception when she is quite lucid and intelligent in other respects. Indeed, the reason anosognosia is so puzzling is that we have come to regard the intellect as primarily propositional in character, and we expect propositional logic to be internally consistent. To listen to a patient deny ownership of her arm and in the same breath admit that it is attached to her shoulder is one of the most perplexing phenomena a neurologist can encounter.

Belief and the Denial of Paralysis

One obvious question is, How deeply does the patient believe his or her own denials and confabulations? Are they simply a surface facade, or perhaps even an attempt at malingering?

The vehemence of LR's denials and her quasi-humorous, euphemistic remarks can themselves be taken as evidence that she is "aware" at some level that she is paralyzed ("Yes, of course, I can use my left hand. In fact, I used it to wash my face this morning," or

"Yeah, I can't wait to get back to two-fisted drinking," or "I've never been very ambidextrous").

The question then becomes, for what sorts of behavior is this tacit knowledge available, if it exists? For example, would it be available for a spontaneous, nonverbal motor response?

I did two experiments to explore this question. In the first, I simply placed a large cocktail tray in front of the patient. (The tray held six plastic glasses containing water.) When normal people reach for the tray to lift it, their right hand goes to the right end of the tray and the left hand to the left side. When I tested hemiplegic patients who did not have anosognosia, their nonparalyzed hand went straight for the middle of the tray near its center of gravity, as expected; but when I tried the same experiment with patients who had anosognosia, their right hand went to the right side of the tray! Obviously, the glasses toppled, but the patients usually made remarks such as, "Oops! How clumsy of me." Thus, even when no direct verbal confrontation is involved, the patient behaves as though the left hand is working normally.

The logic of the second experiment was somewhat different. I gave four patients a choice between a simple unimanual task or a simple bimanual task impossible to perform with one hand. The choice was either to thread a light bulb into a socket that was mounted on a heavy base (unimanual) or to tie a shoelace (bimanual). If the patient threaded the light bulb she would receive a five-dollar reward, and if she tied the shoelace she would receive ten dollars. Remarkably, the patients started trying to tie the laces and kept at it for several minutes without showing any signs of frustration. Even when the patients were given the same choice ten minutes later, they again went invariably for the bimanual task. In one case (LR), the tests were repeated on several consecutive occasions—always with the same result. The patients seem to have no memory of their previous failures.

Thus, my two experiments did not reveal any "tacit" knowledge, but there may be other ways to probe for it. For instance, one could flash words such as "paralysis," "death," or "bitter" on the screen and ask the patient to rate them on a scale of 1 to 10 for "unpleasantness." A normal person would presumably rate death as the most unpleasant. But would patients with anosognosia give the world "paralysis" an especially high rating? Or, indeed, an especially low rating?

What would their galvanic skin response be for the word (compared to that of control patients who are not in denial)?

Clearly, these patients appear not to have tacit knowledge of paralysis; or if such knowledge exists, it is not available for the two tasks described above. The implication is that the denial runs very deep; it is not just a surface facade at a purely verbal level. Another interesting question ensues: Do the patients deny only the immediate consequences of the paralysis, or would they also deny its remote consequences? Are they dimly aware that something is seriously wrong? What if one were to ask them circuitous questions: "Are you doing okay?" "Can you drive home tonight?" "Can you go back to the same job you were holding before?"

I have not explored this approach on a systematic basis, but on the four occasions when I specifically asked such questions, the responses indicated that the patients were indeed unaware of the remote consequences of the paralysis. For instance, a patient might state that she could walk. ("I walked to the restroom this morning, doctor.") I have even seen examples of patients whose job requires the use of two hands, who if asked "Can you go back to your job?" will assert vehemently, "Oh yes, I don't see a problem there." This reply suggests once again that, far from being a mere sensory/motor distortion, the whole range of beliefs about such matters has been radically altered to accommodate the denial (Ramachandran, 1995).

"Repressed" Memories

My next question concerns the patients' memories of their paralysis. As noted, patients with anosognosia will continue vehemently to deny their paralysis even when confronted with contradictory evidence. On some occasions patients will eventually admit that the left arm is "not working," is "weak," or is sometimes even "paralyzed." Even having admitted the paralysis, patients sometimes remain unconcerned about it and display a sort of absentminded indifference. After a patient, upon repeated questioning, has finally admitted that the arm is paralyzed, what if the researcher were to show up again after ten minutes and ask about her left arm? Would she remember her confession?

I have tried this experiment on several occasions and the usual answer seems to be no (Ramachandran, 1994). In other words, if I return to the patient ten minutes later, he or she will once again say, "Oh yes, my left arm is working." There seems to be a selective amnesia of the patient's own earlier admissions. Surprisingly, even on the one occasion when a patient had a "catastrophic reaction," she had no recollection of it a few hours later. One can scarcely get closer to a direct demonstration of what Freudians would call repression.

This amnesia seems to affect only the actions of the left hand, but not other aspects of that hand. On one occasion, a patient was surprised to notice that I had slipped a red hairband on her left hand. After removing the band, I started to question her about the movements of that hand. As expected, she vehemently denied the paralysis but, with repeated questioning, finally admitted that the hand "wasn't working." A few minutes later she had no recollection of this confession, even though she vividly remembered the hairband!

Patients with anosognosia often recover completely after two or three weeks and stop denying that they are paralyzed. Why this happens is still unclear, but it raises another fascinating question. What if one were to go to the patient after she had completely recovered and ask, "When I saw you earlier this week and I asked about your left arm, what did you tell me?" Would she admit that she had been denying the paralysis, or would she also deny the denial (Ramachandran 1994, 1995; Ramachandran and Rogers-Ramachandran, 1996a)?

I have tried this experiment on three patients. One patient, LC, interviewed three days after recovery from anosognosia, vividly recalled that he had denied his paralysis, but (as we shall see) his response was not typical. To my amazement he said, "I could see that it wasn't moving, but my mind didn't want to accept it. I guess I was in denial." The second patient, OS, strongly denied her paralysis on the several occasions that I tested her, but recovered completely from the anosognosia after a month. When I questioned her several months later, she denied her denials and added, "If I denied it, I must have been lying and I am not a liar." The third patient, MG, developed dense anosognosia twelve hours after a right hemisphere stroke. She asserted repeatedly that her left hand was working well. (Indeed, she claimed it was stronger than her right hand.) The next day she recovered completely from the denial and admitted her paralysis. Yet when questioned about the previous day, she said, "You asked me if I could lift a table, and I said I could lift it one inch." "What about your left arm?" I asked. "I said I couldn't use my left arm," she said confidently.

The reason for the difference between LC and the other two patients is unclear. Even after apparently complete recovery from anosognosia, there may be a residual neural defect in the right hemisphere, and the extent to which the patient admits or denies earlier denials may itself depend on the extent of these residual lesions (Ramachandran and Rogers-Ramachandran, 1996a).

Despite the variability, it is evident from these examples that some patients do indeed "deny their denials" even though they are mentally lucid and remember other details quite clearly. Perhaps there is no simple way for a patient to reconcile her current insight into her paralysis with her previous lack of it; consequently, her only recourse is to repress her denials to match her current beliefs. Further experiments may allow us to explore the formation of memory traces—caught in flagrante—and to discover how new items of information are incorporated seamlessly into preexisting cognitive schemata.

What if a patient had a peripheral nerve lesion in her left arm so that her left arm was paralyzed for a few months, and then she developed a right hemisphere stroke rendering her hemiplegic on the left side? Assume, further, that she also had a lesion of the right hemisphere of the kind that normally produces anosognosia. Would she then suddenly say, "Oh, my God, doctor. My arm that had been paralyzed all along is suddenly moving again"? To return to the notion that the patient tends to hold onto his preexisting worldview, does he cling to his updated worldview (Ramachandran, 1995) and therefore say that his left arm is paralyzed, or does he go back to his earlier body image and assert that his arm is in fact moving again? Needless to say, I have yet to see such a patient, but I hope that sooner or later someone will encounter a patient with this problem and ask this question.

Caloric Irrigation

Experiments with anosognosia suggest that information about the paralysis is being held somewhere in the brain, but that access to this information is blocked. To demonstrate this more directly, I took advantage of an ingenious experiment performed by Italian neurologists on a patient with neglect and anosognosia (Bisiach, Rusconi, and Vallar, 1991). They took a syringe filled with ice-cold water and irrigated the woman's left ear canal, a procedure that is usually performed to test vestibular nerve function. Within a few seconds the patient's eyes started to move vigorously (caloric induced nystagmus). When the researchers asked about her arms, she said her left arm was paralyzed. The cold-water irrigation of the left ear brought about an admission of her paralysis.

I tried this same experiment on my patient BM, an elderly woman who had had a right parietal stroke that resulted in left-side paralysis. My purpose was not only to confirm the observation of Bisiach and colleagues, but also specifically to test her memory, something that had not been done before on a systematic basis.

> VSR: Mrs. M, can you walk?
> BM: Yes, I can walk.
> VSR: Can you use your right hand?
> BM: Yes, I can.
> VSR: Are both hands equally strong?
> BM: Yes, of course they're equally strong!

I then irrigated her right ear with cold water and her eyes started moving in the characteristic way. After about a minute I began to question her.

> VSR: How are you doing?
> BM: My ear is cold, but I am fine.
> VSR: Can you use both of your arms?
> BM: Yes, I can use both arms.

The next day, after going through the same questions and eliciting a vehement denial of paralysis, I irrigated the patient's left ear with cold water. I waited until her eyes started moving and then questioned her again about her paralysis.

> VSR: Do you feel okay?
> BM: My ear is very cold, but other than that I am fine.
> VSR: Can you use your hands?
> BM: I can use my right arm but not my left arm. I want to move it, but it doesn't move.
> VSR: Can you use it?

BM: No, it is paralyzed.

VSR: Mrs. M, how long has your arm been paralyzed? Did it start now or earlier?

BM: It has been paralyzed continuously for several days now.

After about eight hours my assistant questioned her.

ASSISTANT: Mrs. M, can you walk?

BM: Yes.

A: Can you use both your arms?

BM: Yes.

A: Can you use your right arm?

BM: Yes.

A: Can you use your left arm?

BM: Yes.

A: This morning, two doctors did something to you. Do you remember?

BM: Yes. They put water in my ear; it was very cold.

A: Do you remember they asked some questions about your arms, and you gave them an answer? Do you remember what you said?

BM: I said my arms were okay.

Thus, even though BM had denied her paralysis every time I saw her in the clinic after her stroke, the information about her failed attempts had nevertheless been getting into her brain. It seems as though the access to these memories is ordinarily blocked, but cold water removes the block. The memories then come to the surface and the patient "confesses" her paralysis. Yet after the effect of the water wears off, the patient flatly denies her earlier admission of paralysis—as though she were completely rewriting her "script." Indeed, it is almost as if we created two separate conscious human beings who were mutually amnesic: the "cold water" BM, who is intellectually honest and acknowledges her paralysis, and the BM without the cold water, who has anosognosia and completely denies her paralysis.

These results suggest once again that anosognosia may provide a new experimental paradigm for studying mnemonic function in the human brain, especially the question of how new memories are seamlessly incorporated into one's preexisting belief system. Such experiments would be especially easy to carry out in conjunction with caloric-induced reversible hyperamnesia, if this effect is confirmed on additional patients. As we have seen, the experiments could also be carried out, even without caloric testing, simply by interviewing the patients repeatedly about their memories as they gradually regain insight.

One has to wonder why cold water produces these apparently miraculous effects, acting almost like a truth serum. One possibility is that it arouses the right hemisphere. Connections from the vestibular nerve project to the vestibular cortex in the right parietal lobe, as well as to other parts of the right hemisphere. Arousal of the right hemisphere makes the patient focus on the left side. Thus, the patient pays attention for the first time to the arm that is lying lifeless and recognizes that she is paralyzed.

This interpretation is probably at least partially correct, but an alternative hypothesis is that the phenomenon is related to rapid-eye-movement (REM) sleep. People spend one third of their lives sleeping; 25 percent of that time their eyes are moving, and that is when they have vivid, emotional dreams. In both the cold-water state and in REM sleep, noticeable eye movements occur and unpleasant memories come to the surface; this may not be a coincidence. Freud believed that while dreaming we pull up material that is ordinarily censored. Perhaps the vestibular stimulation partially activates the same circuitry that generates REM sleep, thereby allowing the patient to recognize unpleasant, disturbing facts about herself—including the paralysis, which is usually repressed when she is awake. I would give this speculative conjecture a 10 percent chance of being correct. (My colleagues would probably give it 1 percent!) But it does lead to a simple, testable prediction; patients with anosognosia should dream that they are paralyzed. In fact, if they are awakened during a REM episode, they may continue to admit their paralysis for several minutes before reverting to denial. (Recall that the effects of caloric-induced nystagmus lasted for at least thirty minutes.)

Phantom Limbs

What is the relevance of phantom limbs to the neurobiology of memory? Before answering this question I will briefly describe other research done on this syndrome.

Phantom limbs have probably been known since antiquity; not surprisingly, an elaborate folklore surrounds them. After Lord Nelson lost his right arm during an unsuccessful attack on Santa Cruz de Tenerife, he experienced compelling phantom-limb pains, including the sensation of fingers digging into his phantom palm. The emergence of these ghostly sensations led Lord Nelson to proclaim that his phantom was a "direct proof of the existence of the soul" (Riddoch, 1941). If an arm can survive physical annihilation, why not the entire person?

The first clinical description of phantom limbs was provided in 1872 by Silas Weir Mitchell (see Melzack, 1992). Despite the hundreds of case studies since then, systematic experimental work began less than ten years ago (Ramachandran, Rogers-Ramachandran, and Stewart, 1992), inspired in part by the demonstration of striking changes in somatotopic maps following deafferentation (Merzenich, et al., 1984; Wall, 1977). Eleven years after dorsal rhizotomy in adult monkeys, the region corresponding to the hand in the cortical somatotopic map (area 3b) could be activated by stimuli delivered to the ipsilateral side of the monkey's face (Pons et al., 1991), direct proof that a massive reorganization of topography had occurred in area 3b. That a similar reorganization occurs in the adult human cortex over distances of 2–3 centimeters was shown by using magnetoencephalography (MEG) (Ramachandran, 1993b, 1996; Yang et al., 1994a, 1994b; Flor et al., 1995). After amputation of an arm, sensory input from the face activated the hand area of the Penfield homunculus. Given this massive reorganization, we wondered what the person would feel if his face were touched. Since the tactile input on the face now activated the hand area of the cortex, we questioned whether the person would feel that he was being touched on his hand as well (Ramachandran, Rogers-Ramachandran, and Stewart, 1992).

Referred Sensations

After testing eighteen patients with either arm amputation or plexus avulsion, we found that eight patients systematically referred sensation from the face to the phantom limb. Many had a topographically organized map of individual fingers on the lower face region and the referred sensations were modality specific. For example, hot, cold, rubbing, vibration, metal, and massage on the face are felt as hot, cold, vibration, metal, and massage at precisely localized points in the phantom. Touching other body parts (torso, legs, chest) usually did not evoke sensation in the phantom, but there was often a second topographically organized map proximal to the amputation stump. The hand area in the Penfield map is flanked on one side by the upper arm and on the other side by the face, precisely the arrangement of points one would expect if the afferents from the upper-arm skin and the face skin were to invade the hand territory from either side.

The fact that stimulating certain trigger points (Cronholm, 1951) can elicit referred sensation in the phantom was noted in the older clinical literature, but the occurrence of a topographically organized map on the face and modality-specific referral from face to phantom were not described. Consequently, no attempt was made to relate these findings to somatotopic brain maps, and the referred sensations were often attributed either to stump neuromas or to activation of a "diffuse neural matrix" (Melzack, 1990). Our own results suggest instead that referred sensations emerge as a direct consequence of the changes in topography following deafferentation—an idea that we refer to as the remapping hypothesis (Ramachandran, 1993a).

That hypothesis also predicts (Ramachandran, 1994) that after trigeminal nerve section one should observe a map of the face on the hand, and this has been shown by Clarke and colleagues (1996). Also, in a patient whose index finger had been amputated, a map of the index finger was found neatly draped across the ipsilateral cheek (Aglioti, Bonazzi, and Cortese, 1994). Finally, our suggestion that these effects derive partly from the unmasking of preexisting connections rather than from sprouting, receives support from our subsequent observation that modality-specific referral from the face to the phantom can occur even a few hours after amputation (Borsook et al., 1998).

These findings provide strong support for the remapping hypothesis. They may allow us to track the time course of perceptual changes in humans and relate them in a systematic way to anatomy. The occurrence of topography and modality specificity rules out any possibility that the referral is due to nonspecific arousal.

Synesthesia

Some patients claim they can vividly experience voluntary movements in their phantom (Melzack, 1992), presumably because reafference signals from motor commands sent to the phantom are monitored in the cerebellum and the parietal lobes. However, with the passage of time the phantom becomes "frozen" or "paralyzed," perhaps because of the continuous absence of visual and proprioceptive confirmation that the commands have been obeyed. Some patients experience excruciatingly painful involuntary clenching spasms in the phantom; like Lord Nelson, they experience their nails digging into the phantom palm and are unable to open the hand voluntarily to relieve the pain.

In one experiment, we placed a vertical saggital mirror on the table in front of a patient. If the patient's paralyzed phantom was, say, on the left side of the mirror, he placed his right hand in an exact mirror-symmetric location on the right side of the mirror. If he looked into the shiny right side of the mirror, the reflection of his own hand was optically superimposed on the felt location of his phantom, so that he had the distinct visual illusion that the phantom had been resurrected. If he then made mirror-symmetric movements while looking in the mirror, he received visual feedback that the phantom limb was actually moving. This was often a source of considerable surprise and delight to the patient (Ramachandran and Rogers-Ramachandran, 1996b).

Indeed, four patients were able to use the visual feedback provided them by the mirror to "unclench" a painfully clenched phantom hand. This action seemed to relieve not only the clenching spasm but associated cramping pain as well. (The burning and lacerating pains in the phantom remained unaffected by the mirror procedure, suggesting that the relief of the clenching probably was not confabulatory in origin.) The elimination of the spasm is a robust effect that was confirmed on several patients. They also pointed out the elimination of the associated pain, but this result requires confirmation with double-blind controls, given the notorious susceptibility of pain to place and to suggestion. In one case, repeated use of the mirror ten minutes a day for three weeks resulted in a permanent and complete disappearance of the phantom arm and elbow (and a "telescoping" of fingers into the stump) for the first time in ten years. The associated pain in the elbow and wrist also vanished. This incident may be the first successful amputation of a phantom limb!

Emergence of "Repressed Memories"

Another poorly understood aspect of phantom limbs concerns the continued existence of "memories" in the phantom (sensations that existed in the limb just prior to amputation) along with the reemergence of long-lost memories pertaining to that limb. For instance, it is well known that patients sometimes continue to feel a wedding ring or a watch band on the phantom. Also, in the first few weeks after arm amputation, many patients report that they experience excruciating clenching spasms in the phantom hand and that these spasms are often accompanied by the unmistakable sensation of nails digging into the palm. It usually takes several minutes—or sometimes even hours— to voluntarily unclench the phantom (unless he uses our mirror device!) but when unclenching eventually does take place, the "nails digging" sensation vanishes as well. The reason is obscure, but one possibility is that when motor commands are sent from the premotor and motor cortex to clench the hand, they are normally damped by error feedback from proprioception. If the limb is missing, such damping is not possible. The motor output is amplified still further, and this overflow or "sense of effort" itself may be experienced as pain.

Why would the "nails digging" sensation also be associated with the spasm? Although this phenomenon is even more difficult to explain, one might suppose that the motor commands to unclench the hand and the sensation of the nails digging are linked in the brain, even in normal individuals, by a Hebbian learning mechanism. Since the motor output is amplified after amputation, it is conceivable that the associated memory of nails digging is correspondingly amplified, giving rise to the excruciating pain. The observation that eliminating the spasms (either by intense prolonged voluntary effort or by use of the mirror) also abolished the digging sensation is consistent with this view. We may, then, be dealing with a primitive form of sensory learning that could conceivably provide an experimental approach to more complex forms of memory and learning in the adult brain.

The reactivation of preamputation memories in the phantom has been noted before (Katz and Melzack, 1990) but little systematic work has been done, and the significance of the findings for an understanding of normal memory appears to have gone largely unrecognized. For example, one of our patients reported that before amputation the arthritic joint pains in her fingers would often flare up when the weather was damp and cold. Remarkably, whenever the air became humid, the same pains would occur in her phantom fingers. Also, when her hand went into a clenching spasm in the evening, the thumb was usually abducted and hyperextended, but on those occasions when it was flexed into the palm, the spasm was accompanied by the distinct feeling of her thumbnail digging into the pad of the fifth digit. The curious implication of this observation is that even fleeting sensory associations may be permanently recorded in the brain; these memory traces may be ordinarily repressed, but normal afferent input may be unmasked by the deafferentation. (Also, surprisingly, the traces may be "gated" by the felt position of the phantom thumb, or even be retrieved on the basis of an unconscious inference: "If my thumb is flexed, it must touch my fifth digit.")

We have also used the mirror procedure on finger-digit amputees with very similar results. One patient had his index finger amputated 1 centimeter distal to the head of the metacarpal about forty years prior to our seeing him. At the time, he had experienced a vivid phantom finger (but no phantom pain) for about a year, but it faded completely after that. Remarkably, when he saw his index finger move in the mirror, he again experienced proprioceptive sensations in his index finger—for the first time in thirty-nine years, which intrigued and delighted him.

Phantom Limbs and Sensory Codes

According to the "labeled lines" theory of sensory coding, every neuron in the sensory pathways (3b or S2 or area 17) has a specific "hardwired" signature; that is, it signals a highly specific percept such as "light touch on my right elbow." It is obvious that sensory coding cannot be based exclusively on an endless hierarchy of labeled lines and maps. At some stage, "pattern coding" (the total spatiotemporal pattern of activity) must take over and determine what the subject actually perceives.

The basic presumption of the remapping hypothesis of referred sensations is that the labeled lines have been switched, so that the same sensory input now activates a novel set of labeled lines (for instance, the face input activates "hand neurons" in S1). As we have seen, this is consistent for both the MEG changes in sensory maps that we observed and the referred sensations reported by many patients (see also Clarke et al., 1996; Kew et al., 1997). But it is possible that the subsequent changes in pattern coding somewhere farther along the nervous system eventually lead to the detection of these anomalous sensations in some patients.

The word "remapping" carries connotations of actual anatomical change, whereas most of the evidence points to unmasking or disinhibition of preexisting pathways (see Borsook et al., 1998; Ramachandran et al., 1992; Ramachandran and Rogers-Ramachandran, 1996b). A more theory-neutral word such as "rerouting" might be preferable, to indicate that information from a specific location on the sensory surface (face or shoulder) is now shunted or rerouted so as to either evoke new patterns of neural activity or activate new anatomical sites that have different perceptual signatures and therefore lead to novel sensations. In either case, the findings imply that there must have been a relatively permanent or stable change in the processing of sensory signals by the adult brain. I would be very surprised if these changes have nothing in common with what we usually call memory and learning.

Capgras Syndrome

The disorder called Capgras delusion is one of the rarest and most colorful syndromes in neurology (Capgras and Reboul-Lachaux, 1923; Young, Reid, Wright, and Hellawell, 1993). Its most striking feature is that the patient comes to regard close acquaintances, typically either parents, children, spouse, or siblings, as impostors. That is, he may claim that the person "looks like" or is even "identical to" his mother but really is not his mother. Although frequently seen in psychotic states, more than a third of the documented cases of Capgras syndrome have occurred in conjunction with traumatic brain lesions, suggesting that the syndrome has an organic basis. These patients are often relatively intact in other respects; they are mentally lucid, their memory is normal, and other aspects of their visual perception are completely unaffected.

What causes this strange disorder? Messages from the face area of the brain are eventually transmitted to the limbic system, concerned mainly with the perception, experience, and expression of emotions. The gateway to the limbic system is the amygdala. Thus, the visual centers of the brain in the temporal lobes send their information to the amygdala, which assesses the emotional significance of the incoming visual input, then transmits it to other limbic structures where these emotions are "experienced."

Is it possible that in Capgras patients there has been a disconnection between the face area of the temporal lobes (IT) and the part of the temporal lobes concerned with the experience of emotion? Perhaps the face area and the amygdala are both intact, but the two areas have been disconnected. As a result, patients can "recognize" people's faces (the feature wherein the syndrome differs from prosopagnosia). But when a patient looks at his mother, even though he realizes that she resembles his mother, he does not experience the appropriate warmth. He therefore says, "Well, if this is my mother, why is it that I'm not experiencing any emotion? This must be some strange person." However bizarre this may seem, it is perhaps the only interpretation that makes sense to a person with this peculiar disconnection. This interpretation of Capgras syndrome is similar to the one proposed by Young et al. (1993), except that they postulate a disconnection between ventral and dorsal "stream" pathways rather than an amygdala-inferotemporal cortex disconnection.

How can a hypothesis of this kind be tested? William Hirstein and I obtained galvanic skin responses from patient DS. When a normal person looks at an emotionally salient object such as his mother or father, this message is transmitted from the visual centers of the brain to the amygdala, where the emotional significance is judged. The message goes to the limbic system, then to the hypothalamus, and from there to the autonomic nervous system, which causes the skin resistance to change (GSR). Most normal people give a strong GSR when they see their mother. Yet when we tested DS, who had Capgras syndrome, we found that when he looked at a photograph of his mother, there was very little change in GSR, supporting the disconnection hypothesis (Hirstein and Ramachandran, 1997; Ramachandran, 1996). Let me emphasize that DS had no problem in seeing that the photograph looked like his mother, and he had no problem experiencing emotions in general. During the interview he felt joy, fear, impatience, boredom, and all the other emotions that one would normally expect a human being to experience—because his limbic system itself was unaffected. What was disturbed was the communication between vision and emotion.

One objection to our interpretation might be that patients with bilateral amygdala lesions do not suddenly develop Capgras syndrome. With the entire amygdala damaged, the patient's brain may have no baseline for comparison; no stimulus evokes a GSR. To develop the Capgras delusion may require a loss of GSR to certain categories of sensory images but not to others. Consistent with this, DS showed a normal GSR to threat gestures and loud noises, so his amygdala was probably intact.

Capgras syndrome is a striking example of how a bizarre, seemingly incomprehensible psychiatric syndrome can be at least partially understood in terms of the known neuroanatomy of the temporal lobes. The concept can be tested via a relatively simple technique, GSR, to show what might in fact be happening in the brain.

What is the relevance of Capgras syndrome to an understanding of human memory? The disorder defies the conventional intuition about memory, since it seems to imply that "recognition" and "familiarity" are dissociable. A moment's reflection, however, dispels this implication. We have all had the experience of, say, running into a colleague in another city and not recognizing her—yet realizing that she is familiar. (Or someone has just shaved; he looks inexplicably strange, yet you recognize him.) Perhaps what is seen in Capgras is an extreme exaggeration of this dissociation. A similar dissociation, of course, occurs in temporal lobe epilepsy when patients experience déja vu (familiar but not recognized) and jamais vu (unfamiliar but recognized). Such observations may imply the existence of a special-purpose mechanism in the brain that generates a "glow of familiarity" which allows successive episodes of the same object or person to be linked.

Let us return now to patient DS. One intriguing aspect of his delusion is that it was *modality specific;* he had no trouble recognizing his father or mother over the phone! A possible explanation for this specificity is that there might be separate pathways from the auditory and visual cortex to the amygdala, and that only the latter were damaged by his head injury.

Given the many well-known physiological functions of the amygdala, I wondered whether other deficits would emerge in DS if we were to study him more intensively. In particular, physiologists recording cell responses in the amygdala have found that, in addition to responding to facial expressions and emotions, the cells also respond to the direction of eye gaze.

This fact is not surprising, given the important role that gaze direction plays in primate social communication—the averted gaze of guilt, shame, or embarrassment. We tend to forget that emotions, even though privately experienced, often involve interaction with other people, and that one way we interact is through eye contact. Given this link between gaze direction, familiarity, and emotions, I set out to determine if DS's ability to judge the direction of gaze would be impaired.

I prepared a series of images, each showing the same model either looking directly at the camera lens or at a point an inch or two to the right or left of the lens. DS's task was simply to signify whether the model was looking straight at him or not. While normal individuals can detect tiny shifts in gaze with uncanny accuracy, DS was hopeless at the task. Only when the model's eyes were looking way off to one side was DS able to discern correctly that she was not looking at him.

This finding in itself is interesting but not altogether unexpected, given the known role of amygdala and temporal lobes in detecting gaze direction. But on the eighth trial of looking at these photos, DS did something completely unexpected; he exclaimed that the model's identity had changed. He was looking at a new person who merely resembled the "first."

"This one is older," DS said firmly. He stared hard at both images. "This is a lady, the other one is a girl." Later in the sequence, DS made another duplication: one model was old, one young, and a third one even younger. At the end of the test session he continued to insist that he had seen three different people. Two weeks later he reacted the same on a retest with images of a completely new face.

How could DS look at the face of one person and claim that she was actually three different people? Why did simply changing the direction of gaze lead to this profound inability to link successive images? The answer might lie in the mechanics of how we form memories, in particular our ability to create enduring representations of faces.

Suppose you go to the grocery store one day and a friend introduces you to a new person, Joe. You form a memory of that episode and tuck it away in your brain. Two weeks go by and you run into Joe in the library. He tells you a story about your mutual friend, you share a laugh, and your brain files a memory about this second episode. Another few weeks pass and you meet Joe again in his office—he is a medical researcher and is wearing a white lab coat—but you recognize him instantly from earlier encounters. More memories of Joe are created during this time, so that you now have in your mind a "category" called Joe. This mental picture becomes progressively refined and enriched each time you meet Joe, aided by an increasing sense of familiarity that creates an incentive to link the images and the episodes. Eventually you develop a robust concept of Joe—he tells great stories, works in a lab, makes you laugh, knows a lot about gardening, and so forth.

Now consider what happens to individuals with anterograde amnesia caused by damage to the hippocampus. Such patients are completely unable to form new memories, even though they have reasonable recollection of all events in their lives that took place before the hippocampus was injured. The logical conclusion is that memories are not actually stored in the hippocampus (hence the preservation of old memories), but that the hippocampus is vital for the acquisition of new memory traces in the brain. When one of these patients meets a new person (Joe) on three consecutive occasions—the supermarket, the library, and the office—he will not remember ever having met Joe before. He will simply not recognize him. He will insist each time that Joe is a complete stranger, no matter how many times they have interacted, talked, exchanged stories, and so forth.

But is Joe really a complete stranger? Rather surprisingly, experiments show that such amnesia patients partially retain the ability to form new categories that transcend successive Joe episodes. If our patient met Joe ten times and each time Joe made him laugh, he would tend to feel vaguely jovial or happy on the next encounter, but still would not know who Joe is. There would be no sense of familiarity whatsoever—no memory of each Joe episode—yet the patient would acknowledge that Joe makes him happy. The amnesia patient, unlike

DS, can link successive episodes to create a new concept (an unconscious expectation of joy) even though he forgets each episode. DS remembers each episode but fails to link them.

Thus, DS is in some respects the mirror image of an amnesia patient. When he meets a total stranger such as Joe, his brain creates a file for Joe and the associated experiences he has with Joe. But if Joe leaves the room for thirty minutes and returns, DS's brain, instead of retrieving the old file and adding to it, sometimes creates a completely new file.

Why does this happen in Capgras syndrome? It may be that, to link successive episodes, the brain relies on a specific signal from the limbic system. If this "glow" or sense of familiarity is missing, the brain cannot form an enduring category over time. The brain sets up separate categories each time, which is why DS asserts that he is meeting a new person who merely resembles the person he met a half-hour ago. Cognitive psychologists and philosophers often make a distinction between tokens and types, saying that all experience can be classified into general categories or types as opposed to specific exemplars or tokens. Our experiments with DS suggest that this is not just an abstract academic distinction; that it is embedded deep in the architecture of the brain.

As we continued to test DS, we noticed that he had certain other quirks and eccentricities. For instance, he sometimes seemed to have a problem with visual categories. All of us make mental taxonomies or groupings of events and objects: ducks and geese are birds, but rabbits are not. Our brains set up these categories even without formal education in zoology, presumably to facilitate memory storage and to enhance our ability to access these memories at a moment's notice.

DS, on the other hand, often made remarks hinting that he was confused about categories. For example, he had an almost obsessive preoccupation with Jews and Catholics, and he tended to label a disproportionate number of recently encountered people as Jews. This propensity reminded me of another rare syndrome called Fregoli, in which a patient keeps seeing the same person everywhere: in walking down the street, nearly every woman's face may look like his mother's face, or every young man may resemble his brother. (I hypothesize that instead of having severed connections from face recognition areas to the amygdala, the Fregoli patient may have an *excess* of such connections. Every face is imbued with familiarity and "glow," causing him to see the same face over and over again.)

Observations on DS and other patients like him offer insights into how each of us constructs narratives about our life and the people who inhabit it. In a sense, one's life—one's autobiography—is a long sequence of highly personal episodic memories about one's first kiss, prom night, wedding, birth of a child, fishing trips, and so on. But it is much more than that. Clearly, a personal identity, a sense of a unified "self," runs like a golden thread through the fabric of our existence.

The Scottish philosopher David Hume drew an analogy between the human personality and a river—the water in the river is ever changing, yet the river itself remains constant. What would happen, he asked, if a person were to dip his foot into a river, then dip it in again after half an hour—would it be the same river or a different one? If you find this a silly semantic riddle, you are correct; for the answer depends on the definition of "same" and "river."

Silly or not, one thing is clear. For DS, given his difficulty with linking successive episodic memories, there may indeed be two rivers. To be sure, this tendency to make copies of events and objects was most pronounced when he encountered faces—DS did not often duplicate objects. Yet on occasion he would run his fingers through his hair and call it a "wig," partly because his scalp felt unfamiliar owing to scars from the neurosurgery he had undergone. On rare occasions DS even duplicated countries, claiming at one point that there were two Panamas (he had recently visited there during a family reunion). In this regard, Capgras syndrome blends imperceptibly into a class of memory disorders called the reduplicative paramnesias.

Most remarkable of all, DS sometimes duplicated himself. The first time it happened, I was showing DS pictures of himself from a family photo album. I pointed to a snapshot of him taken two years before the accident.

"Whose picture is this?" I asked.

"That's another DS," he replied. "He looks just like me, but it isn't me." I couldn't believe my ears. DS may have detected my surprise, since he reinforced his point by saying, "You see? He has a mustache; I don't."

This delusion did not occur when DS looked at himself in a mirror. Perhaps he was sensible enough to realize that the face in the mirror could not be anyone's other than his. But his tendency to duplicate himself—to regard himself as a distinct person from a former DS— sometimes emerged spontaneously during conversation. To my surprise, he once volunteered, "Yes, my parents sent a check, but they sent it to the other DS."

Philosophers have argued for centuries that if any one thing about our existence is completely beyond question, it is the simple fact that "I" exist as a single human being who endures in space and time. But even this axiomatic foundation of human existence is called into question by DS.

Conclusion

I have in this article considered three curious disorders: anosognosia, phantom limbs, and Capgras syndrome. Although all three have been known for seven or eight decades, their relevance to understanding the neurobiology of memory appears to have gone largely unnoticed. Perhaps the preliminary results reported in this chapter will provide a stimulus for further inquiry.

References

Aglioti, S., Bonazzi, A., and Cortese, F. (1994). Phantom lower limb as a perceptual marker of neural plasticity in the mature human brain. *Proceedings of the Royal Society of London, Series B, 255,* 273–278.

Alkon, D. L., Collin, C., Ito, E., Lee, C. J., Nelson, T. J., Oka, K., Sakakibara, M., Schreurs, B. G., and Yoshioka, T. (1993). Molecular and biophysical steps in the storage of associative memory. *Annuals of the New York Academy of Science, 20,* 500–504.

Babinski, J. (1914). Contribution a l'étude des troubles mentaux dans l'hémiplégie organique cérébrale (anosognosie). *Revue Neurologique, 27,* 845–847.

Bailey, C. H., and Kandel, E. R. (1995). Molecular and structural mechanisms underlying long-term memory. In M. S. Gazzaniga (Ed.), *The cognitive neurosciences* (pp. 19–36). Cambridge, MA: MIT Press.

Bartlett, F. C. (1932). *Remembering: A study in experimental and social psychology.* Cambridge: Cambridge University Press.

Bisiach, E., Rusconi, M. L., and Vallar, G. (1991). Remission of somatoparaphrenic delusion through vestibular stimulation. *Neuropsychologia, 29,* 1029–31.

Borsook, D., Becerra, L., Fishman, S., Edwards, A., Jennings, C. L., Stojanovic, M., Papinicolas, L., Ramachandran, V. S., Gonzalez, R. G., and Breiter, H. (1998). Acute plasticity in the human somatosensory cortex following amputation. *Neuroreport, 9,* 1013–17.

Capgras, J., and Reboul-Lachaux, J. (1923). L'illusion de "soisies" dans un délire systématise chronique. *Bulletin de la Société Clinique de Médicine Mentale, 2,* 6–16.

Clarke, S., Regli, L., Janzer, R. C., Assal, G., and de Tribolet, N. (1996). Phantom face: Conscious correlate of neural reorganization after removal of primary sensory neurones. *Neuroreport, 7,* 2853–7.

Cronholm, B. (1951). Phantom limbs in amputees: A study of changes in the integration of centripetal impulses with special reference to referred sensations. *Acta Psychiatry and Neurology Scandinavia (supplement), 72,* 301–310.

Flor, H., Elbert, T., Knecht, S., Wienbruch, C., Pantev, C., Birbaumer, N., Larbig, W., and Taub, E. (1995). Phantom-limb pain as a perceptual correlate of cortical reorganization following arm amputation. *Nature, 375,* 482–484.

Freud, A. (1946). *The ego and the mechanisms of defense.* New York: International Universities Press.

Freud, S. (1996). *The standard edition of the complete works of Sigmund Freud,* Vols. 1–23. London: Hogarth Press.

Goldstein, K. (1940). *Human nature.* Cambridge, MA: Harvard University Press.

Hirstein, W., and Ramachandran, V. S. (1997). Capgras syndrome: A novel probe for understanding the neural representation of the identity and familiarity of persons. *Proceedings of the Royal Society of London Series B, 264,* 437–444.

Katz, J., and Melzack, R. (1990). Pain "memories" in phantom limbs: Review and clinical observations. *Pain, 43,* 319–336.

Kew, J. J., Halligan, P. W., Marshall, J. C., Passingham, R. E., Rothwell, J. C., Ridding, M. C., Marsden, C. D., and Brooks, D. J. (1997). Abnormal access of axial vibrotactile input to deafferented somatosensory cortex in human upper limb amputees. *Journal of Neurophysiology, 77,* 2753–64.

Lynch, M. A. (1989). Mechanisms underlying induction and maintenance of long-term potentiation in the hippocampus. *Bioessays, 10,* 85–90.

Melzack, R. (1990). Phantom limb and the concept of a neuromatrix. *Trends in Neuroscience, 13,* 88–92.

Melzack, R. (1992). Phantom limbs. *Scientific American, 266,* 120–126.

Merzenich, M. M., Nelson, R. J., Stryker, M. P., Cynader, M. S., Schoppmann, A., and Zook, J. M. (1984). Somatosensory cortical map changes following digit amputation in adult monkeys. *Journal of Comparative Neurology, 224,* 591–605.

Milner, B., Corkin, S., and Teuber, H. L. (1968). Further analysis of the hippocampal amnesic syndrome: Fourteen-year follow-up study of H.M. *Neuropsychologia, 6,* 215–234.

Mishkin, M. (1978). Memory in monkeys severely impaired by combined but not separate removal of amygdala and hippocampus. *Nature, 273,* 297–298.

Pons, T. P., Garraghty, P. E., Ommaya, A. K., Kaas, J. H., Taub, E., and Mishkin, M. (1991). Massive cortical reorganization after sensory deafferentation in adult macaques. *Science, 252,* 1857–60.

Ramachandran, V. S. (1993a). Filling in gaps in perception: Part II. Scotomas and phantom limbs. *Current Directions in Psychological Science, 2,* 56–65.

Ramachandran, V. S. (1993b). Behavioral and MEG correlates of neural plasticity in the adult human brain. *Proceedings of the National Academy of Science (USA), 90,* 10413–20.

Ramachandran, V. S. (1994). Phantom limbs, neglect syndromes, repressed memories, and Freudian psychology. In O. Sporns and G. Tononi (Eds.), *Selectionism and the brain: International review of neurobiology,* Vol. 37 (pp. 291–333). San Diego: Academic Press.

Ramachandran, V. S. (1995). Anosognosia in parietal lobe syndrome. *Consciousness and Cognition, 4,* 22–51.

Ramachandran, V. S. (1996). What neurological syndromes can tell us about human nature: Some lessons from phantom limbs, Capgras syndrome, and anosognosia, *Cold Spring Harbor Symposia on Quantitative Biology, 61,* 115–134.

Ramachandran, V. S., and Rogers-Ramachandran, D. (1996a). Denial of disabilities in anosognosia. *Nature, 382,* 501.

Ramachandran, V. S., and Rogers-Ramachandran, D. (1996b). Synaesthesia in phantom limbs induced with mirrors. *Proceedings of the Royal Society of London, Series B, 263,* 377–386.

Ramachandran, V. S., Rogers-Ramachandran, D., and Stewart, M. (1992). Perceptual correlates of massive cortical reorganization. *Science, 258,* 1159–60.

Riddoch, G. (1941). Phantom limbs and body shape. *Brain, 64,* 197.

Schacter, D. L. (1996). *Searching for memory: The brain, the mind, and the past.* New York: Basic Books.

Squire, L. R. (1987). *Memory and brain.* New York: Oxford University Press.

Stanton, P. K., and Sejnowski, T. J. (1989). Associative long-term depression in the hippocampus induced by hebbian covariance. *Nature, 339,* 215–218.

Wall, P. D. (1977). The presence of ineffective synapses and the circumstances which unmask them. *Philosophical Transactions of the Royal Society of London, Series B, 278,* 361–372.

Weir Mitchell, S. (1872). *Injuries of nerves, and their consequences.* Philadelphia: Lippincott.

Weiskrantz, L. (1987). Neuroanatomy of memory and amnesia: A case for multiple memory systems. *Human Neurobiology, 6,* 93–105.

Yang, T. T., Gallen, C. C., Ramachandran, V. S., Cobb, S., Schwartz, B. J., and Bloom, F. E. (1994a). Noninvasive detection of cerebral plasticity in adult human somatosensory cortex. *Neuroreport, 5,* 701–704.

Yang, T. T., Gallen, C., Schwartz, B., Bloom, F. E., Ramachandran, V. S., and Cobb, S. (1994b). Sensory maps in the human brain. *Nature, 368,* 592–593.

Young, A. W., Reid, I., Wright, S., and Hellawell, D. J. (1993). Face-processing impairments and the Capgras delusion. *British Journal of Psychiatry, 162,* 695–698.

Acknowledgments

I thank J. Bogen, P. Churchland, F. H. C. Crick, W. Hirstein, D. Rogers, and the late J. Salk for stimulating discussions, and the NIMH for support.

The Role of Memory in the Delusions Associated with Schizophrenia

4

Chris Frith
Raymond J. Dolan

This chapter will cover three areas: the variety of false beliefs reported by patients with schizophrenia; the kinds of abnormal cognitive processes that might give rise to such false beliefs; brain imaging studies that indicate how cognitive processes which relate to delusions might be instantiated in the brain.

False Perceptions and False Beliefs

The most striking psychological abnormalities associated with schizophrenia are hallucinations and delusions. Hallucinations are false perceptions ("hearing voices when no one is there"); delusions are false beliefs. Table 4.1 gives examples of hallucinations and delusions reported by patients and shows their traditional labeling by psychiatrists.

While a description of false perceptions is relatively straightforward, the definition of false beliefs in psychiatric settings is more problematic. Delusions are traditionally defined as idiosyncratic false beliefs that are held firmly in spite of evidence to the contrary. This definition suggests that if enough people believe something false, then it is not a delusion. In practice, as can be seen from Table 4.1, many of the false beliefs reported by schizophrenic patients are sufficiently bizarre that there is little argument about their abnormality. Further, the distinction between a false perception and a false belief is not always clear-cut. A symptom such as thought broadcasting, in which

Table 4.1   Hallucinations and delusions associated with schizophrenia

1. I hear a voice saying, "You're not going to smoke the cigarette the way you want to."	Second-person auditory hallucination
2. I hear a voice saying, "He is an astronomy fanatic. Here's a taste of his own medicine. He's getting up now. He's going to wash. It's about time."	Third-person auditory hallucination
3. It was like my ears being blocked up and my thoughts shouted out.	Thought broadcasting
4. Thoughts are put into my head like "Kill God." It's just like my mind working, but it isn't. They come from this chap, Chris; they're his thoughts.	Thought insertion
5. The force moved my lips. I began to speak. The words were made for me.	Delusions of control
6. I saw someone scratching his chin, which meant that I needed a shave.	Delusions of reference
7. People at work are victimizing me. A bloke at work is trying to kill me with some kind of hypnosis.	Delusions of persecution

Source: Examples from Leff, 1982, and Cutting, 1992.

the patient reports hearing his thoughts spoken aloud as he thinks them, is obviously an abnormal perception. Likewise, the patient who claims that his colleagues at work are trying to poison him using hypnosis certainly has a false belief.

Many symptoms, however, are not so easy to classify. Examples are delusions of control and thought insertion. The patient with delusions of control reports that his actions are being "made for him" by some external force. Note that, for identification of this symptom, it is not sufficient for the patient to say something like "The government is controlling my actions." The patient must describe his experience of an actual force that induces him to carry out the actions (Wing, 1978). Likewise the patient with thought insertion will describe his sensation of thoughts that are not his own coming into his mind. In both of these cases a strong perceptual quality is evident in what the patient reports. The symptoms seem to lie in the middle of a continuum that runs from false perceptions to false beliefs. This middle ground of abnormal psychological experience suggests that perceptions and beliefs are not necessarily distinct categories. Rather, the data from psychotic patients indicate interactions between these two domains of cognition. In psychotic patients it seems that not only can a vivid and unusual perception alter a belief system, but also a very strong belief can modify perceptual experience (Kraupl Taylor, 1979).

Common cognitive mechanisms underlie both perceptual experience and belief formation. William James has commented that "whilst part of what we perceive comes though our senses from the object before us, another part always comes out of our mind" (James, 1890). His statement encapsulates the view that perceptions are partly a function of prior knowledge. This prior knowledge, which must be a form of memory, is often expressed as beliefs. It follows that both perceptions and beliefs must be intimately related to the operations of memory.

What is the role of prior knowledge in perceptual experience? Prior knowledge enables the sensory input to be organized, recognized, interpreted, and understood (Frith and Dolan, 1997). At the same time, our knowledge base is continuously updated on the basis of sensory experience. If the sensory input is sufficiently unusual, the updated knowledge that results may be incompatible with that of other people (or even with other areas of knowledge within the same individual), leading to false beliefs. Consequently, one explanation of the false beliefs reported by schizophrenic patients is that they are derived in a rational manner from the experience of false perceptions (Mahler, 1974). In other words, beliefs are reasonable inferences, involving some central system, from an impoverished sensory input.

Consider, for example, the report of the patient shown in Example 4.1. The patient describes false perceptions typical of schizophrenia. He hears voices, but cannot identify their source. The voices comment on his actions. He also hears the voices repeating his thoughts aloud (thought echo). He tries to explain these experiences. These people can speak to him at a distance and read his thoughts because they have inherited occult powers. They must be using some naturally occurring electricity or magnetism that may involve the iron in their blood.

Given the remarkable nature of the perceptions of this patient, such explanations are not so far-fetched. Some fifty years after the patient wrote this letter, functional magnetic resonance imaging is being developed by neuroscientists to study mental activity (at a distance) using the magnetic properties of the blood!

Example 4.1

The Experience
I was . . . startled by these same pursuers. I could catch part of their talk, but . . . could see them nowhere. I heard one of them say, "You can't get away from us. We'll get you after a while." To add to the mystery, one of them repeated my thoughts aloud, verbatim. I tried to elude them, but I heard the voices of these pursuers as close as ever.

The Patient's Explanation
Among these pursuers are some brothers and sisters who inherited astounding occult powers. Besides being able to tell a person's thoughts, they are able to project their magnetic voices a distance of a few miles without talking loud. This power . . . seems to be due to their natural bodily electricity . . . Maybe the iron contained in their blood corpuscles is magnetized.

Source: From a letter written by L. Percy King in the 1940s, reproduced in Kaplan, 1964, pp. 134–135.

Disorders of Central Monitoring

If false beliefs can arise from a reasonable attempt to explain false perceptions, then our primary problem is to explain the origin of false perceptions. By definition, false perceptions are not based on external sensory input. Therefore, they must be based on aberrant information arising within the patient's own mind or brain. For some symptoms the patient is clearly aware of the internal origin of the abnormal perceptions. In thought broadcasting the patient knows these are his *thoughts,* but hears them as if spoken aloud. For other symptoms there seems to be only partial awareness. With delusions of control, the patient recognizes that he is moving his arm, but experiences this movement as caused by some other agent. With thought insertion, the patient recognizes that the thoughts are in his own mind but experiences them as alien (not his). With auditory hallucinations, there is often no recognition of the internal origin of the experience. From the patient's perspective, the voice is that of another.

In the early part of this century the German psychopathologist Karl Jaspers said that these kinds of reports were so far outside the range of normal experience as to be unexplainable in psychological terms (Jaspers, 1913). His argument seems to have been that it was impossible to see how anything in the patient's past experience could lead to such phenomena. Today our approach is very different. We are not so much interested in explaining the content of symptoms, but instead we place emphasis on their form. This change of emphasis is no doubt strongly influenced by the success of cognitive neuropsychology in explaining some of the consequences of brain lesions (Shallice, 1988). The major lesson to be learned from studies of brain-damaged patients is the massive parallel nature of the brain which contains multiple independent modules and pathways that can be damaged independently of one another. The kinds of disorders that ensue are frequently best characterized in terms of the discrepancies between damaged and intact components.

A particularly interesting example, discussed in Chapter 3, is provided by explanations of Capgras syndrome (Ellis and Young, 1990; Hirstein and Ramachandran, 1997). Patients with this disorder have bizarre false beliefs which involve the conviction that someone close to them, usually a husband or wife, has been replaced by a double (Capgras and Reboul-Lachaux, 1923). This symptom is occasionally seen in patients with schizophrenia but can also occur after brain damage or in patients with Alzheimer's disease (Burns, Jacoby, and Levy, 1990).

Capgras is part of a wider group of symptoms called reduplicative delusions. Some patients, for example, claim that it is their house, rather than their spouse, which has been replaced by a exact copy (Kapur, Turner, and King, 1988). Capgras syndrome is surely an example of a bizarre false belief, but our explanation of it assumes that it reflects a *perceptual* disorder; the face of the spouse is experienced as being different in such a way as to lead to the conclusion that it cannot be the face of the "real" spouse. It is proposed that Capgras syndrome is the mirror of another neurological disorder called prosopagnosia (Damasio, Damasio, and Van Hoesen, 1982; Meadows, 1974).

Prosopagnosia is a straightforward perceptual disorder. The patient can no longer recognize the identity of faces. She knows she is looking at a face, but cannot identify whose face it is. Recent research has shown, however, that information concerning the identity of a face is nevertheless available to the patient. In particular, such a patient shows greater autonomic responses to the faces of familiar people even though she fails to recognize them (Bruyer, 1991). This observation suggests that at least two independent routes normally operate in face perception. The first leads to recognition of identity; the second, largely unconscious, leads to an emotional response to the face that includes the feeling of familiarity. In prosopagnosia the first route is damaged while the second remains intact. It is proposed that in Capgras syndrome there is an intact route to identity, whereas the route to familiarity and emotional evaluation is damaged. The patient recognizes the face of his wife, but gets neither the expected emotional response nor a feeling of familiarity. Something is definitely wrong with this perception overall: the face looks like that of his wife but is devoid of the essential qualities that make it really her. The altered quality of perceptual experience leads the patient to infer that it is not really his wife and must therefore be a double.

On the basis of the lesions and cognitive processes associated with both prosopagnosia and Capgras syndrome respectively, it is possible to get an idea of the brain regions associated with the two proposed routes involved in face perception. Recognition of facial identity depends to a large extent on regions of the inferior temporal cortex, particularly on the right (De Renzi, 1996; Dolan et al., 1997). In contrast, emotional responses depend on pathways that involve components of the limbic system (Bauer, 1984). These distinctions between pathways for identity and those for emotional evaluation have been confirmed by more recent brain imaging studies in normal volunteers. Many studies confirm that facial identity is associated with activity in the inferior temporal cortex (Allison et al., 1994; Dolan et al., 1997; Haxby et al., 1994).

We recently attempted to determine the route involved in emotional responses to faces by scanning volunteers who had been conditioned (using an aversive noise) to have an emotional response to previously unknown neutral or happy faces. After conditioning, the enhanced processing of these faces, based on a change in their emotional value, involved regions in a number of limbic areas including amygdala, basal forebrain, and orbital frontal cortex (Morris, Friston, and Dolan, 1997). It is the functioning of this route that may be damaged in Capgras syndrome.

A number of studies suggest that encounters with objects, as well as with people, engage processes that lead not only to identity but also to emotional evaluation. These are parallel and reciprocal processes. The absence of the emotional evaluation process would lead to an alteration of the quality of experience in our encounters with the world. This could trigger a reassessment of information derived from perceptual systems in such a manner as to engender false beliefs.

Perceptual Delusions in Schizophrenia

Delusions of Control

Let us for the moment accept that the belief that a person's being replaced by a copy is a reasonable explanation of a perceptual mismatch between the identity and the emotional evaluation of a face. Can we apply the same analysis to symptoms typically associated with schizophrenia? One symptom we have considered in some detail is known as a delusion of control; the patient describes his actions as not under his own control, but initiated by some external force: "My fingers pick up the pen, but I don't control them. What they do has nothing to do with me" (Mellors, 1970). In the case of these kinds of false perceptions associated with schizophrenia, our problem is to explain how an internally generated event comes to be experienced as coming from the outside. We have proposed that the problem arises because of a disconnection between the normal coupling of intention and action (Frith, 1996). I feel my arm moving, but there is no intention to move it; the movement must be caused by an external force.

We are saying that the patient no longer has conscious access to, or memory for, his motor intentions. Experimental evidence exists to support this proposition. In the study in question, patients were required to draw simple patterns on a computer screen using a joystick. In one condition the movements of the joystick were not displayed on the screen. Subjects had to remember what they had done without relying on a visual display on the screen as in the other condition. We found that, in the absence of visual feedback, patients with symptoms such as delusions of control were impaired in remembering the drawing they had made (Mlakar, Angel, Hampton, and Berger, 1982). We have also found that, again in the absence of visual feedback, patients with delusions of control had difficulty in correcting movement errors (Frith and Done, 1989). The problem is consistent with the concept that these patients have difficulty monitoring their own movement intentions and are therefore overreliant on visual feedback.

In our original formulation we suggested that patients with delusions of control and other passivity experiences have difficulty with self-monitoring (see also Chapter 2). In certain contexts they are unaware of their intentions and therefore interpret the actions they are performing as the result of outside forces. More recent developments in the theory of motor control have provided a more complete account along similar lines (Wolpert, Ghahramani, and Jordan, 1995). In order to monitor the effects of our own actions we have to be able to predict the sensory consequences of those actions (the forward model). The motor codes used to generate the action must be converted into sensory codes representing the predicted consequences. If something goes awry with this system (such as a faulty prediction), a mismatch occurs between the predicted and the actual sensory consequences of the action. This result is analogous to the mismatch experienced by the Capgras patient between the perception of the identity of a face and the perception of its familiarity. We propose that it is this perception of an unexpected quality of an action that leads the patient to believe that the action is not fully under his control.

The mirror disorder of the types of delusions of control we have been describing would be certain kinds of anosognosia. In these cases the patient is unaware of her own disabilities (see Chapter 3), which have usually been brought about by a right hemisphere stroke. Such a patient may claim to have moved her paralyzed left arm when no movement has actually occurred. The patient is aware of her intention to move her arm, but is unaware that the predicted sensory consequences of this movement have not occurred. She mistakenly, but firmly, asserts that the movement has occurred.

These data indicate that representations of motor intentions are stored independently of parameters that guide actual movements. The key brain regions involved can be inferred from studies in animals that indicate that cells in the parietal cortex, which represent the position of the arms and the eyes, are updated by an intention to move the arm as well as by actual movements (Snyder, Batista, and Andersen, 1997). Abnormal functioning of the parietal cortex has been observed in patients with delusions of control (Spence et al., 1997). In this study brain activity was measured while subjects made a paced sequence of movements with a joystick. In the target condition these movements were intentional (or willed) in the sense that the subjects chose for themselves precisely which of four possible movements to make each time the pacing signal was given. Such willed movements are associated with activity in the frontal, anterior cingulate, and parietal cortex. Patients experiencing delusions of control showed abnormal overactivity in the parietal cortex of the right hemisphere. This overactivity was observed in two separate comparisons, relative to normal volunteers and to other schizophrenic patients not experiencing these types of delusions of control. In addition, the overactivity disappeared when patients were retested after their delusions had ceased—strong evidence that the presence of this particular delusion is associated with parietal overactivity. This overactivity can be interpreted as a concomitant of the experience of unexpected changes in the position of the hand, which is represented in the parietal cortex.

Considerable evidence is available that unexpected stimuli give rise to more neural activity than expected ones (Blakemore, Rees, and Frith, 1998; Shafer, Amochaev, and Russell, 1981). A simple mechanistic account of this observation is that activity in the relevant sensory region can be damped down on the basis of expectations. When a limb is moved, the sensory consequences are predicted on the basis of the commands used to generate the movement (the forward model). Information about the sensory consequences can be used to attenuate activity in precisely the regions that will be activated by the movement (Paus, Marrett, Evans, and Worsley, 1995; Rushton, Rothwell, and Craggs, 1981). Failure in this system will therefore lead to overactivity in the area representing hand position and the experience of movements that have not been self-generated.

Auditory Hallucinations

We can apply the same analysis to auditory hallucinations, which are among the most characteristic symptoms of schizophrenia. Auditory hallucinations take many forms. During *thought broadcasting* the patient hears his own thoughts being spoken aloud. The thoughts are recognized as the patient's own, but are experienced as coming from outside. During *thought insertion* (technically a delusion) the patient experiences thoughts coming into his mind that are not his own. The thoughts are in his mind, but they are not self-generated. During *auditory hallucinations* the patient hears voices talking to him or about him. In a few cases the content of the hallucinations can be shown to correspond directly to the contents of subvocal speech produced by the patient (see Example 4.2).

As with delusions of control, the patient's subvocal speech or thought is perceived as not self-generated, but as coming from some other source. Applying the same explanation to auditory hallucinations, we propose that this response arises because the thought or subvocal speech is unexpected through lack of awareness of the intention to speak or think. At the physiological level, we have observed overactivity in the left temporal cortex of schizophrenic patients while they perform a word generation task (Fletcher, Frith, Grasby, Friston, and Dolan, 1996; Frith et al., 1995). This region is relevant to the language system, just as the parietal lobe is relevant to the limb movement system. We have yet to show, however, that this overactivity is

---

Example 4.2

The patient, RW, reported hearing a female voice . . . addressing statements to him or referring to him as "he."

RW, whisper: If you're in his mind, you come out of there, but if you're not in his mind, you won't come out of there. You want to stay there.

Examiner: Who said that?

RW, normal speech: Er, she said . . .

RW, whisper: I said that.

RW was challenged that he talked to himself.

RW, normal voice: No I don't. *(aside)* What is it?

RW, whisper: Mind your own business, darling, I don't want him to know what I was doing.

RW, normal voice: See that, I spoke to ask her what she was doing and she said mind your own business.

Source: Green and Preston, 1981, p. 206.

specifically related to auditory hallucinations. Furthermore, in most cases the symptom is associated with actions such as thinking, which do not lead to overt sensory consequences. It remains to be seen whether it is possible to provide a plausible mechanism whereby a mismatch can occur between intentions and consequences when no overt behavior and hence no sensory changes are involved.

Abnormal Perceptions and Abnormal Beliefs

We have given an account of how some of the strange perceptions associated with psychosis may arise when the sensory input no longer matches expectations based on prior knowledge. We shall now consider whether the occurrence of these false perceptions is sufficient to explain the bizarre false beliefs that many psychotic patients report.

Consider a patient with Capgras syndrome. He sees a woman who looks exactly like his wife but does not evoke in him an emotional response or a feeling of familiarity. Is the conclusion that she has been replaced by an alien really the first explanation that springs to mind? Such an explanation, taken at face value, seems too extreme. It simply does not fit with our knowledge or beliefs about the world (see Chapter 3). In addition, patients with bizarre delusions of this kind firmly adhere to their strange beliefs despite much evidence to the contrary. We are assuming that beliefs are derived to a large extent from semantic and episodic memories. Normally there is considerable coherence between what we believe and the contents of semantic and episodic memories. The explanations that some psychotic patients give for their strange perceptions seem no longer to be properly constrained by their knowledge of the world. We also have to remember that many patients apparently develop unusual beliefs in the absence of any strange perceptions.

We have obtained direct evidence that strange perceptions are not sufficient to evoke delusions. If perceptual symptoms like hallucinations and delusions of control arise from a mismatch between the actual and the expected consequences of our own actions, then we can artificially create these weird experiences in the laboratory. We did so by using special-effects equipment to distort the sound of the subject's voice (Cahill, Silbersweig, and Frith, 1996). The signal from a throat microphone was fed into special-effects equipment. The pitch of the voice was distorted, then instantaneously fed back to the subject through earphones in real time. We engaged people in conversation while they were attached to this equipment with the special-effects box out of sight. We asked them to comment on what they thought was going on, and observed what happened to their appraisals as we distorted the pitch of their voice to varying degrees.

Our first observation was that normal people did not produce bizarre accounts of their perceptions. They correctly inferred that we were distorting the sound of their voice. Precisely the same comments were made by patients in a chronic phase of their illness when they were no longer experiencing hallucinations or delusions, but only displaying negative features of the disorder. Very different comments were made by patients in an acute phase of their illness, particularly if they were prone to experience delusions. These patients made comments such as "Any time I speak, it speaks with me" or "I think it's an evil spirit speaking when I speak." The likelihood of attributing the voice to another speaker increased with the degree of distortion and also with the severity of their current delusions.

These results clearly show that weird perceptions are not sufficient to engender bizarre explanations in normal people, or even in people who have had delusions in the past. However, weird perceptions do elicit bizarre explanations in people in an acute phase of schizophrenia who already report other false beliefs.

Memory Impairment

We have suggested that individuals may arrive at bizarre beliefs if these beliefs are not sufficiently constrained by semantic and episodic memories. Is there, then, a more general problem with semantic and episodic memory associated with schizophrenia? It has long been known that schizophrenic patients perform poorly on tests of memory recall. McKenna and his colleagues have shown that some patients can even be classified as amnesic on the basis of the discrepancy between performance on memory tests and other intellectual abilities (McKenna et al., 1990). Unlike amnesia deriving from damage to medial temporal lobe structures, the psychotic patients seem to have inordinate problems with semantic memory. What this seems to mean is that the psychotic patients are little concerned about the "meaningfulness" of their replies.

Upon investigating memory recall in a group of patients who were relatively well at the time of testing and had normal IQs, we found evidence for confabulation in addition to poor memory (Nathaniel-James and Frith, 1996). The patients heard short stories derived from Aesop's fables and were subsequently asked to recall them. In nearly every case confabulations were produced, in the sense that incidents or ideas were recalled that had not actually occurred in the stories. Such errors almost never happened in our control group. Many of the confabulations were bizarre. For example, one story described how a rich man involved in a shipwreck had to swim for his life with the other passengers. One patient recalled that "a rich man had gone on a swimming expedition, had stopped swimming in the middle of the sea, and was hailed by a passing ship." He seems to have used the fragments he could remember from the story in an attempt to reconstruct it, but this reconstruction was not properly constrained by knowledge of the world and what sort of events are likely. Rich men do not usually go on swimming expeditions and stop in the middle of the sea. The result was not simply the consequence of the patient's memory impairment. He was not simply filling the gaps with a somewhat outlandish reconstruction. When we took subgroups of patients and controls matched for the number of items correctly recalled, the patients still showed significantly more confabulations.

The delusional memories reported by some patients resemble this sort of confabulation, in that events are recalled that could not have occurred on the basis of the patient's knowledge of the real world (David and Howard, 1994). There is little difference between these delusions about what happened in the past and full-blown psychotic delusions about the present state of the world.

For example, Baddeley and his colleagues have described a patient who believes that he is a rock guitarist and a Russian chess grand master, in spite of the fact that he cannot play the guitar or chess and does not speak Russian (Baddeley, Thornton, Chua, and McKenna, 1996). "But if you don't speak Russian, isn't that rather odd for a Russian chess player?" "Yes, well, I don't speak Russian, but I think its possible that I've been hypnotized to forget things like the fact that

I can speak Russian." Clearly, his beliefs on these particular topics are no longer properly constrained by his knowledge about the world and his past—just as the recollections of the confabulating patient are no longer constrained by his knowledge of the world. We can speculate therefore that the processes involved in retrieval of long-term memories and the processes underlying the formation of beliefs overlap. Delusions result when something goes wrong with these processes.

The Neural Basis of Recollection

Among the many brain imaging studies of retrieval from long-term memory (see Chapter 7), there is considerable unanimity suggesting that the main brain areas activated during retrieval are in the right prefrontal cortex and in the medial parietal cortex or precuneus (Buckner and Tulving, 1994). Lesion studies suggest that the medial temporal cortex including the hippocampal complex also has a role, but it has been much more difficult to demonstrate with imaging. In part this may be because the hippocampal complex is involved in both acquisition and retrieval and is often activated by "control" tasks, during which subjects are not required to remember anything (Rugg, Fletcher, Frith, Frackowiak, and Dolan, 1996). The activity observed in the right prefrontal cortex has been variously associated with retrieval attempt (Kapur, Craik, Brown, Houle, and Tulving, 1995), effort (Schacter et al., 1996), and success (Rugg, Fletcher, Frith, Frackowiak, and Dolan, 1996).

The most recent evidence suggests that this right frontal activity is associated with intentional retrieval and may reflect the attempt to reconstruct an image of the original episode on the basis of partial cues. Right frontal activity can also be seen in studies using event-related potentials (ERPs; see Chapter 2) and endures for an extended number of seconds after successful recognition has occurred (Wilding and Rugg, 1997). We speculate that the underlying processes are involved in ensuring that the reconstructed episode is consistent with our knowledge of the world and of ourselves.

The types of "surveillance" or monitoring processes associated with right prefrontal activity need not apply only to long-term memory. We have observed right frontal activity in situations where perceptions were anomalous and did not fit with previous knowledge of the world. We asked volunteers to move their hands in opposition (Luria's alternation task) while observing the movement in a mirror in the sagittal plane (see Chapter 3). The volunteer sees what appear to be a left hand and a right hand, even though one is actually a reflection of the other. When the volunteer alternately makes a fist with each of the two hands, he sees the hands moving in synchrony; but from his kinesthetic sensation and his knowledge of movement intentions he knows that this visual perception is false. In this situation, where there is incompatibility between different sources of knowledge (veridical proprioceptive and false visual), activity increases in the right prefrontal cortex (Fink et al., 1999).

We suggest that in this experiment the right frontal activity reflects an attempt to reconcile current perceptions with actual expectations about the world based on prior knowledge of actual intentions and confirmatory proprioceptive feedback. The result is equivalent to that in the memory retrieval experiment, where the right frontal activity reflects the attempt to reconcile retrieved memories of past perceptions with current perceptual and semantic cues.

The role of the activity in the medial parietal cortex is far less understood. It has been shown that this area is more active when highly imageable material is being recollected, suggesting that the region may be involved with visual imagery (Fletcher et al., 1995). However, activity in this area has been observed in a number of studies that did not involve long-term memory retrieval. In one of our studies volunteers were shown pictures so impoverished that the objects represented could not be recognized (Dolan et al., 1997). The objects could, however, be perceived and recognized if the picture had previously been seen in an unimpoverished version.

It was found that successful perception of the impoverished view was associated with activity in the posterior medial parietal cortex and, furthermore, that this region interacted with areas in the inferior temporal cortex associated with recognition of the particular class of object being presented (right fusiform for faces). In this study, perception of an impoverished picture was possible because of an interaction between the impoverished sensory input and prior knowledge. We suggest that this interaction occurs in the inferior temporal cortex, an area specialized for object recognition in general. The medial parietal cortex would seem to hold prior knowledge about the object in a form suitable for providing the top-down signal that modifies activity in the inferior temporal cortex to enable a "mind's eye" reconstruction of a face percept. Perhaps the retrieval of episodic memories also depends on the "tuning up" of impoverished perceptions on the basis of this low-level prior knowledge. In the study of Dolan and his colleagues the impoverished objects were seen irrespective of the intentions of the subjects. No right prefrontal activity was seen, in contrast to cases where retrieval was intentional (Dolan et al., 1997).

The results of these brain imaging studies suggest an overlap between brain systems involved in perception (abnormalities of which can lead to hallucinations) and systems involved in long-term memory retrieval (abnormalities of which can lead to delusions). This link involves the constraining effects of our prior knowledge of the world.

Psychogenic Amnesia as a Mirror of Delusions

A delusion arises when our representation of a state of affairs in the world is not properly constrained by our more general knowledge of the world. There is a close relationship between a delusion and a false memory in which the recollection and reconstruction of a past event fails to be properly constrained by our more general knowledge of the world. Just as prosopagnosia is the mirror disorder of the Capgras delusion, we suggest that pure retrograde amnesia (often thought to be psychogenic) is the mirror of the delusional memory. The patient with pure retrograde amnesia has no memory of certain past events. We propose that a recollection is rejected as a reflection of a past event because the patient falsely concludes that it does not fit with his more general knowledge base.

We scanned a patient with pure retrograde amnesia (associated with a small frontal lesion and a series of major and distressing life events) as he was shown pictures of family and friends (Costello, Fletcher, Frith, Dolan, and Shallice, 1998). There were three conditions: (a) pictures from outside the amnesic period for which he recollected the event, (b) pictures of events from the amnesic period, which he failed to recollect, and (c) pictures of events at which he had not been present and so could not recollect. Activity associated with pictures from the amnesic period differed from that in both of the other conditions in that it was higher in the medial parietal cortex and lower in the right prefrontal cortex, both areas normally associated with memory retrieval.

We can speculate that the reduced activity in the right prefrontal cortex reflected the premature termination of an attempt to reconstruct the episode and the conclusion that no such episode was available in memory. One possibility is that the depressed affect associated with the amnesic period attenuated frontal function and thus caused premature termination of the reconstructive processes. We are not aware of studies in which retrieval of delusional memories associated with psychosis has been studied. However, Schacter and his colleagues have studied retrieval of false memories in normal volunteers (Schacter et al., 1996). They found that retrieval of illusory memories was associated with greater right frontal activation than was retrieval of veridical memories.

Conclusion

On the basis of our imaging studies, we propose that the right prefrontal cortex is particularly associated with integrating current perceptions, ideas, and memories with prior knowledge in both the semantic and the episodic domains. Memories have to be integrated with long-term knowledge systems, while current sensations have to be integrated with current plans and intentions. Whether different regions within the right prefrontal cortex are involved in these various domains of integration remains to be discovered. Some of the strange beliefs and experiences reported by psychotic patients may reflect abnormalities within these integrative processes.

References

Allison, T., Ginter, H., McCarthy, G., Nobre, A. C., Puce, A., Luby, M., and Spencer, D. D. (1994). Face recognition in human extrastriate cortex. *Journal of Neurophysiology, 71*, 821–825.

Baddeley, A., Thornton, A., Chua, S. E., and McKenna, P. (1996). Schizophrenic delusions and the construction of autobiographical memory. In D. C. Rubin (Ed.), *Remembering our past: Studies in autobiographical memory* (pp. 384–428). Cambridge: Cambridge University Press.

Bauer, R. M. (1984). Autonomic recognition of names and faces in prosopagnosia: A neuropsychological application of the guilty knowledge test. *Neuropsychologia, 22,* 457–469.

Blakemore, S. J., Rees, G., and Frith, C. D. (1998). How do we predict the consequences of our actions? A functional imaging study. *Neuropsychologia, 36,* 521–529.

Bruyer, R. (1991). Covert face recognition in prosopagnosia: A review. *Brain and Cognition, 15,* 223–235.

Buckner, R. L., and Tulving, E. (1994). Neuroimaging studies of memory: Theory and recent PET results. In J. Boller and J. Grafman (Eds.), *Handbook of neuropsychology* (10th ed.). Amsterdam: Elsevier.

Burns, A., Jacoby, R., and Levy, R. (1990). Psychiatric phenomena in Alzheimer's disease. II: Disorders of perception. *British Journal of Psychiatry, 157,* 76–81.

Cahill, C., Silbersweig, D., and Frith, C. D. (1996). Psychotic experiences induced in deluded patients using distorted auditory feedback. *Cognitive Neuropsychiatry, 1,* 201–211.

Capgras, J., and Reboul-Lachaux, J. (1923). L'illusion de "soisies" dans un délire systématise chronique. *Bulletin de la Société Clinique de Médicine Mentale, 2,* 6–16.

Costello, A., Fletcher, P. C., Dolan, R. J., Frith, C. D., and Shallice, T. (1998). The origins of forgetting in a case of isolated retrograde amnesia following a haemorrhage: Evidence from functional imaging. *Neurocase, 4,* 437–446.

Cutting, J. (1992). *The right cerebral hemisphere and psychiatric disorders.* Oxford: Oxford University Press.

Damasio, A. R., Damasio, H., and Van Hoesen, G. W. (1982). Prosopagnosia: anatomical basis and behavioural mechanisms. *Neurology, 32,* 331–341.

David, A. S., and Howard, R. (1994). An experimental phenomenological approach to delusional memory in schizophrenia and late paraphrenia. *Psychological Medicine, 24,* 515–524.

De Renzi, E. (1996). Current issues in prosopagnosia. In H. Ellis, M. Jeeves, and F. Newcombe (Eds.), *Aspects of face processing.* Dordrecht: Martinus Nijhoff.

Dolan, R. J., Fink, G. R., Rolls, E., Booth, M., Holmes, A., Frackowiak, R. S. J., and Friston, K. J. (1997). How the brain learns to see objects and faces in an impoverished context. *Nature, 389,* 596–599.

Ellis, H. D., and Young, A. W. (1990). Accounting for delusional misidentification. *British Journal of Psychiatry, 157,* 239–248.

Fink, G. R., Marshall, J. C., Halligan, P. W., Frith, C. D., Driver, J., Frackowiak, R. S. J., and Dolan, R. J. (1999). The neural consequences of conflict between intention and the senses. *Brain, 122,* 497–512.

Fletcher, P., Frith, C. D., Baker, S., Shallice, T., Frackowiak, R. S. J., and Dolan, R. J. (1995). The mind's eye—activation of the precuneus in memory related imagery. *Neuroimage, 2,* 196–200.

Fletcher, P. C., Frith, C. D., Grasby, P. M., Friston, K. J., and Dolan, R. J. (1996). Local and distributed effects of apomorphine on fronto-temporal function in acute unmedicated schizophrenia. *Journal of Neuroscience, 16,* 7055–62.

Frith, C. D. (1996). The role of the prefrontal cortex in self-consciousness: The case of auditory hallucinations. *Proceedings of the Royal Society of London B, 351,* 1505–12.

Frith, C. D., and Dolan, R. J. (1997). Brain mechanisms associated with top-down processes in perception. *Philosophical Transactions of the Royal Society: Biology, 352,* 1221–30.

Frith, C. D., and Done, D. J. (1989). Experiences of alien control in schizophrenia reflect a disorder in central monitoring of action. *Psychological Medicine, 19,* 359–363.

Frith, C. D., Friston, K. J., Herold, S., Silbersweig, D., Fletcher, P., Cahill, C., Dolan, R. J., Frackowiak, R. S. J., and Liddle, P. F. (1995). Regional brain activity in chronic schizophrenic patients during the performance of a verbal fluency task. *British Journal of Psychiatry, 167,* 343–349.

Green, P., and Preston, M. (1981). Reinforcement of vocal correlates of auditory hallucinations by auditory feedback: A case study. *British Journal of Psychiatry, 139,* 204–208.

Haxby, J., Horwitz, B., Ungerleider, L. G., Maisog, J. M., Pietrini, P., and Grady, C. L. (1994). The functional organisation of human extrastriate cortex: A PET-rCBF study of selective attention to faces and locations. *Journal of Neuroscience, 14,* 6336–53.

Hirstein, W., and Ramachandran, V. S. (1997). Capgras syndrome: A novel probe for understanding the neural representation of the identity and familiarity of persons. *Proceedings of the Royal Society of London B, 264,* 437–444.

James, W. (1890). *The principles of psychology.* New York: Holt.

Jaspers, K. (1913). *General psychopathology* (English trans. 1962). Manchester: Manchester University Press.

Kaplan, B. (Ed.). (1964). *The inner world of mental illness.* New York: Harper and Row.

Kapur, N., Turner, A., and King, C. (1988). Reduplicative paramnesia: Possible anatomical and neuropsychological mechanisms. *Journal of Neurology, Neurosurgery and Psychiatry, 4,* 579–581.

Kapur, S., Craik, F., Brown, G. M., Houle, S., and Tulving, E. (1995). Functional role of the prefrontal cortex in memory retrieval: A PET study. *Neuroreport, 6,* 1880–84.

Kraupl Taylor, F. (1979). *Psychopathology.* Surrey, UK: Quartermaine House.

Leff, J. P. (1982). Acute syndromes of schizophrenia. In J. K. Wing and L. Wing (Eds.). *Handbook of psychiatry* (pp. 8–12). Cambridge: Cambridge University Press.

Mahler, B. (1974). Delusional thinking and perceptual disorder. *Journal of Individual Psychology, 30,* 98–113.

McKenna, P. J., Tamlyn, D., Lund, C. E., Mortimer, A. M., Hammond, A., and Baddeley, A. D. (1990). Amnesic syndrome in schizophrenia. *Psychological Medicine, 20,* 967–972.

Meadows, J. C. (1974). The anatomical basis of prosopagnosia. *Journal of Neurology, Neurosurgery and Psychiatry, 37,* 489–501.

Mellors, C. S. (1970). First-rank symptoms of schizophrenia. *British Journal of Psychiatry, 117,* 15–23.

Mlakar, R. C., Angel, R. W., Hampton, B., and Berger, P. A. (1982). Impaired central error correcting behaviour in schizophrenia. *Archives of General Psychiatry, 39,* 101–107.

Morris, J., Friston, K. J., and Dolan, R. J. (1997). Neural responses to salient visual stimuli. *Proceedings of the Royal Society of London B, 264,* 769–775.

Nathaniel-James, D., and Frith, C. D. (1996). Confabulation in schizophrenia: Evidence of a new form. *Psychological Medicine, 26,* 391–399.

Paus, T., Marrett, S., Evans, A. C., and Worsley, K. (1995). Neurophysiology of saccadic suppression in the human brain. *IBRO World Congress of Neuroscience, 478* (abstract).

Rugg, M. D., Fletcher, P. C., Frith, C. D., Frackowiak, R. S. J., and Dolan, R. J. (1996). Differential activation of the prefrontal cortex in successful and unsuccessful memory retrieval. *Brain, 119,* 2073–83.

Rushton, D. N., Rothwell, J. C., and Craggs, M. D. (1981). Gating of somatosensory evoked potential during different kinds of movement in man. *Brain, 104,* 465–491.

Schacter, D. L., Réiman, E., Curran, T., Yun, L. S., Bandy, D., McDermott, K. B., and Roediger, H. L. (1996). Neuroanatomical correlates of veridical and illusory recognition memory revealed by PET. *Neuron, 17,* 267–274.

Shafer, W. P., Amochaev, A., and Russell, M. J. (1981). Knowledge of stimulus timing attenuates human cortical evoked potentials. *Electroencephalography and Clinical Neuroscience, 52,* 9–17.

Shallice, T. (1988). *From neuropsychology to mental structure.* Cambridge: Cambridge University Press.

Snyder, L. H., Batista, A. P., and Andersen, R. A. (1997). Coding of intention in the posterior parietal cortex. *Nature, 386,* 167–170.

Spence, S. A., Brooks, D. J., Hirsch, S. R., Liddle, P. F., Meehan, J., and Grasby, P. M. (1997). A PET study of voluntary movement in schizophrenic patients experiencing passivity phenomena (delusions of alien control). *Brain, 120,* 1997–2011.

Wilding, E. L., and Rugg, M. D. (1997). Event-related potentials and the recognition memory exclusion task. *Neuropsychologia, 35,* 119–128.

Wing, J. K. (1978). Clinical concepts of schizophrenia. In J. K. Wing (Ed.), *Schizophrenia: Towards a new synthesis* (pp. 1–30). London: Academic Press.

Wolpert, D. M., Ghahramani, Z., and Jordan, M. I. (1995). An internal model for sensorimotor integration. *Science, 269,* 1880–82.

Conscious and Nonconscious Aspects of Memory and Belief: From Social Judgments to Brain Mechanisms

Implicit Stereotypes and Memory: The Bounded Rationality of Social Beliefs | 5

Mahzarin R. Banaji
R. Bhaskar

The constructs of *belief* and *memory* have become closely intertwined in contemporary research on stereotyping. Yet even a few decades ago psychology's treatment of belief (stereotype) and memory moved along trajectories so disconnected that a link between the two might have seemed implausible. The theme of this book prompts a glance at the consequences of the relationship between belief and memory in experimental social psychology, the field that laid claim to a rigorous understanding of how beliefs about social groups shape judgments of their members.

Stereotyping and Prejudice

In the connection that developed between the social psychological study of belief and the cognitive study of memory, the concept of stereotype came to be demystified in two fundamental ways. First, the link between belief and memory allowed stereotyping and its uglier cousin, prejudice, to be viewed as ordinary in origin and pervasive in the sweep of its contagion.[1] Instead of considerations of the inherently evil nature of humans that produced prejudice and resulting group conflict, social psychology came to understand these phenomena as rooted in the very nature of how knowledge is acquired and used— that is, in the ordinary, constrained operations of an information processing system. Second and more recently, discoveries of the implicit aspects of memory have exposed the substantial unconscious component of social beliefs as well. In contrast to the first hundred years of research, which conveyed a view of memory and beliefs as operating exclusively in a conscious mode, the past two decades have shown increasingly that both memory and belief also operate implicitly in powerful yet unconscious ways, outside the actor's awareness or control (Greenwald and Banaji, 1995; Schacter, 1987).

This chapter draws on both developments, exploring the premise that the *ordinary* and *implicit* character of stereotypes and prejudice provides a more accurate representation of their nature, and reveals their full influence in human affairs. Together the properties of ordinariness and implicitness raise questions about how the limits on human thought and preferences diminish the rationality of stereotyped beliefs and prejudicial judgments. Conventionally, boundedly rational behaviors have been viewed as cognitive curiosities that influence human thought. Our purpose however, is to emphasize that cognitive acts are social acts and inherently have moral dimensions. This simple extension from ordinary and implicit social judgments to their moral consequences changes the scope of social cognition's view of stereotyping and prejudice in deep and permanent ways.

The Ordinary Nature of Stereotyping and Prejudice

The classic tract *The Authoritarian Personality* (Adorno, Frenkel-Brunswik, Levinson, and Sanford, 1950) provides the clearest statement of the intuitive position that stereotypes and prejudice are rooted in the structure of the prejudiced personality of special individuals. As averred in the preface to the book, "The central theme of the work is a relatively new concept—the rise of an 'anthropological' species we call the authoritarian type of man. In contrast to the bigot of the older style he seems to combine the ideas and skills which are typical of a highly industrialized society with irrational or antirational beliefs" (p. xi). The mission of *The Authoritarian Personality* was to identify and understand "the *potentially fascistic* individual, one whose structure is such as to render him particularly susceptible to antidemocratic propaganda" (p. 1; emphasis in original). This was a remarkable book providing a complex theory that merged psychoanalytic thinking with social science findings, and it encouraged a great deal of research. Although its central message was never formally challenged and is still endorsed in some quarters, it failed to have permanent theoretical impact. It was another volume, containing ideas quite ahead of their time, that stood waiting for academic psychology to catch up. In a beloved and now widely cited book, *The Nature of Prejudice,* Gordon Allport offered a radically different view of prejudice as reflecting "[man's] normal and natural tendency to form generalizations, concepts, categories, whose content represents an oversimplification of his world of experience" (1954, p. 27).

In the decades since Allport's book, and especially since the emphasis on social cognition in the mid-1970s, a steady transformation has occurred in thinking about stereotypes and prejudice, removing from them associations of unnaturalness and uniqueness. At least in their academic discourse, social psychologists have moved from the view that stereotypes and prejudice reflect the warped beliefs and preferences of distasteful individuals who threaten harmonious social existence, to the view that such processes are best considered the unhappy and even tragic outcomes of the ordinary workings of human cognition. As a consequence, a fundamental interconnectedness between the cognitive processes of memory, perception, attention, categorization, and reasoning on the one hand and the social processes of stereotyping and prejudice on the other became permanently established (see Banaji and Greenwald, 1994; Hamilton, 1981).[2]

Research has borne out Allport's (1954) claim that "categories have a close and immediate tie with what we see, how we judge, and what we do. In fact, their whole purpose seems to be to facilitate perception and conduct—in other words, to make our adjustment to life speedy, smooth, and consistent. This principle holds even though we often make mistakes in fitting events to categories and thus get ourselves in trouble" (p. 21). In this chapter we agree with Allport's prescient view that stereotypes and prejudice are rooted in the ordinary mechanisms of perception and categorization, and our data will provide evidence in support. We treat these mistakes as not only "getting ourselves in trouble," but as quite systematically getting others in trouble as well. Fortunately, we have access to an additional forty-five years of empirical research and national debate about intergroup relations, and these are the backdrop against which we discuss the implications of ordinary prejudices for imagining the ideal of a just society.

The Unconscious Nature of Stereotyping and Prejudice

A second shift in thinking has allowed yet another link between stereotypes and memory to emerge; this one stems from the inclusion of unconscious processes. Abelson's (1986) comment that "beliefs are like possessions" captured the idea that psychological beliefs are capable of evoking the feelings of ownership, endowment, and attachment typically elicited by material possessions. As if referring to tangible entities, we speak of acquiring, inheriting, and adopting beliefs, or of losing, disowning, and abandoning them. Such metaphors reveal in our language a view of beliefs as entities that are available to conscious awareness and responsive to conscious control (for instance, "I used to be an atheist, but I gave it up for Lent").[3] Such an understanding of beliefs as residing largely within conscious awareness and control is not only intuitive, but its widespread acceptance within the scientific community has determined methods of research used through the first century of experimental social psychology (see Banaji and Greenwald, 1994; Greenwald and Banaji, 1995).

Without debating the assumption that beliefs are consciously available and deployed, we worked with the assumption that the opposite of well-worn truths may also be true (cf. McGuire, 1973). For the past several years, one of us (MRB) has been interested in the discovery of the unconscious or implicit operation of beliefs and preferences.[4] This goal has involved creating in research participants the effortless articulation of stereotypes and prejudice, in some instances without their conscious awareness of such use or without conscious control over their expression. The research is part of a wide range of experiments designed to show the many ways in which stereotypes can be automatically activated and utilized even by actors who may intend a quite different response (Banaji, 1997; Chen and Bargh, 1997; Devine, 1989; Fazio, Jackson, Dunton, and Williams, 1995; Greenwald and Banaji, 1995; see Fiske, 1998, for a review).

The main message of this new body of research is the inevitability of unconscious stereotyping and prejudice. The best of intentions do not and cannot override the unfolding of unconscious processes, for the triggers of automatic thought, feeling, and behavior live and breathe outside conscious awareness and control. Again, Allport (1954) predicted the empirical findings decades in advance and in surprisingly modern language: "A person with dark brown skin will activate whatever concept of Negro is dominant in our mind. If the dominant category is one composed of negative attitudes and beliefs we will automatically avoid him, or adopt whichever habit of rejection is most available to us" (p. 21).

In the remainder of this chapter we champion two views, one directly reflecting the state of the science, the other a speculation about what the discoveries imply for social justice. Our position is that all humans are implicated to varying degrees in the operation of implicit stereotypes and prejudice. The pervasiveness of such expressions has been underestimated because large portions occur outside the awareness and control of both perceivers and targets. Based on evidence of the ways in which perception, attention, categorization, and memory operate to produce biases in judgment, stereotyping and prejudice too must be viewed as the outcome of ordinary and automatic thinking and feeling (Allport, 1954; Banaji and Greenwald, 1994; see Hamilton, 1981, for many chapters that include this assumption).

Such a position is allied more generally with psychological research that has offered a humbling view of human thought and rationality (Nisbett and Ross, 1980; Simon, 1983; Tversky and Kahneman, 1974). In contrast to a traditional nineteenth-century assumption that behavior is rational, the established modern view is that humans are boundedly rational, having "neither the facts nor the consistent structure of values nor the reasoning power at their disposal" to make decisions in line with subjective expected utility, "a beautiful object deserving a prominent place in Plato's heaven of ideas, . . . [but] impossible to employ . . . in any literal way in making actual human decisions" (Simon, 1983). Over the past few decades, such a depiction of decisionmaking has forced an acceptance of bounded rationality as the proper characterization of stereotyping and prejudice.[5]

Second, when stereotypes are unconsciously activated and used, two direct challenges to the implementation of fairness are posed: (a) perceivers and targets are often unaware of the steady and continuous rendering of judgments, and (b) judgments are based on beliefs about targets' social groups rather than on targets' actions. Such issues concerning fairness are not inventions of twentieth-century concepts of justice. Resolutions of the concerns they raise were implemented in relatively ancient systems. When judgments about humans are made, it is a fundamental principle of justice, now almost a thousand years old in Anglo-American jurisprudence (Assize of Clarendon, 1166), that targets of judgment should be made aware of the judgment. The main modern purpose of this rule, is, of course, to ensure that judgments are not based on factual error—although a deeper principle is also involved, that justice is better served when an opportunity to be heard exists (Ptahotep scrolls, 2400 B.C.). An unaware judge subverts this principle, because targets of judgment are denied the opportunity to contest, contradict, or modify the judgment.

Further, it is an equally hoary and fundamental principle of justice that judgments about individuals must be based on the individuals' own behavior, involving specific acts of commission and omission. Societies in which punishment was based on association (as when families of traitors were beheaded in seventh-century T'ang China) are regarded as barbaric by the standards of contemporary democracies. In this century, social science research in which beliefs about groups have been shown to influence judgments of individuals has been increasingly interpreted as representing bias. This interpretation arises not from a concern with the correctness of perceivers' beliefs about the group, but because the application of group-level knowledge (some X are Y) to individuals (X is Y) is deemed incorrect.[6]

The purpose of presenting the experimental evidence that follows is largely to help deconstruct an opposing view of stereotyping as correct and rational. This perspective is perhaps expressed most infelicitously by McCauley, Jussim, and Lee (1995), who endorse with evident approval the decision of a taxi driver not to stop for "a lone Black male at midnight in a bad neighborhood" (pp. 300–301). Such a view is so commonly held in contemporary American culture that the legitimacy of group-based judgments brings us up against a troubling tension between what is so socially prevalent as to be self-evident and what is correct upon sustained reflection. We will argue in the concluding section of this chapter that stereotypic behaviors of the sort endorsed by McCauley and colleagues may well be termed reasonable in the narrow sense that "reasonable" people in the same circumstances would exhibit the same behavior (Hart, 1976), which is nevertheless (a) inconsistent with logic, practice, intention, and assessment of similar outcomes in other domains, and (b) irrational in the classical, axiomatic sense of subjective expected utility theory (Arrow, 1963; Savage, 1972).

Overview of Experiments

Memory is regarded as the petri dish in which one can view the movements of particular forms of stereotypes and prejudice. Such a use of memory to study stereotypes is not new (see Hamilton, 1981), but research on implicit memory has allowed the even more prominent use of memory to examine stereotypes (see Banaji and Greenwald, 1994; Greenwald and Banaji, 1995). Implicit memory measures are those that do not require conscious recollection of a prior episode (Schacter, 1987). In line with such a definition, Greenwald and Banaji (1995) defined implicit stereotypes to be "the introspectively unidentified (or inaccurately identified) traces of past experience that mediate attributions of qualities to members of a social category" (p. 15).

Of the many potential connections between belief and memory, our focus has been on *beliefs about social groups as revealed through implicit or automatic memory*. Beliefs that serve as the building blocks of this research program concern characteristics of social groups that are widely endorsed, at least in the United States at the turn of the twenty-first century. Such beliefs may or may not be accurate descriptions of social groups, and while the limit on their accuracy is itself of interest, that is not an issue of primary concern here. For the purpose of this research, we work with beliefs that are simply endorsed with wide consensus, and we track their unwitting use in the judgment of individual members of social groups. Examples of the type of beliefs about social groups whose effects we might observe are that men are more likely to be famous than women; that the elderly are less alert mentally than younger adults; that women are emotional, nurturing, and submissive, but men are aggressive, competent, and strong; that the poor are more likely to be black than white; that women have less talent for leadership than men; that East Asians are intelligent but passive; and that gay men are feminine.

In one line of research, we examined how a subset of such beliefs about gender and race are expressed in judgments of individual members of these groups. Experimentally, individuals were created to be equally associated or dissociated with characteristics such as fame, criminality, aggression, or dependence, and situations were designed to measure the extent to which beliefs about the social groups of these individuals were unconsciously used in judging them. By creating conditions under which conscious awareness or control was reduced, we found that implicit memory reveals the implicit operation of stereotypes and prejudice.

In these experiments we have also discovered that implicit expressions of beliefs and attitudes are unrelated to explicit versions of the same beliefs and attitudes. Here college students are the theoretically appropriate population for study, for we are keenly interested in individuals known to consciously hold egalitarian beliefs and nonprejudicial attitudes. Showing the operation of implicit stereotypes and prejudices in individuals who consciously disavow their presence captures a dissociation in which we are interested, that between conscious and unconscious social judgment. Our interest is driven by a relatively straightforward concern. Dissociations between implicit and explicit beliefs are fundamentally important in understanding their nature, the relationship of each to the other, and the consequences of each. Further, it is necessary to acknowledge that there are indeed consequences of implicit and unintended expressions of beliefs because of their power to reward and punish on the basis of group membership.

Verifications of beliefs about social groups are so pervasive, frequent, and fleeting as to be quite unnoticed in the course of everyday life. A glimpse of John revving a tow truck, Jane walking with a brood of kindergartners, Tyrese slam-dunking a basketball, Mary Cheng playing a violin—these actions are ordinary enough that they may not evoke conscious contemplation of their meaning or cause. But they are automatically added to the cumulative mental record of social experience, with each episode strengthening a particular association—that between the psychological attributes signified by the act and the social group to which the actor belongs. Such exposures strengthen the belief that males are strong, that females are nurturant, that young black men are athletic, that Asian Americans have musical talent.

The consequences of such learning interest us here, for it is the well-learned and automatically activated associations between psychological qualities and social groups that can short-circuit the consciously espoused goal of assuring mental due process in social judgment, that is, that a person be judged not by color of skin, but by content of character. If this is indeed an espoused goal, then the findings from recent experiments in social psychology suggest that in social interaction such a goal of fair and equal treatment is largely ephemeral (see Bargh, Chen, and Burrows, 1996). A substantial and growing literature shows that exposure to specific behaviors automatically leads to inferences about the abstract psychological qualities that underlie the behaviors (Uleman, 1987), and that generalization from observation or experience with single individuals to other members of the group may be swift and unconscious (Henderson-King and Nisbett, 1996; Lewicki, 1986). Further, such beliefs can actually produce behavior consistent with the activated belief, demonstrating that implicit stereotypes have self-fulfilling consequences (Chen and Bargh, 1997). Beliefs about qualities such as intelligence and ability, toughness and softness, and the capacity for good and harm are implicitly and lawfully applied to individual members of groups, whether consciously endorsed or not, and whether consciously deemed morally appropriate or not.

In some experiments we have analyzed the computational circumstances that give rise to implicit stereotyping and prejudice. That the speed of mental computation can provide insight into social processes is not a new idea, although explicit appreciation of its value is not easily available in discussions of social cognition (Banaji, 1995). We have examined the automatic activation of beliefs and attitudes about social groups by measuring the time required to produce them under conditions of varying cognitive constraints. We use the time it takes to produce a decision about a person (in the presence of associated or dissociated beliefs or evaluative information) as a measure of the strength of the stereotype or attitude (cf. Fazio, Sanbonmatsu, Powell, and Kardes, 1986). For instance, gender-stereotypic words such as "mechanic" or "secretary" are presented for approximately 250 milliseconds, then replaced by a male or female name (John, Jane). Participants must judge whether the second item is a male or female name. The speed of judging male and female names in the presence of stereotypic items can reveal the strength of such stereotypes and provide an individual difference measure of the strength of such beliefs. By varying the constraints under which the judgments are made, we can speak more directly about the mechanisms that limit the application of conscious intention and deliberate strategy. Such constraints serve theoretically to vary the bounds on the rationality of participants' output.

To describe the subterranean connections between belief and memory, we proceed by summarizing the research procedures and major findings obtained in a single laboratory, with some experiments demonstrating the effects of implicit beliefs without conscious *awareness*, and others showing evidence of their operating outside conscious *control*. Together they serve as the empirical basis of our claims about the belief-memory relationship, and allow consideration of broader questions regarding the moral implications of implicit beliefs and preferences.

The Experiments

Selective Application of Activated Beliefs

Some of our research revealed how exposure to behaviors that automatically activate beliefs about social groups can implicitly and selectively influence judgment. In particular, we examined the consequences for targets who were judged during a state of temporary activation of stereotypes in the perceiver.

In one series of studies, we activated abstract knowledge about beliefs associated with women and men, such as *dependence* and *aggressiveness*, by presenting sentences that captured relevant behaviors which participants had to unscramble (T never goes alone; P kicked the dog). In a later session, one that participants believed to be unrelated to the prior task, we obtained the judgments of two individuals, Donna and Donald, who performed identical actions (Banaji, Hardin, and Rothman, 1993). After exposure to behaviors about dependence (T never goes alone), a female but not a male target was expected to suffer from the perception of greater dependence, while after exposure to behaviors about aggression (P kicked the dog), a male but not a female target was expected to be punished because of the perception of greater aggressiveness. Even more strongly than predicted, results revealed that the temporary activation of a belief did not influence person judgment when the target did not belong to the stereotyped group—say, when a male target was judged after exposure to dependence-related information and when a female target was judged after exposure to aggression-related information. Targets were judged more harshly only when the activated stereotyped belief and the targets' group membership were stereotypically matched; that is, when a female target was judged after exposure to behaviors depicting dependence, and a male target was judged after exposure to behaviors depicting aggression. In other words, activated beliefs about social groups are differentially sticky with regard to whom they are applied to in social judgments.

Temporary exposure to behaviors that activate a belief associated with social groups appears to shift the judgment of targets who merely belong to the social group associated with the activated belief. Interestingly, these data reveal both the ease with which shifts in judgment are possible and their limits. Belief activation appears to be necessary for producing stereotyped judgments, for no change from baseline was observed in the no-activation condition. In other words, men and women were not judged to be differentially aggressive or dependent when a belief was not activated prior to judgment.[7]

The conclusion about the relationship between belief and memory is obvious: judgments of individuals are shifted in a more extreme direction when they follow activation of a belief about the target's social group. Participants are not aware of such shifts and would perhaps even deny that such influences on their judgment are possible. From other experiments we know that individuals who employ stereotypes implicitly have no prior intention of doing so, and would consider such use to be unjust. Yet such ordinary and implicit influences occur and threaten the goal of fair and equal interpersonal treatment (Chen and Bargh, 1997).

Unequal Standards for Judgment

We tested whether the established link between gender and fame (for instance, that men as a group are more likely to be considered famous than women) would increase the assignment of (false) fame to nonfamous men when compared with equally nonfamous women. Participants in the research were exposed to a list of names, famous and nonfamous, male and female. Later they were presented with the same names in addition to new (previously unseen) names with similar characteristics. The task was to identify whether each name was the name of a famous person or not. Jacoby, Kelley, Brown, and Jasechko (1989) predicted and found that when faced with this task, people are poised to make a particular error detected in the form of false alarms on nonfamous names. Unable to separate varying sources of familiarity for a name (that is, familiarity from recent exposure versus familiarity from fame), participants were twice as likely to incorrectly judge a familiar (nonfamous) name "famous" than an unfamiliar (nonfamous) name.

The rationale for our experiments was that a belief about greater male fame ought to predispose participants toward greater incorrect identification of male than female names when implicit memory for nonfamous names still lingered as a function of prior exposure. Indeed, in four experiments we found a greater propensity for false alarms (identification of nonfamous names as famous) for familiarized male than female names, with no difference found on unfamiliarized names (Banaji and Greenwald, 1995). Using signal detection statistics, we found that this effect was located in the component of bias (β) and revealed itself in a more lenient criterion for judging male than female fame. In other words, an accurate belief about the differential fame of two social groups translated into differential standards for judging individuals equally (un)deserving of fame. Here ordinary conditions of familiarity were sufficient to justify greater assignment of fame to men than to women. Again, the ordinary and implicit nature of social judgment is the basis of a threat to fair and equal social treatment.

False Memories Created by Race Beliefs
We have also used a variant of the gender-fame task to examine errors that may occur under a more stark set of conditions (Walsh, Banaji, and Greenwald, 1995). Male names were varied in race between European American and African American (Frank Smith and Adam McCarthy or Tyrone Washington and Darnell Jones).[8] We suggested

to the participants that they might have memory for these names, some of which were those of criminals. In fact, none of the names were names of criminals. Participants were told that some of the names on the list might seem familiar because they had appeared in the media. The task was to identify each name as criminal or noncriminal. In five experiments, we found that on average subjects "remembered" 1.7 times as many black than white names as criminals.

This finding was obtained with various proportions of white and black names (85:10; 50:50), and within and between subject designs. Additional experiments varied instructions that pointed to the race of the targets with varying degrees of explicitness, and in one case even informed participants that "people who are racist identify more black than white names; please do not use the race of the name in making your judgment." Such experiments have continued to reveal the bias. Our assessment is that participants who show the race bias believe their judgment to be based on a genuine memory for each identified name, black or white, and also believe that their assessment is not influenced by the race of the name. Yet belief produces a memory and, consistent with research on false memory (Roediger and McDermott, 1995), it leads in these circumstances to the greater false identification of black men as criminals.

More than any other experimental result from our laboratory, this finding has provoked a "rationality" defense of our participants' behavior. We report a relevant experimental variation here, simultaneously pointing out that the term "rational" as used in informal questions about this research has generally been innocent of any rigorous definition.[9] In the absence of other knowledge about the individual in question, it is rational, the argument goes, to use existing knowledge about the link between race and crime in completing the task at hand. In other words, the rational choice, it is argued, lies in using group membership in judgment.

If identifying proportionally more black than white names as criminal is indeed rational, then conditions allowing fuller access to cognitive resources should produce even greater rational behavior (that is, the greater identification of criminals on the basis of group membership) than conditions under which such access is restricted. In a separate study we did not find this to be the case. Subjects were asked to identify criminal names in a 2×2 design. One factor varied an instruction regarding racism: the control group was given no instruction, and the experimental group was alerted that "people have been found to associate criminality with African Americans more than with whites, Asians, or other ethnic groups. This is true for people who believe they have race prejudices (people who are racist) as well as for those of us who believe we are not prejudiced. Please try not to be influenced by the race of the name in making your judgments." The other factor varied the time available to complete the task. Participants were either self-paced throughout or were informed that they had only one minute to complete the task. The task actually took about one minute to complete, so the time-pressure instruction created only the expectation of a constraint.

When no instruction to avoid using the race of the name was offered, both the self-paced and the time-pressure conditions produced the familiar race bias. In other words, having greater access to cognitive resources in the self-paced condition failed to produce the putatively more rational response of greater criminal identification of black than white names. When the instruction to avoid using race of the name was in place, participants equalized their identification of black and white names as criminals in the self-paced condition, but still continued to show race bias in the time-pressure condition. Those who assume that a race bias is rational must concede that rationality apparently gives way to what would be considered the less rational response (of no race bias) when instructions to be fair and a perceived time constraint are present. That an instruction to achieve a prescribed goal (in this case of unbiased responding) and the availability of sufficient resources can change behavior (a race bias in criminal judgment) illustrates a fundamental characteristic of boundedly rational behavior: the domain dependence of these bounds and their malleability within specific problem contexts.

For decades, civil rights legislation has been premised on the assumption that to discriminate on the basis of group status (race, religion, sex) in decisions about individuals is unacceptable. When the decision is a judgment of criminality, when such judgments do not reflect an explicit prejudice on the part of the actor, and when the decision is based on cultural knowledge that is widely shared however dubious its origin, the consequences are deeply disturbing. Participants in our experiments are neither racist in the accepted sense of the term nor inclined to cause harm intentionally to the individuals they identify. In fact, explicit measures of racism and belief in the fairness of the criminal justice system show participants to be consciously egalitarian and fair-minded. Nonetheless, their behavior reveals the influence of beliefs on (false) memory about vital attributes of a person's character.

It is important that performance on explicit measures is not related to the magnitude of the race bias. Implicit and explicit stereotypes may be quite dissociated, as seen in these experiments, although they may come to be associated under other circumstances. We are still far from understanding the nature of the association between explicit and implicit attitudes and beliefs, and it is clear from more recent data (Lepore and Brown, 1997) that their relationship is by no means a simple one (see Blair, forthcoming).

In summary, the experiments on personality, fame, and criminality judgments demonstrate that ordinary conditions of judgment reveal the complex interaction of stereotypic beliefs and memory. In the gender-fame studies, participants were seduced by the familiarity of names to give males the greater benefit of fame implicitly, even when no such privilege was earned. In the personality experiments, harsher assessments of aggression and dependence were applied along gender-stereotypic lines, even when the differentially judged men and women had performed identical actions. In the race-crime studies, the costly judgment of criminality was levied disproportionately on nonguilty black men because of a false memory generated with surprising ease.

In spite of their ordinary and implicit operation, such judgments are not without consequence, for they clearly reveal the inequitable distribution of punishment and reward along lines of group membership. The impact of such judgments is seen to be even greater when their ordinary and implicit character reveals the ubiquity of their influence in everyday social interaction, and the slim opportunities that exist for self-doubt or disbelief about the poverty of the underlying mental due process.

Automatic Activation of Gender

Small differences in time can make large differences in the behavior of complex systems. If the sea of quarks had taken 10^{-30} instead of 10^{-35}

seconds to form, the shape and form of the universe would have been vastly different—if one had formed at all. The significance of small amounts of time, here on the order of milliseconds, is visible in many activities involving skill, such as music, cooking, and baseball. For example, expert opinion about the difference between a "not bad" and a "good" judgment on a catcher's release time is 9/100ths of a second (Will, 1990).[10] In the equally skilled game of social perception, differences in response latencies can reveal how the interaction of specific social experiences and a boundedly rational cognitive architecture jointly shape thought and behavior.

In some experiments we have taken small differences in the time to complete a social computation as an indicator of the strength of social beliefs, that is, the association between social groups and the qualities ascribed or denied to them. Time to respond to associations between social groups and physical or psychological qualities has allowed us to measure a particular component of unconscious thought: the lack of control over expressions of stereotypic beliefs and prejudicial attitudes (Banaji and Hardin, 1996; Blair and Banaji, 1996).

Our assumption is a simple and powerful one—that the speed of response to one stimulus in the context of another stimulus (related or unrelated) is an indicator of the underlying strength of association (semantic or evaluative) between the two (Meyer and Schvaneveldt, 1971; Neely, 1977). Such automatic responses capture thoughts and feelings that are deployed without conscious control, and our procedure has served well in exploring the strength of automatically activated beliefs by measuring their association in memory. Using a variation of a standard semantic priming technique, we presented gender-stereotypic words (emotional, aggressive, skirt, cigar) for short durations of approximately 300 milliseconds followed by male and female first names (Ann, Lisa, David, George). The speed of rapidly judging names to be either male or female was taken to be a measure of the strength of association in memory between these social groups and associated concepts (see also Dovidio, Evans, and Tyler, 1986).

A central feature of unconscious processes is the notion of control. A growing literature demonstrates that social actors' ability to control and modify their beliefs, judgments, and behavior is constrained by variables such as the awareness of inappropriate influences on judgments and behavior, the availability of cognitive resources to make spontaneous corrections, and the knowledge of suitable strategies to implement such corrections. The greater the degree of conscious deliberation that can be exerted over an action, a thought, or a feeling, the greater the assumed control over it.

Among the most fundamentally learned social categories is that of gender. Children show evidence of knowledge about gender and its associations at an early age (Fagot and Leinbach, 1989; Martin and Little, 1990). From our experiments we have solid evidence of the ability to classify gender-related information into female-male categories: first names (Jane, John), traits (nurturant, competitive), occupations (nurse, doctor), kinship (sister, brother), and verbal or pictorial representations of physical attributes (lipstick, cigar). Presenting prime-target pairs for approximately 300 milliseconds, we have shown that feminine primes strongly facilitate judgments of female over male names and that, analogously, masculine primes strongly facilitate judgments of male compared to female names. In other words, prime-target pairings whose gender association is congruent facilitate judgment when compared with pairings that do not share the property of gender (Banaji and Hardin, 1996; Blair and Banaji, 1996).

Implicit Attitudes

In a more recently developed task, Greenwald, McGhee, and Schwartz (1998) used an interference task, namely control, to capture the same process of unconscious judgment. The procedure, called the *implicit association test* (IAT), was devised to measure the strength of attitudes by assessing the extent to which two concepts (for instance, black–good/white–bad versus black–bad/white–good) are associated. The task requires participants to classify items from two categories (*black* names and *unpleasant* words) on a computer key while at the same time classifying items from two contrasting categories (*white* names and *pleasant* words) on a different key. Response latencies to perform this task are compared with trials in which the opposite categories are paired, that is, when black names/pleasant words are assigned to a single response key and white names/unpleasant words are assigned to a contrasting key. The underlying assumption is that if two concepts are evaluatively congruent (black-bad and white-good), trials that involve such pairings should be relatively easier than pairings that associate incongruent or less congruent concepts (black-good and white-bad). The difference in response latencies in the two types of pairings provides a measure of automatic attitude toward the group black compared with the group white.

In fact, Greenwald and colleagues (1998) showed that the IAT task is a quite powerful indicator of automatic attitudes toward nonsocial categories such as insects versus flowers and weapons versus musical instruments, with the vast majority of participants showing favorable attitudes toward flowers and instruments. In measuring social attitudes, this group found that independent of explicitly expressed attitudes toward social groups, white and Asian participants showed negative attitudes toward black Americans, and Korean Americans and Japanese Americans showed greater implicit liking for their respective ingroups compared with the outgroup.

The implicit association test permits measurement of attitudes and beliefs in a wide range of categories. We are currently conducting experiments that measure (a) automatic liking of male and female leaders with an interest in predicting voting behavior (Carpenter and Banaji, 1997); (b) automatic gender identity, gender attitude, and their relationship to each other (Lemm and Banaji, 1998); (c) automatic gender attitudes toward science and math versus language and arts, links between academic orientation and self-concept, and the developmental course of such preferences (Nosek, Banaji, and Greenwald, 1998); (d) the relationship between automatic self-esteem, group esteem, and group identity (Rosier, Banaji, and Greenwald, 1998); and (e) dissociated attitudes toward a single object (Mitchell, Nosek, and Banaji, 1998).

Taken together, the experiments on uncontrollable beliefs and attitudes demonstrate the difficulty in curbing unconscious associations between social groups and activation of stereotypic beliefs and prejudicial feelings toward them. In the automatic gender-stereotyping studies described earlier, we found that the absence of sufficient cognitive resources and a well-defined strategy disallowed conscious attempts at correction. The same was true in the experiments using the IAT. Subjective awareness of inability to perform as fast in the incompatible condition as in the compatible condition often accompanies in-

ability to control automatic preferences and beliefs among participants, who include in their number the experimenters themselves.

The Bounded Rationality of Implicit Social Beliefs

The gender-fame experiments, the race-criminality experiments, and
the experiments to measure automatic preferences apparently pose a
tension between two positions that we refer to as *guilt by association*
and *guilt by behavior.*[11]

On the one hand, it has been argued that the use of knowledge
about social groups to make decisions about individual humans is appropriate and defensible. (We refer to this as the guilt-by-association
position.) For instance, in a rousing defense of the accuracy of stereotyped judgments, McCauley, Jussim, and Lee (1995) say: "In this case
[when no individuating information is available], the stereotype of the
group is likely to dominate the evaluation of the stereotyped target (*as
normatively it should*)" (p. 301; emphasis added). Often proponents
of guilt-by-association decisions compare them to selection decisions
about inanimate objects such as computers or restaurants. If, for example, the task is to pick the better of two working models of a mechanical gadget such as a computer, it would be quite appropriate to
pick the manufacturer with the lower failure rate. Likewise, if the task
is to identify criminals, the guilt-by-association position holds that the
greater identification of black than white names in the race-criminality
experiments is rational and defensible on grounds of base-rate information.

On the other hand, many personal and social codes of ethics hold
that judgments about individuals should be based on an individual's
own behavior without attention to group membership. According to
this guilt-by-behavior position, it is implausible or incorrect to infer
that the parents of murderers are more likely to be murderers because
they belong to the same social group—family. Or that because police
officers are convicted of crimes at a higher rate than the general population (Uviller, 1996), Officer X is a criminal.

This belief that guilt by association is morally repugnant is so fundamental that it has occupied a central place in all codes of justice
from Ptahotep (Ptahotep, 2300 B.C.) to Hammurabi to Asoka (259

B.C.; see Nikam and McKeon, 1958) to the Assize of Clarendon (1166; see Plucknett, 1956) to all modern constitutions (with a small number of European exceptions in this century).[12]

The guilt-by-association position perhaps rests on a particular confusion between what most individuals are likely to do in a given situation and what is considered rational. The ordinary expression of a stereotype takes the form, Many Xs have property A, x is an X, therefore x has property A. Such routine inferences are exactly that—they are routine, and hence perhaps mistakenly assumed to be rational. As every schoolchild knows, behavior that is routine and seemingly reasonable need not be rational. For a decision to be rational, it must conform to the axioms of rationality in the sense of Savage (1972) or Arrow (1963).[13] For the axioms to be valid descriptors of behavior, the existence of a global utility function that captures all possible choices over time is a necessary and sufficient condition. Rational choice consists of decisions that always maximize this global utility function.

It can be shown that the requirements of these axioms are quite constraining (Debreu, 1971). In general, preferences cannot always be articulated, and when they are, they are not always consistent or necessarily stable over time. Additionally, most tasks cannot be readily represented within the confines of a global utility function, and information about the consequences of actions that allow rational choice is not always available. In the remainder of the chapter, our use of the word "rational" is restricted to this classic, axiomatic sense.[14]

Rational behavior, with this axiomatic import, has an all-or-none flavor. Behavior is either rational or irrational and, by definition, rational behavior is always correct. Our arguments about the bounded rationality of our subjects' behavior rely on the fundamental premise that *behavior that seems reasonable can be irrational and therefore incorrect.* Judging a single individual on the basis of information about her or his group can seem statistically justifiable, but cannot be justified by an appeal to rationality. We will demonstrate exactly how participants' behavior is not classically rational and how the departure from rationality can be explained by understanding the information-processing constraints that drive the behavior.

In addition, we suggest that the guilt-by-association position is based on a particular fallacy: two identical decision processes are seen to be equally acceptable even when their outputs have differential moral consequences—incalculable moral consequences can follow misjudgments of humans, whereas no difficulties accrue to an unselected computer. We argue that decision processes should be compared not on the basis of structural similarity alone, but also by taking a consequentialist approach attendant on the benefit or harm produced by the decision.

We devote the remainder of the chapter to assessing the kinds of judgments that the preceding experiments have highlighted. Specifically, our assessment will be based on two standards of good judgment (see Hastie and Rasinski, 1988). According to the first standard, judgments are considered to be correct, appropriate, justified, and ultimately defensible if they fit a coherent theory such as the axioms of probability or rationality. As an example, decisions in the classic "Linda problem" are considered to be incorrect when they fail to meet the conjunction relation—that is, $P(A)$ and $P(B)$ are both always greater than $P(A, B)$. By the second standard, judgments are considered to be good if they fit the data, that is, are empirically verified. For example, a weather forecaster's performance can be assessed by comparing predictions to actual weather. We show that the judgments under scrutiny in this chapter may be considered vulnerable to both standards. In other words, judgments of the sort produced in these experiments are not consistent with either theory-fitting or data-fitting standards.

We further demonstrate how participants' behavior is not classically rational in that it adheres to other accepted criteria of incorrect or problematic judgments. Such behavior is shown to conform to the computational characteristics that exemplify boundedly rational behavior.

Not Classically Rational

Following nearly fifty years of research in psychology, we demonstrate that the behavior of participants in our experiments shows no evidence of classic rationality. Table 5.1 gives a partial list of the many utility functions that participants might choose (if they were rational). Inspection suggests why all of them are unlikely descriptors of behavior. Not only do the utility functions require computations that are

Table 5.1 Possible utility functions for participants in race-criminality experiments

---

1. Minimize [(black names/white names)$_{sample}$ − (black names/white names)$_{population}$]
2. Minimize [(black names/white names)$_{sample}$ − (black names/white names)$_{arrested}$]
3. Minimize [(black names/white names)$_{sample}$ − (black names/white names)$_{convicted}$]
4. Minimize [(black names/white names)$_{sample}$ − (black names/white names)$_{incarcerated}$]
5. Minimize [(criminal proportion)$_{sample}$ − (criminal proportion)$_{population}$]
6. Minimize [(criminal proportion)$_{sample}$ − (criminal proportion)$_{arrested}$]
7. Minimize [(criminal proportion)$_{sample}$ − (criminal proportion)$_{convicted}$]
8. Minimize [(criminal proportion)$_{sample}$ − (criminal proportion)$_{incarcerated}$]

Note: Utility functions 1 through 4 are race-conscious utility functions. Utility functions 5 through 8 are race neutral. All the utility functions require awareness of the properties of names in the general population (absolute and relative numbers of criminals and noncriminals, and so on). Each utility function also requires a participant to decide how many names to circle based on these ratios, using criteria that are extrinsic to the problem representation (such as which of the particular names to select, given the numerical outcome of a utility function).

too complex to be performed by subjects without a calculator, they also require data that even subjects keenly aware of the domain are unlikely to have (relative frequency of blacks and whites in America as a whole, of blacks and whites convicted of crimes, of arrested blacks and whites, of incarcerated blacks and whites, of black and white names in news reports, number of Type I and Type II errors in news reports, and the like). We do not dwell on this argument, its conclusions fortunately being in tune with decades of research showing that human behavior is not classically or axiomatically rational (March and Simon, 1958; Newell and Simon, 1972; Simon, 1955, 1976, 1983; Tversky and Kahneman, 1974).

In addition, specific findings from the experiments challenge the consistency of preference structures demanded by classic rationality, with participants' utility functions being malleable in a wide variety of experimental circumstances. In the gender-personality experiments, extremity of ratings (of aggression and dependence) shifted as a function of prior exposure to behaviors related to the personality concepts. In the gender-fame studies, false identifications increased after prior exposure to names. Similarly, in the race-criminality studies, the rate of misidentification was influenced by experimental manipulations of instruction, time pressure (Walsh, Banaji, and Greenwald, 1998), and mood state (Park and Banaji, 1998). Neither argument, based on plausibility and on experimental data, challenges the idea that the observed behaviors are reasonable, but they do not permit the assessment that the behaviors are rational. Bounded rationality is a more appropriate characterization of the behaviors we have encountered here.

Other Standards of Judgment

Disciplines vary in their methods for determining error. To show that using knowledge about a group (however correct it may be) to make judgments about individual members is best characterized as erroneous, we broadly define four criteria: universality of social practice, logic, intention, and analogy.

Social Practice.   Across time and culture social practice has universally recognized the moral discomfort inherent in category-based social judgments. Our oldest and most remote example is the apocryphal story of how the sixth-century philosopher Sankara, Hinduism's most rigorous thinker, reached his epiphany into nondualism as the direct result of a category-based social judgment. Leaving the river after his ritual sacred bath, he (a Brahmin) brusquely ordered a man, obviously an untouchable, to step aside so as to avoid any possibility of physical contact. Sankara's shame at the discovery of his prejudice, when it turned out that the untouchable was a deep thinker, influenced the development of the important philosophy of *Advaita* (Iyer, 1964).

Less remotely, concerns with category-based social judgments have been a part of the American political psyche. In the last century, Justice Harlan's dissent in *Plessy* v. *Ferguson* (1897), among the most-cited opinions of the Supreme Court, states eloquently that category-based judgments involving race are immoral and cannot be the basis of public policy. In his dissent he wrote:

> Our constitution is color-blind, and neither knows nor tolerates classes among citizens . . . The law regards man as man, and takes no account of his surroundings or of his color when his civil rights as guaranteed by the supreme law of the land are in-

volved. It is therefore to be regretted that this high tribunal, the final expositor of the fundamental law of the land, has reached the conclusion that it is competent for a state to regulate the enjoyment by citizens of their civil rights solely upon the basis of race. In my opinion, the judgment this day rendered will, in time, prove to be quite as pernicious as the decision made by this tribunal in the Dred Scott Case.

American history since has revealed the majority opinion's moral bankruptcy, but we cite Justice Harlan here to ask whether what appeared distasteful in 1897 for public policy might seem unacceptable in 1997 for interpersonal and intergroup social judgments.[15]

In the first half of this century, Walter Lippmann (1922) and Gordon Allport (1954) both emphasized the ordinary cognitive foundations of category-based judgments, yet their writings clearly reveal their recognition of the failures inherent in such judgments. Most poignantly, Gunnar Myrdal (1944) noted that Americans experience a moral dilemma, "*an ever-raging conflict between, on the one hand, the valuations preserved on the general plane which we shall call the 'American Creed,' where the American thinks, talks, and acts under the influence of high national and Christian precepts, and on the other hand, . . . group prejudice against particular persons or types of people . . . dominate his outlook*" (p. xlvii; emphasis in original). A half-century later, Devine's work strikingly shows the continued existence of the moral dilemma in the form of heightened guilt among American students confronting their prejudice (Devine, Monteith, Zuwerink, and Elliot, 1991; Zuwerink, Devine, Monteith, and Cook, 1996). It is surprising that with the backdrop of a history such as this from Harlan to Devine, McCauley and colleagues (1995) believe that to make category-based judgments is "normatively as it should be."

Logic. The inference, logically considered, that black-sounding names are more likely to be names of criminals is fallacious. When stating a stereotype in the form of a logical proposition, the appropriate logical quantifier is "some," "several," "many," or "a few," but almost never "all." The type of logical deduction revealed by experimental participants is of the following kind: "Some members of the set X have characteristic α. Object #<22310> is a member of the set X. Therefore object #<22310> has characteristic α." This deduction violates an elementary rule of Aristotelian logic, treating the proposition "Some members of the set X have characteristic α," as though it were the same as "All members of the set X have characteristic α."

Confusing the logical quantifier "some" with the logical quantifier "all" is the kind of error known in logic as a confinement law error (Kalish and Montague, 1964). Psychologists have labeled such errors in syllogistic reasoning as the atmosphere effect (Woodworth and Sells, 1935). Premises containing "some" create an atmosphere for accepting inferences that actually deserve the answer ". . . can't say—*no specific* conclusion follows from the premises. If a person accepts a specific conclusion for an invalid syllogism, that is an error in reasoning, and such errors frequently conform to predictions based on the atmosphere hypothesis" (Bourne, Dominowski, and Loftus, 1979, p. 277). To defend inferences based on stereotypes as accurate (Jussim, McCauley, and Lee, 1995) is thus to challenge a hitherto uncontested rule of Aristotelian logic.

Intention. Here we focus on a different argument, the thesis being that, under many circumstances, an outcome is considered incorrect if it is inconsistent with that which is intended.[16] Intending to draw a cube and having a cylinder emerge instead is obviously an error. Intending to drive on the right side of the road but ending up on the left is likewise an error. In a similar way, intending to feel and behave in line with one's values, but failing to do can be considered an error. In fact, recognizing the inconsistencies between "ought" and "actual" is apparently what accounts for the discomfort expressed when a mismatch between desired feelings and behaviors versus actual feelings and behavior is highlighted (Devine et al. 1991).

Unawareness of the discrepancy between intention and behavior as well as the discomfort that accompanies awareness of such discrepancies cannot justify the characterization of these errors as anything but errors. How a society should choose to deal with such errors and their consequences is a separate question and one that is beyond the scope of this chapter. Our purpose is to emphasize that conclusions about decisionmaking that are disturbing ought not to be mischaracterized as benign or correct.

Analogy.   A final argument for considering the experimental results as representing error can be made by analogy. In other areas where criteria of incorrectness similar to those in our experiments are met, the behavior is routinely classified as an error. For example, the long history of research on perceptual illusions (errors) contains many examples of identical objects that nevertheless violate all perceptual experience that they are so. When two objects that are identical in shape and size (such as tabletops in Shepard's parallelogram illusion, 1990, p. 48) are perceived to be dissimilar, we regard the resulting misperception as a remarkable error. Explanations concerning the origin of the perceptual error do not produce a desire to recategorize the error as reflecting a correct judgment.

Likewise, when two behaviors are identical (one performed by Donna, the other by Donald) but are not judged to be so, we must regard the resulting misperception as an error. Interest in false memory led Roediger and McDermott (1995) to replicate an earlier finding that presenting lists of words related to a concept (for example, sleep-related words such as "dream" or "pillow") can produce a false memory for the word "sleep," an item which never appeared on the list.

As the label "false memory" itself suggests, the obtained misidentifications are considered to be false by definition, and scientists who study memory do not become confused about whether to regard such false memories as revealing error. Likewise, mistakenly "remembering" a person who is not a criminal as a criminal is an error by definition, and the apparent confusion it creates about whether to regard it as an error or not may most charitably be understood as reflecting a desire to avoid confronting the seamy side of decisionmaking that accompanies such social judgments.

Computational Characteristics of Bounded Rationality
We have seen how participants' behavior fails to meet conventional criteria for classic rationality and criteria for correctness. Now we use a computational approach to show how the ordinary and implicit cognitive processes that underlie stereotyping can collectively produce

behavior that is boundedly rational. We do so by discussing how errors can arise when representations of problems in one domain are mistakenly applied to superficially similar but substantively distinct problems in another domain. We noted previously that the behavior is boundedly rational by demonstrating how computational constraints can be significant determinants; for instance, relaxing a particular constraint such as time can produce a change in the behavior.

In studies of human problem solving, an established finding concerns the inability to represent superficially similar but substantively different problems as distinct. The assumption of similarity can lead to the use of inappropriate methods to solve the problem at hand.[17] For example, Bhaskar and Simon (1977) showed that a problem was misclassified as a thermodynamics problem rather than a physics problem because a copy of steam tables (sometimes necessary for solving thermodynamics problems, but never necessary for solving physics problems) was made available. This caused a lengthy detour, resulting in approximately thirty minutes as opposed to five minutes to solve the problem. Similarly, Hinsley, Hayes, and Simon (1977) reported that subjects skilled at algebra word problems spent large amounts of time on nonsense problems worded similarly to real problems, even though a superficial examination would have revealed the nonsensical character of the alleged problem. Such experiments have confirmed that humans sometimes represent problems inappropriately by failing to see real differences between them. Such misconstrual is a central feature of boundedly rational behavior, and here we describe how it may be implicated in the errors of stereotyping we have observed.

When confronting the task of criminal identification, what is the alternative representation that participants might use? As mentioned before, a task that has informally but frequently been raised as analogous is the task of identifying poorly performing models of a mechanical object such as a computer. It has been proposed that just as it is reasonable to select a functioning computer over a dysfunctional one based on manufacturer history, it is also reasonable to identify more black than white names as criminals.

Signal detection theory offers a useful way to represent a problem solver's decisionmaking on both of these tasks. The goal of the hypothetical computer identification task is to identify dysfunctional computers (poorly performing models); the goal of participants in our experiments is to identify dysfunctional humans (criminals). In one case, the information that is supplied is the manufacturer's name, in the other case it is the person's race. For the computer identification task, the immediate goal is to identify as many poorly performing computers as possible. *Hits* represent poor models correctly identified as such, *misses* represent poor models identified as good ones, *false alarms* represent good models incorrectly identified as poor models, and *correct rejections* represent identification of good models as good. *In the computer selection task, misses have a high cost.* That is, incorrectly labeling a poor model as good can result in one's ending up with a computer that breaks down often. A false alarm, which simply implies that one may have rejected a good computer, is essentially costless. This is because the problem solver's basic objective, which presumably is to "acquire a good model by ruling out all poor models from the candidate set," is not frustrated by false alarms. That is, a false alarm cannot lead to the selection of a poor computer.

Such a representation is consistent with the task performed by our subjects. Analogous to the computer task, hits represent criminals being correctly identified as criminals, and correct rejections involve correctly identifying noncriminals as noncriminals. False alarms represent noncriminals misidentified as criminals, and misses represent the misidentification of criminals as noncriminals. In the criminal selection task, as in the computer selection task, misses are costly (incorrectly labeling a criminal as noncriminal can lead to a criminal's going free). The similarity between the two tasks ends here. *In the criminal identification task, false alarms have an incalculably high cost.*

This difference in the false-alarm costs of the two tasks is sufficiently significant that a representation for one task is inappropriate for the other. For example, the computer selection task involves minimizing misses while producing an unlimited number of false alarms. In contrast, the criminal identification task requires that both misses and false alarms are to be managed because of the high costs of both, and especially those of false alarms. The two tasks are quite distinct. Yet, as the false alarms (on both black and white names) suggest, participants did not use a rule strict enough to prevent *any* false alarms, the only correct outcome. Although the two problems of computer and criminal identification may seem to be the same, the failure to recognize their difference is no different from the misidentification of the physics problem as a thermodynamics problem; only the consequences are graver.

Why is the cost of false alarms high in the criminal identification task? Our society, and most liberal societies, generally proceed on the principle that it is important not to declare the innocent to be guilty. When we consider the many possible objectives of criminal punishment—deterrence, incapacitation, just punishment, and rehabilitation (U.S. Sentencing Commission, 1996, p. 1)—we see that the possible innocence of the punished frustrates every social objective. A decision procedure that ignores the cost of false alarms, however plausibly or excusably, violates basic and almost universally accepted concepts of justice and fairness. Such cost is only more profound when we consider that the incorrect application of guilt is selectively leveled against particular social groups. Thus, the computational path from ordinary cognition to ordinary prejudice ultimately reveals the extraordinary moral burden imposed by human bounded rationality.

Conclusion

In the past, stereotypic beliefs and prejudicial attitudes were largely conceived of as conscious and were treated as outside the interpretive scope of ordinary cognition. Decades of research in social psychology have refuted both myths. It is now evident that the computational and unconscious character of stereotypes and prejudice does not require appeal to the operation of unique processes or unique persons. Rather, as the sample data presented here show, stereotyped beliefs and prejudicial attitudes multifariously reveal their presence through ordinary biases rooted in memory. Social psychology's refutation of these myths has come at a price—the perception that demonstrating the ordinary computational nature of stereotyping and prejudice dissociates it from its moral impact. We have argued to the contrary, that the bounded rationality of human social cognition reveals the hitherto unrecognized but deeply moral quality intrinsic to theories of human judgment and decisionmaking.

References

Abelson, R. P. (1986). Beliefs are like possessions. *Journal for the Theory of Social Behavior, 16,* 223–250.

Adorno, T. W., Frenkel-Brunswik, E., Levinson, D., and Sanford, R. N. (1950). *The authoritarian personality.* New York: Harper.

Allport, G. W. (1954). *The nature of prejudice.* Cambridge, MA: Addison-Wesley.

Anderson, J. R. (1990). *The adaptive character of thought.* Hillsdale, NJ: Lawrence Erlbaum.

Armour, J. D. (1997). Hype and reality in affirmative action. *University of Colorado Law Review, 68,* 1173–1210.

Arrow, K. J. (1963). *Social choice and individual values.* New Haven: Yale University Press.

Ashmore, R. D., and Del Boca, F. K. (1981). Conceptual approaches to stereotypes and stereotyping. In D. L. Hamilton (Ed.), *Cognitive processes in stereotyping and intergroup behavior* (pp. 1–36). Hillsdale, NJ: Lawrence Erlbaum.

Banaji, M. R. (1995). The significance of an 8 millisecond effect. Paper presented to the Society of Experimental Social Psychology, Washington, DC.

Banaji, M. R. (1997). Introductory comments. *Journal of Experimental Social Psychology, 33,* 449–450.

Banaji, M. R., and Greenwald, A. G. (1994). Implicit stereotyping and unconscious prejudice. In M. P. Zanna and J. M. Olson (Eds.), *The psychology of prejudice: The Ontario symposium,* Vol. 7 (pp. 55–76). Hillsdale, NJ: Lawrence Erlbaum.

Banaji, M. R., and Greenwald, A. G. (1995). Implicit gender stereotyping in judgments of fame. *Journal of Personality and Social Psychology, 68,* 181–198.

Banaji, M. R., and Hardin, C. (1996). Automatic stereotyping. *Psychological Science, 7,* 136–141.

Banaji, M. R., Hardin, C., and Rothman, A. J. (1993). Implicit stereotyping in person judgment. *Journal of Personality and Social Psychology, 65,* 272–281.

Bargh, J. A., Chen, M., and Burrows, L. (1996). Automaticity of social behavior: Direct effects of trait construct and stereotype activation on action. *Journal of Personality and Social Psychology, 71,* 230–244.

Bhaskar, R., and Simon, H. A. (1977). Problem solving in semantically rich domains: An example from engineering thermodynamics. *Cognitive Science, 2,* 192–215.

Billig, M. (1996). *Arguing and thinking: A rhetorical approach to social psychology* (2nd ed.). Cambridge: Cambridge University Press.

Blair, I. V. (Forthcoming). Implicit stereotypes and prejudice. In G. Moskowitz (Ed.), *Future directions in social cognition.*

Blair, I., and Banaji, M. R. (1996). Automatic and controlled processes in stereotype priming. *Journal of Personality and Social Psychology, 70,* 1142–63.

Bourne, L. E., Jr., Dominowski, R. L., and Loftus, E. F. (1979). *Cognitive processes.* Englewood Cliffs, NJ: Prentice-Hall.

Carpenter, S. J., and Banaji, M. R. (1997). Implicit attitudes toward female leaders. Paper presented at the annual meeting of the Midwestern Psychological Association, Chicago.

Chen, M., and Bargh, J. A. (1997). Nonconscious behavioral confirmation processes: The self-fulfilling consequences of automatic stereotype activation. *Journal of Experimental Social Psychology, 33,* 541–560.

Debreu, G. (1971). *A theory of value.* New York: Wiley.

Devine, P. G. (1989). Stereotypes and prejudice: Their automatic and controlled components. *Journal of Personality and Social Psychology, 56,* 5–18.

Devine, P. G., Monteith, M., Zuwerink, J. R., and Elliot, A. J. (1991). Prejudice with and without compunction. *Journal of Personality and Social Psychology, 60,* 817–830.

Dovidio, J. F., Evans, N. E., and Tyler, R. B. (1986). Racial stereotypes: The contents of their cognitive representations. *Journal of Experimental Social Psychology, 22,* 22–37.

Fagot, B. I., and Leinbach, M. D. (1989). The young child's gender schema: Environmental input, internal organization. *Child Development, 60,* 663–672.

Fazio, R. H., Jackson, J. R., Dunton, B. C., and Williams, C. J. (1995). Variability in automatic activation as an unobtrusive measure of racial attitudes: A bona fide pipeline? *Journal of Personality and Social Psychology, 69,* 1013–27.

Fazio, R. H., Sanbonmatsu, D. M., Powell, M. C., and Kardes, F. R. (1986). On the automatic activation of attitudes. *Journal of Personality and Social Psychology, 50,* 229–238.

Fiske, S. T. (1998). Stereotyping, prejudice, and discrimination. In D. T. Gilbert, S. T. Fiske, and G. Lindzey (Eds.), *The handbook of social psychology* (4th ed.), (pp. 357–411). New York: McGraw-Hill.

Gewirth, A. (1996). *The community of rights.* Chicago: University of Chicago Press.

Greenwald, A. G., and Banaji, M. R. (1995). Implicit social cognition: Attitudes, self-esteem, and stereotypes. *Psychological Review, 102,* 1–27.

Greenwald, A. G., McGhee, D. E., and Schwartz, J. L. (1998). Measuring individual differences in implicit cognition: The implicit association test. *Journal of Personality and Social Psychology, 74,* 1464–80.

Hamilton, D. L. (1981). *Cognitive processes in stereotyping and intergroup behavior.* Hillsdale, NJ: Lawrence Erlbaum.

Hart, H. L. A. (1976). *The concept of law.* New York: Oxford University Press.

Hastie, R., and Rasinski, K. A. (1988). The concept of accuracy in social judgment. In D. Bar-Tal and A. W. Kruglanski (Eds.), *The social psychology of knowledge* (pp. 193–208). New York: Cambridge University Press.

Henderson-King, E. I., and Nisbett, R. E. (1996). Anti-black prejudice as a function of exposure to the negative behavior of a single black person. *Journal of Personality and Social Psychology, 71,* 654–664.

Hinsley, D., Hayes, J. R., and Simon, H. A. (1977). From words to equations: Meaning and representation in algebra word problems. In P. Carpenter and M. A. Just (Eds.), *Cognitive processes in comprehension* (pp. 89–106). Hillsdale, NJ: Lawrence Erlbaum.

Iyer, M. K. V. (1964). *Advaita Vedanta according to Sankara.* New York: Asia Publishing House.

Jacoby, L. L., Kelley, C. M., Brown, J., and Jasechko, J. (1989). Becoming famous overnight: Limits on the ability to avoid unconscious influences of the past. *Journal of Personality and Social Psychology, 56,* 326–338.

Jussim, L. J., McCauley, C. R., and Lee, Y-T. (1995). Why study stereotype accuracy and inaccuracy? In Y. T. Lee, L. J. Jussim, and C. R. McCauley (Eds.), *Stereotype accuracy: Toward appreciating group differences* (pp. 3–27). Washington, DC: American Psychological Association.

Kalish, D., and Montague, R. (1964). *Symbolic logic: Techniques of formal reasoning.* New York: Harcourt Brace Jovanovich.

Kotovsky, K., and Fallside, D. (1989). Representation and transfer in problem solving. In D. Klahr and K. Kotovsky (Eds.), *Complex information processing: The impact of Herbert Simon.* Hillsdale, NJ: Lawrence Erlbaum.

Lemm, K. M, and Banaji, M. R. (1998). Implicit and explicit gender identity and attitudes toward gender. Paper presented at the annual meeting of the Midwestern Psychological Society, Chicago.

Lepore, L., and Brown, R. (1997). Category and stereotype activation: Is prejudice inevitable? *Journal of Social and Personality Psychology, 72,* 275–287.

Lewicki, P. (1986). *Nonconscious social information processing.* New York: Academic Press.

Lippmann, W. (1922). *Public opinion.* New York: Harcourt Brace.

Lombardi, W. J., Higgins, E. T., and Bargh, J. A. (1987). The role of consciousness in priming effects on categorization: Assimilation versus contrast as a function of awareness of the priming task. *Personality and Social Psychology Bulletin, 13,* 411–429.

March, J. G., and Simon, H. A. (1958). *Organizations.* New York: Wiley.

Martin, C. L., and Little, J. K. (1990). The relation of gender understanding to children's sex-typed preferences and gender stereotypes. *Child Development, 61,* 1427–39.

McCauley, C. R., Jussim, L. J., and Lee, Y-T. (1995). Stereotype accuracy: Toward appreciating group differences. In Y-T. Lee, L. J. Jussim, and C. R. McCauley (Eds.), *Stereotype accuracy: Toward appreciating group differences* (pp. 293–312). Washington, DC: American Psychological Association.

McGuire, W. J. (1973). The yin and yang of progress in social psychology: Seven koan. *Journal of Personality and Social Psychology, 26,* 446–456.

Meyer, D., and Schvaneveldt, R. (1971). Facilitation in recognizing pairs of words: Evidence of a dependence between retrieval operations. *Journal of Experimental Psychology, 90,* 227–234.

Mitchell, J., Nosek, B., and Banaji, M. R. (1998). Dissociated attitudes. Paper presented at the annual meeting of the American Psychological Society, Washington, DC.

Myrdal, G. (1944). *An American dilemma: The Negro problem in modern democracy.* New York: Harper.

Neely, J. (1977). Semantic priming and retrieval from lexical memory: Roles of inhibitionless spreading activation and limited-capacity attention. *Journal of Experimental Psychology: General, 106,* 226–254.

Newell, A., and Simon, H. A. (1972). *Human problem solving.* Englewood Cliffs, NJ: Prentice-Hall.

Nikam, N. A., and McKeon, R. (1958). *Asoka, king of Magadha.* Chicago: University of Chicago Press.

Nisbett, R. E., and Ross, L. (1980). *Human inference: Strategies and shortcomings of social judgment.* Englewood Cliffs, NJ: Prentice-Hall.

Nosek, B., Banaji, M. R., and Greenwald, A. G. (1998). Gender differences in implicit attitude and self-concept toward mathematics and science. Paper presented at the annual meeting of the Midwestern Psychological Association, Chicago.

Nozick, R. (1993). *The nature of rationality.* Princeton: Princeton University Press.

Park, J., and Banaji, M. R. (1998). The influence of positive mood on implicit stereotyping. Paper presented at the annual meeting of the American Psychological Society, Washington, DC.

Plessy v. Ferguson, 163, U.S. 537 (1897).

Plucknett, T. F. T. (1956). *A concise history of the common law.* Boston: Little, Brown.

Ptahotep (2300 B.C.). *The instruction of Ptahotep (6th Dynasty) 2300–2150 B.C.*

Rawls, J. (1971). *A theory of justice.* Cambridge, MA: Belknap Press, Harvard University Press.

Roediger, H. L., and McDermott, K. B. (1995). Creating false memories: Remembering words not presented in lists. *Journal of Experimental Psychology: Learning, Memory, and Cognition, 21,* 803–814.

Rosier, M. D., Banaji, M. R., and Greenwald, A. G. (1998). The implicit association test, group membership and self esteem. Paper presented at the annual meeting of the Midwestern Psychological Association, Chicago.

Savage, R. (1972). *The foundations of statistics.* New York: Dover.

Schacter, D. L. (1987). Implicit memory: History and current status. *Journal of Experimental Psychology: Learning, Memory, and Cognition, 13,* 501–518.

Shepard, R. N. (1990). *Mind sights.* New York: Freeman.

Simon, H. A. (1955). A behavioral model of rational choice. *Quarterly Journal of Economics, 69,* 99–118.

Simon, H. A. (1976). *Administrative behavior.* 3rd ed. New York: Macmillan.

Simon, H. A. (1983). *Reason in human affairs.* Palo Alto, CA: Stanford University Press.

Simon, H. A., and Ando, A. (1961). Aggregation of variables in dynamic systems. *Econometrika, 29,* 111–138.

Strack, F., Schwarz, N., Bless, H., Kubler, A., and Wanke, M. (1993). Awareness of the influence as a determinant of assimilation versus contrast. *European Journal of Social Psychology, 23,* 53–62.

Tversky, A., and Kahneman, D. (1974). Judgment under uncertainty: Heuristics and biases. *Science, 185,* 1124–31.

Uleman, J. S. (1987). Consciousness and control: The case of spontaneous trait inferences. *Personality and Social Psychology Bulletin, 13,* 337–354.

U.S. Sentencing Commission. (1996). *Federal sentencing guidelines.* St. Paul, MN: West Publishing Company.

Uviller, H. R. (1996). *Virtual justice: The flawed prosecution of crime in America.* New Haven: Yale University Press.

Walsh, W., Banaji, M. R., and Greenwald, A. G. (1995). *A failure to eliminate race bias in judgments of criminals.* New York: American Psychological Society.

Walsh, W., Banaji, M. R., and Greenwald, A. G. (1998). The misidentification of black men as criminals. Manuscript, Yale University.

Wegener, D. T., and Petty, R. E. (In press). Flexible correction processes in social judgment: The role of naive theories in corrections for perceived bias. *Journal of Personality and Social Psychology.*

Will, G. (1990). *Men at work.* New York: G. K. Hall.

Woodworth, R. S., and Sells, S. B. (1935). An atmosphere effect in formal syllogistic reasoning. *Journal of Experimental Psychology, 18,* 451–460.

Zuwerink, J. R., Devine, P. G., Monteith, M. J., Cook, D. A. (1996). Prejudice toward blacks: With and without compunction? *Basic and Applied Social Psychology, 18,* 131–150.

Notes

1. This chapter is concerned with beliefs about social groups, namely stereo-types. As a result, a natural theoretical connection is extended to the construct, prejudice. Following convention, by *stereotype* we refer to the cognitive component, or beliefs about social groups (for example, Politicians are crooks) and by *prejudice* to the affective component, or attitudes about social groups (I dislike politicians).

2. For a resistance to the view that stereotyping and prejudice are not acts of ordinary cognition, but in some sense reflect special processes, see Billig (1996, pp. 158–170).

3. Paraphrased from Max Klinger of *MASH*.

4. The experiments reported in this chapter involve a continuing collaboration with Tony Greenwald, and research with several students past and present, mostly notably Irene Blair, Siri Carpenter, Buju Dasgupta, Jack Glaser, Aiden Gregg, Curtis Hardin, John Jost, Kristi Lemm, Jason Mitchell, Brian Nosek, Jai Park, Marshall Rosier, Alex Rothman, and Wendi Walsh.

5. Bounded rationality and the information-processing approach to psychology have been the defining, paradigm-shifting concepts of modern psychological and social science. As is all too common with such sweeping transformations, it is entirely possible that a new generation of readers does not have a clear sense of the meaning of the term *bounded rationality*. When we declare behavior to be boundedly rational, we deem it to have the following characteristics (March and Simon, 1958, p. 169): (a) behavior is satisficing rather than optimizing; (b) alternatives for actions are explored through sequential processes; (c) these sequential processes largely use specialized, domain-specific knowledge, rather than general, domain-independent problem-solving strategies; (d) each sequential process is restricted in the scope of problems it can deal with; and (e) the collections of processes are largely independent of one another, so that the memory and problem-solving system is best viewed as a collection of loosely coupled, "nearly decomposable" units (Simon and Ando, 1961).

6. See Ashmore and Del Boca (1981) and Banaji and Greenwald (1994) for comments about the historical transformation in definitions of stereotypes, from treating them as exaggerations and incorrect judgments to focusing on the application of group knowledge (accurate or inaccurate) to judgments of individuals.

7. Data from other investigators suggest that the stereotyping effects obtained in our studies may have been removed or reversed in the presence of awareness of the activating or priming event (see Lombardi, Higgins, and Bargh, 1987; Strack, Schwarz, Bless, Kubler, and Wanke, 1993; Wegener and Petty, 1997).

8. Names used in these experiments were generated by the experimenters and by research participants. Each name was then judged by a new group of participants for the likelihood that it was a European-American or African-American name (on a five-point scale). Selected names in each category were those judged to be high in the likelihood of being African American (or European American) *and* low in likelihood of being European American (or African American).

9. We will shortly discuss the question of why our participants do not meet axiomatic criteria of rationality.

10. We thank John Jost for bringing this source to our attention.

11. It should be obvious that positive judgments that confer benefits on recipients (instead of guilt), if they are differentially administered as a function of group membership, have a similar discriminatory effect.

12. Guilt by association is to be carefully distinguished from punishment by association. Even in T'ang China, when family members of traitors were executed it was not assumed that they were guilty. The punishment was most likely for reasons of deterrence and retribution.

13. These axioms are as follows:

  1. Given any pair of outcomes A and B, it is always true that A *is preferred to* B (A ≥ B), B *is preferred to* A (B > A), or one is *indifferent* between A and B (A ⊁ B and B ⊁ A).
  2. Preferences are transitive (if A > B and B > C, then A > C).
  3. If action a_1 leads to A, and action a_2 leads to B, and A > B, then $a_1 > a_2$.

14. Such an axiomatic characterization of rationality is generally agreed to be somewhat sterile, a perception that has spawned alternative conceptions of rationality that are descriptively plausible (Anderson, 1990; Gewirth, 1996; Nozick, 1993; Rawls, 1971). Such accounts have generally been more successful in capturing a commonsense conception of rationality, simultaneously discarding some of the more implausible, unpersuasive aspects of classic axiomatic rationality (global consistency and utility functions, universally specified preference structures, and the like).

In spite of its sterility, the classic axiomatic conception of rationality provides a syntactic framework that can house many of the alternatives that have been suggested. Even when the requirement of global consistency is abandoned, every alternative descriptive conception of rationality relies on representing it as adaptive behavior (see Anderson, 1990, p. 28). This takes the form, typically, of representing behavior as constrained optimization. (By "constrained optimization" we imply the conventional sense used in mathematics, economics, or operations research: the objective is to maximize or minimize the numerical value of some mathematical functions, while each of a number of other mathematical functions—the constraints—are required not to fall below or exceed some other specified value. Much of the success of modern social science derives from the generality of this representation.)

We will see that every alternative conception of rationality considered to be less sterile and more descriptively plausible can be cast in the form of utility functions that must be maximized, subject to certain constraints. Within the stereotyping context, we show that the utility functions and constraints that might represent rationality in any of these other more descriptively plausible senses require the participants in our experiments to either (a) use knowledge that they are unlikely to have, or (b) make assumptions that cannot meet their own expressed moral beliefs and standards. Demonstrating the difficulty of using classic axiomatic rationality as a valid descriptor of participants' behavior serves therefore as a vehicle for simultaneously demonstrating the same difficulty with these more substantive and plausible conceptions of rationality.

15. We point out the applicability of judicial decisions to discussions about interpersonal decisions. On the other hand, legal scholars (see Armour, 1997) have applied the evidence about biases in interpersonal judgment to matters of public policy such as affirmative action.

16. Not all failures to implement intended behavior are errors. To pick an extreme example, intending to kill someone and not being able to follow through would hardly be seen as an error.

17. Conversely, sometimes superficially dissimilar problems that are substantively the same are not recognized as such (Kotovsky and Fallside, 1989).

Acknowledgments

The research and writing of this chapter were supported in part by NSF Grant SBR-9422241, a triennial leave from Yale University, and fellowships from the John Simon Guggenheim Foundation and Cattell Fund to M. R. Banaji. We thank John Bargh, Wil Cunningham, Nilanjana Dasgupta, Robyn Dawes, Jack Glaser, Richard Hackman, Reid Hastie, Jason Mitchell, Brian Nosek, Peter Salovey, Daniel Schacter, Yaacov Schul, Wendi Walsh, and Bernd Wittenbrink for their comments on a previous version.

Belief and Knowledge as Distinct Forms of Memory

6

Howard Eichenbaum

J. Alexander Bodkin

In this chapter we approach the phenomena of belief and knowledge as distinct forms of memory, from the perspectives of cognitive neurobiology and neuropsychiatry. Our approach is necessarily reductionist, consequent to making assumptions about belief and knowledge that permit their dissection by the techniques of experimental cognitive neurobiology. In this analysis we focus on identifying distinct neural pathways that are critical to these different forms of memory, on characterizing how the relevant brain pathways encode information differently for use as belief versus knowledge, and on elucidating how these distinct forms of memory interact to influence behavior. In addition, we briefly examine aberrations in belief and knowledge encountered in specific mental disorders, as these shed light on the normal interactions of belief and knowledge in guiding behavior.

The structure of our presentation is as follows:

1. We begin by defining *belief* and distinguishing it from *knowledge*.
2. We take the strong and admittedly simplistic position that belief and knowledge are distinct forms of memory, or uses of memory, and we suggest that they are mediated by different brain systems.
3. We support these hypotheses with data from animal models of cognition and memory, and from neuropsychological studies of human amnesia.

176

4. We connect the experimental literature on neurobiological bases of memory and the clinical literature on psychiatric diseases, attempting to show how cognitive abnormalities consequent to some brain disorders can be viewed as aberrations in belief and knowledge.

5. Having conceptually separated these two forms of memory, we explore how belief and knowledge interact seamlessly in normal memory processing.

Belief and Knowledge

Philosophers have generally defined *knowledge* as justified *true belief* (Chisholm, 1966), and have seen knowledge and belief as reflecting essentially the same mental phenomenon. According to this view, whether in a particular instance this mental phenomenon rises to the status of knowledge depends in large part on facts external to the knower or believer, that is, whether the relevant facts in the outside world are in actuality as they are proposed or conceptualized by the subject. We depart from this fairly conventional view to propose that knowledge and belief may instead reflect distinct processing modes of the brain, that they utilize memory differently and reflect the activity of different brain systems. The distinction we make between knowledge and belief turns on the concept that knowledge is, as it were, *justified* through a particular type of representation and processing, whereas belief is not.

For purposes of this discussion, both belief and knowledge are considered to be fully reflected in dispositions to behave in a specifiable purposeful manner. Thus, for example, either the knowledge or the belief that a desired goal can be achieved by acting in a certain manner will lead to an organism's tending to behave in that manner. We propose that the difference between knowledge and belief in their purest forms is that knowledge is a disposition to behave that is constantly subject to corrective modification and updating by experience, while belief is a disposition to behave in a manner that is resistant to correction by experience. Extensive interactions take place in nature between knowledge and belief; but in their purest forms we consider this distinction to hold. Accordingly, our general position is that the neural processing systems and mechanisms underlying knowledge are of a nature that is continuously influenced by testing and reinforcement, whereas the neural processing systems and mechanisms underlying belief are of a nature that is resistant to modification by reinforcement or lack of reinforcement. Our main aims are to identify these systems in brain pathways and to characterize their processing mechanisms.

These distinctions between knowledge and belief are supported by common definitions. For example, the Oxford American Dictionary defines *belief* as "the feeling that something is real or true." Central to this characterization is the implication that belief involves an acceptance or conviction of something as true without reference to any specific facts or to episodes in which directly relevant information was gathered. By contrast, the same dictionary defines *know* as "to have in one's mind or memory as a result of experience or learning or information." Knowing involves being cognizant of new information and being able to recollect old information, and is thus characterized as involving inquiry and observation in specific episodes. Moreover, knowing at its fullest involves being conversant with, and having a command of, a body of facts and principles. Thus, knowing involves bringing to consciousness, either during experience or through explicit recall, specific facts and instances, and being able to manipulate mentally the information about these facts and instances to make effective judgments and decisions. Beliefs, when they appear to function in this way, are functioning as knowledge, making it frequently difficult—to our constant dismay—to distinguish which is operative in daily life.

From the outset we emphasize that we do not mean to imply that beliefs are weak forms of knowledge. Beliefs can involve very strong convictions or behavioral dispositions, even without the ability to refer to any confirming fact or instance, as in cases of religious or political belief. And beliefs may in fact be accurate representations, though they do not have to be. We do not claim that beliefs cannot be based on learned facts or direct experience, but only that such specific confirming information is not required and need not be referred to in having a belief about something and acting accordingly. Thus *belief* is sometimes used in everyday life when one bases a conclusion on previous experiences, but lacks or does not seek a full understanding of the causal connections among them.

We recognize that the separation between belief and knowledge is not complete. Surely the use of previous experience influences both belief and knowledge, but the former leads to a feeling, acceptance, or conviction; the latter leads to refinement through continuous accumulations of information, and manipulation of information involving inferences and generalizations. Knowledge involves continuous testing and updating of our organization of information, and using these information structures to guide new decisions and insights. But beliefs can "drive" knowledge processing as well, in that a belief will guide the recall of specific instances or facts that support the belief, and a belief can be used to manipulate and take command of a set of facts and rules. Thus, we think of belief-driven and knowledge-driven information processing as fundamentally interactive rather than operating in parallel. How knowledge and belief processes occur simultaneously, and how they interact in conditions of mental disorder as well as in normal conditions, will be considered last.

The Psychology of Knowledge

Ideas about the fundamental cognitive mechanisms that mediate knowledge can be found in both early and modern accounts of the psychology of memory. A brief review of these readings further clarifies our characterization of knowledge as involving two major features, a systematic organization of information and the ability to compare and contrast new and old information to make inferences and generalizations from a knowledge structure.

At the very origins of modern experimental psychology, William James (1890) strongly related his views of memory to the concept of knowledge, defining memory as "the *knowledge* of an event, or fact, of which meantime we have not been thinking, with the additional consciousness that we have thought or experienced it before" (p. 648; emphasis added). He indicated that knowledge is derived by thinking over one's experiences and weaving them into systematic relations with one another. He argued that our ability for conscious recollection is related to the number and diversity of associative connections within the network organization of knowledge. In practical terms, James suggested that one could not optimize memory performance simply by attempting to strengthen traces, but rather by increasing the number of divergent associations: "all improvement of the memory lies in the line of elaborating the associates of each of the several things to be remembered" (James, 1890, p. 663; see Chapter 1 of this volume). From such a network of associations arises the ability to recollect and express memories across many circumstances.

Additional historical insights can be found in accounts by other early experimentalists who explored memory. Sir Fredric Bartlett (1932) examined the recall of mythical and surreal narratives, observing that people omitted or made more realistic those details that were inconsistent with the conventional social structure and experiences of his subjects. He proposed that remembering is guided by a systematic mental representation of experiences or "an active organization of past reactions" into what he called a schema, which we take to be identical with our view of a knowledge structure.

Modern investigations on the active nature of schema-based processing emphasize the application of inferential organization of material to fit the schematic representation. Edward Tolman (1932) provided complementary insights from studies of maze learning in rats, in which he distinguished different types of learning and focused on the representation of spatial environments by "cognitive maps." He distinguished such maps from the acquisition of "habits" by both the contents of the representation and the flexibility with which memories could be expressed. He argued not only that organisms learn to anticipate particular stimuli, but also that the interconnected elements of the cognitive map make possible the ability to take appropriate shortcuts and roundabout routes in maze solution, that is, to make navigational inferences.

Based on evidence from early neurophysiological studies, Donald Hebb (1949) offered a brain circuit level theory for associational networks and inferential memory expression. He suggested that groups of neighboring neurons called cell assemblies process specific percepts and can be activated in an ordered fashion, a "phase sequence," such that "two concepts may acquire a latent 'association' without ever having occurred together in the subject's past experience" (p. 132).

In sum, the collective work of James, Bartlett, Tolman, and Hebb addressed the issues of memory in ways consistent with the notion of knowledge presented here. Their accounts focused on conscious memory as an elaborate network of associations (that is, a knowledge structure) that can be used with great flexibility for comparing and relating items not specifically experienced together during learning. Moreover, this kind of memory can support new associations and inferences that allow us to express memory in novel ways.

Role of the Hippocampus

The Hippocampus and Knowledge

Experimental findings support the existence of a system in the brain for the acquisition, manipulation, and expression of knowledge. Studies on the neuropsychology of memory have revealed both the anatomical location of what can be called knowledge-processing pathways and some of the fundamental cognitive processes mediated in support of knowledge. These studies focus both on the phenomenology of human amnesia and on studies of learning and memory in animals with experimental brain damage.

In studies of human amnesia, our understanding has come mainly from the discovery that "declarative" or "explicit" memory can be dissociated from "procedural" or "implicit" memory (Cohen and Eichenbaum, 1993; Schacter, 1987; Squire, Knowlton, and Musen, 1993). The terms *declarative* and *explicit* refer to the fact that this kind of memory is retrieved through direct inquisition and conscious recollection, and that these memories are revealed through verbal declaration or other direct forms of expression. Most would see these processes and their outcomes as very similar to our everyday memory for facts and events, and it is this kind of memory that is selectively lost after damage to the hippocampal region of the brain.

Understanding of declarative memory from a neuropsychological perspective began with studies of patient HM who, after removal of most of the hippocampal formation and its associated medial temporal-lobe structures, suffered a profound impairment in new learning that was remarkable in its severity and selectivity (Scoville and Milner, 1957). For more than a decade, HM had suffered from increasingly severe and frequent seizures that were refractory to pharmacological treatment, leading finally to bilateral surgical resection of the medial temporal lobe to remove the focus of seizure activity. This surgery, in combination with pharmacological treatment, did greatly alleviate the seizures, but left HM's memory severely impaired. His amnesia was global, in that the deficit was equally severe across all forms of learning materials and modalities of their presentation. Yet the amnesia was also highly selective to some aspects of memory processing. HM showed normal retention of most of the memories he had acquired years before the surgery, including his childhood. In addition, he demonstrated intact primary-memory or immediate-memory capacity. What was absent was his capacity to bridge the gap between immediate and long-term memory.

These observations of preserved remote and immediate memory capacities led investigators to conclude that it was indeed his memory that was impaired, not his perceptual, cognitive, linguistic, and motor capacities, and they showed that different kinds of memory processing can be distinguished in amnesia. The case of HM also made it clear that the hippocampus is not the final repository of memories, because his remotely acquired knowledge was intact. It has come to be generally accepted that this knowledge storehouse is in the cerebral cortex and that the hippocampus only modifies cortical processing of memories through its bidirectional interactions with widespread areas of the cortex. Nevertheless, from the perspective taken here, HM's impairment can be viewed as a deficit in knowledge processing, specifically in the ability to integrate new information into his existing knowledge structure. Specifically how the hippocampal region contributes to knowledge processing will be considered next, in a review of some relevant findings derived from animal models of amnesia.

The Hippocampus and Relational Representation

Conscious recollection and explicit memory expression are operationalized relatively easily for studies on human subjects. However, the underlying cognitive or associational mechanisms that support these phenomena in humans are not obvious. To address this gap, one of us (HE) has been involved in a program of experiments aimed at identifying the fundamental processes of declarative memory in animal species, where the contents of learning can be exquisitely controlled, and where neurobiological studies can be performed with a level of anatomical resolution not possible in studies of humans.

Studying declarative memory in animals of course presents a problem: animals do not express their memories by verbal declaration.

Also, whether or not they have a capacity for conscious recollection is a matter of philosophical debate. And it is not clear what "explicit" expression means in the context of animal testing paradigms.

Despite these limitations, many of the characterizations from James, Bartlett, Tolman, and Hebb offer clues about how to operationalize properties of memory that would be equally applicable to animals and humans. In particular, based on these previous accounts and on more recent discoveries about human amnesia (Cohen and Squire, 1980), Eichenbaum and N. J. Cohen developed the hypothesis that declarative memory is supported by a *relational representation,* that is, an encoding of memories according to relevant relationships among the items (Cohen and Eichenbaum, 1993; Eichenbaum, 1997; Eichenbaum, Otto, and Cohen, 1992, 1994). Furthermore, a central property of this type of memory is its *representational flexibility,* a quality that permits inferential use of memories in novel situations. Conversely, nondeclarative memories involve *individual representations* such that memories are isolated and are encoded only within the brain modules in which perceptual or motor processing is engaged during learning. These individual representations are *inflexible* in that they can be revealed only through reactivation of those modules within the restrictive range of stimuli and situations in which the original learning occurred. We have tested these hypotheses within the general conceptual framework which assumes that damage to the brain structures shown to be critical for declarative memory in HM should likewise impair the expression of the equivalent mode of memory representation in animals.

Here we focus on a single experiment that directly measured the capacity for development and flexible expression of a relational representation. Our assessments involved testing transitive inference, a cognitive function first described by Jean Piaget in his studies of human cognitive development (Piaget, 1928). The term *transitive inference* signifies the ability to infer a relationship between items that have not been presented together, based on previous learning of a set of overlapping premises. For example, if presented with the premises "the blue rod is longer than the red rod" and "the red rod is longer than the green rod," one can infer that the blue rod is longer than the green rod. The capacity for inferential judgment in this test is interpreted as prima facie evidence of the representation of orderly relations, and therefore a specimen of the kind of knowledge structure we wish to investigate.

The capacity for transitive inference is acquired in children by the age of seven, according to Piaget, as much as three years earlier if the ability to remember the premises has developed. More recently, tests of transitive inference have also been employed to determine whether animals are capable of relational representation and inferential judgment (Dusek and Eichenbaum, 1997). Subjects are first trained on a series of two-item discriminations called premise pairs (A > B, B > C, C > D, D > E; where each letter stands for a stimulus element and ">" describes the relationship "should be selected over"). Each of the discriminations could be learned individually or represented as an orderly hierarchy that includes all five items (A > B > C > D > E).

To examine which of the representations is employed, animals are given probe tests derived from pairs of nonadjacent elements, specifically B versus D and A versus E. An appropriate choice between the two nonadjacent and nonend elements, B and D, provides unambiguous evidence for transitive inference. Conversely, the choice between end elements A and E can be guided entirely by the independent reinforcement histories of these elements, because choices of A during premise training are always rewarded and choices of E are never rewarded. Thus the combination of the probe tests B versus D and A versus E provide the strongest assessment of capacities for making novel judgments guided by inferential expression of the orderly organization or by reward history of the individual elements, respectively. Several studies have shown that apes, monkeys, and even rats are capable of transitive inference. In the following section we present the details of our own experiment, which sought to identify the role of the hippocampal system in transitive inference.

In our version of the transitive inference task, we used rats as experimental subjects and common odors as the memory cues. Furthermore, the format in which rats were trained exploited their natural investigatory activities during food-searching behavior. The odor cues were mixed into cups filled with sand, and animals were rewarded for selecting the correct odor by obtaining a tasty Froot Loop buried in the sand of the correct cup (Figure 6.1A).

We compared the performance of normal rats with those whose pathways to and from hippocampus had been disconnected in one of two ways (a fornix transection or ablation of the perirhinal and entorhinal cortex). Animals were initially trained on the series of premise pairs, using a trial-blocking method that introduced the pairs

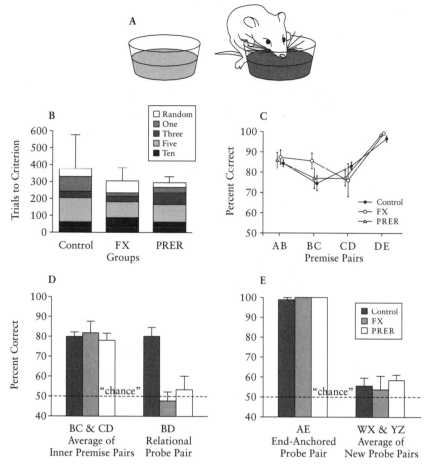

Figure 6.1 Performance on the transitive inference task by normal (control) rats and rats with disconnection of the hippocampus either by transection of the fornix (FX) or ablation of the perirhinal-entorhinal cortex (PRER).

A. The stimulus cups filled with odorized sand.

B. The mean number of trials required to reach a performance criterion on each of several phases of premise training, during which each premise pair was presented repeatedly in a block of the specified number of trials before presentation of the succeeding premise. Error bars represent standard error (S.E.) above the mean. Groups did not differ statistically in the rate of acquisition of the premise pairs.

C. Mean response accuracy (± S.E.) on each of the four premise pairs during the probe test sessions. Performance was better on the end-anchored premises (AB and DE), but groups did not differ significantly in performance on individual premise pairs during testing.

D. Mean response accuracy (+ S.E.) for the average performance on premise pairs BC and CD and for the critical test pair BD during the test sessions. Control subjects performed as well on BD as on the inner premise pairs, but rats with either type of hippocampal damage were severely impaired, performing no better than chance on the BD judgment.

E. Response accuracy (+ S.E.) for control probe pair AE and the average response accuracy for new control pairs (WX and YZ). Performance was near perfect for all groups on AE and near chance for all groups in learning new pairs in this testing format. (Reproduced from Dusek and Eichenbaum, 1997.)

and their correct responses gradually. Ultimately, however, they were presented with premise pairs in random order. After achieving solid performance on the premise pairs, probe trials containing the critical BD choice and the control AE choice were presented, intermingled with repetitions of the premise pairs. On these probe trials animals were rewarded for the "correct" (transitive) selection, in order to avoid dissuading them from making transitive choices and maintaining performance on the probe trials. In order to minimize new learning of the BD pair, probes were presented only twice per test session and widely spaced among repetitions of premise pairs. In addition to testing for possible contamination by new learning of the BD pair, all animals were subsequently tested for their ability to learn about new odor cues presented in the probe test format.

Normal rats, as well as rats with hippocampal damage, achieved criterion performance very rapidly on each training phase (Figure 6.1B). In addition, all rats readily reached criterion with randomly presented premise pairs in an equivalent number of trials. In probe testing all rats continued to perform well on the premise pairs during the test sessions (Figure 6.1C). Indeed, all groups demonstrated a serial position curve such that performance was best on pairs that included one of the end items. On the critical BD probe test, normal subjects demonstrated robust transitive inference. Their performance on BD trials significantly exceeded chance level and was not different from their performance on premise pairs that included items B and D (Figure 6.1D). In striking contrast, the rats with hippocampal damage did not perform better than chance on the BD probe, and thus their performance on BD was much lower than that on the premise pairs that included B and D (the BC and CD pairs), and much worse than the performance of normal animals on the test of transitivity.

A further analysis of transitivity examined performance on the very first presentation of the BD pair, which may be considered a "pure" test of inferential responding uncontaminated by food reinforcements given on repeated probe trials. Of the normal subjects, 88 percent chose correctly on the first BD presentation, whereas only 50 percent of the rats with hippocampal damage were successful on the initial BD judgment. Thus, by several measures the data strongly indicate that rats with hippocampal damage have no capacity for transitive inference even though they could learn each of the premise problems as well as normal subjects.

Analyses of performance on other types of probe trials demonstrated the selectivity of the deficit in transitive inference in rats with hippocampal region damage. All rats performed extremely well on the AE trials, which can be solved without a transitive judgment (Figure 6.1E), and no group differences in performance were noted on this test. Conversely, all groups showed minimal evidence of learning during presentations of the new odor pairs (WX and YZ), and there were no group differences in performance on these tests.

The contrast between robust performance on BD over new odor pairs in normal rats strongly indicates their judgments on the BD pairs reflected inferential capacity. Conversely, the absence of a significant difference on this comparison, combined with intact performance on the AE pair, emphasizes the selective loss of the capacity for transitive inference in rats with hippocampal damage. The striking dissociation between fully intact performance on the premise pairs and no capacity for transitivity suggests that rats with hippocampal damage learned the premise pairs in a way that did not involve orderly relations among the odor cues. This learning is impressive in that the solutions somehow resolved the ambiguities of reward associations for each item (for instance, B is good when paired with C but not when paired with A) without reference to the relational organization.

Memory-without-Knowledge: A Selective Impairment in Memory Expression

The above-described experiment indicates the devastating limitations on memory resulting from a nonfunctional hippocampal region. At the same time, however, one is struck by the extent of intact learning capacity of these same animals. In the transitive inference task, rats with hippocampal damage performed at least as well as normal subjects in learning a series of four partially conflicting problems (Figure 6.1B), and they continued to perform well in extended random-order testing (Figure 6.1C). Similarly, animals with hippocampal damage are surprisingly successful in learning many simple discrimination problems, and even complex spatial problems, albeit in each case with limitations on the flexibility of memory expression they can employ. Let us further explore these aspects of memory-without-knowledge with two more examples from our laboratory.

In one study we examined the effects of hippocampal damage on spatial learning using the Morris water-maze task, which in some ways replicates the demands of natural spatial navigation (Eichenbaum, Stewart, and Morris, 1990). The apparatus was a large circular swimming pool filled with an opaque water solution and containing an escape platform slightly submerged at a fixed location relative to salient extra-maze visual cues (Figure 6.2A). In the standard version of this task, rats were released into the water at different starting points on successive trials, a manipulation that strongly encouraged the rats to develop a representation of spatial relations among the extra-maze cues. Under this condition, intact animals rapidly learned the location of the platform, demonstrating their memory by escaping with progressively shorter latencies. In contrast, rats with hippocampal damage failed to learn the escape locus. When we eliminated the demand for learning spatial relations by releasing the rats from a constant start position on each trial (the starting point shown in Figure 6.2A), rats with hippocampal damage learned to escape nearly as rapidly as normal animals. We ascertained that the representation of hippocampally lesioned rats was based on the extramaze cues, as was the case for normal rats.

Then, to assess the flexibility of the spatial memory representation supporting accurate performance on this version of the water-maze task, we presented rats with different types of probe trials, each involving an alteration of the cues or starting points, intermixed within a series of repetitions of the instruction trial. In one of our probes we required animals to navigate guided by the same cues, but beginning each swim from a novel start location (Figure 6.2B). Normal rats found the platform on probe trials as rapidly as on repetitions of the instruction trials. By contrast, rats with hippocampal damage required considerably longer to find the platform from novel locations (Figure 6.2C). Examination of the swim paths on individual probe trials showed that intact rats swam directly to the platform regardless of the starting position, whereas rats with hippocampal damage swam in various directions, sometimes never locating the platform (Figure 6.3).

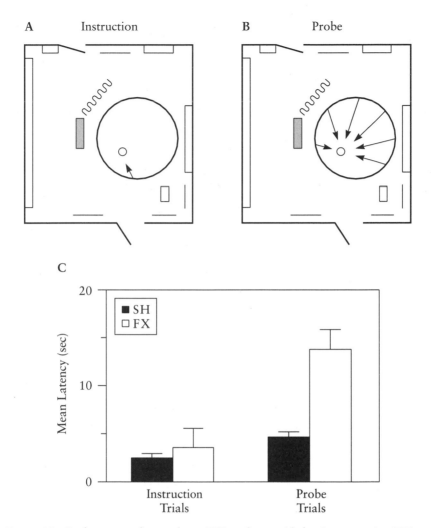

Figure 6.2 Performance of normal rats (SH) and rats with fornix transection (FX) on the Morris water-maze task.

A. A schematic diagram of the test room, and symbols representing a variety of room cues that could be seen from inside the swimming pool. The location of the escape platform is shown as a small circle within the pool, but it was submerged below the cloudy water and could not be seen during swimming. The starting position and ideal direct trajectory of the rats in the constant-start training version of the task is indicated by the arrow.

B. Arrows indicate the starting positions and direct trajectories of swims from starting locations used in the probe trials.

C. Mean latency (+ standard error) to find the escape platform during repetitions of the instruction trial and during probe, all trials. Rats with hippocampal damage did not differ statistically from intact rats on instruction trials, but were substantially and significantly slower to find the platform on probe trials. (From Eichenbaum et al., 1990.)

Thus, the hippocampus is critical when learning relations among cues is emphasized. Even when learning is successful, spatial memory expression in rats with hippocampal damage is limited to repetition of the training path. As found in our study on transitive inference, the hippocampus is a critical component of the brain pathway for the flexible expression of memory from an organized knowledge structure.

Another useful example comes from our research on simple olfactory discrimination learning (Eichenbaum, Fagan, Mathews, and Cohen, 1988; Eichenbaum, Mathews, and Cohen, 1989). We found that rats with damage to the hippocampal system actually outperformed normal rats in learning to discriminate two odor cues presented in separate trials and for which no choice between the cues had

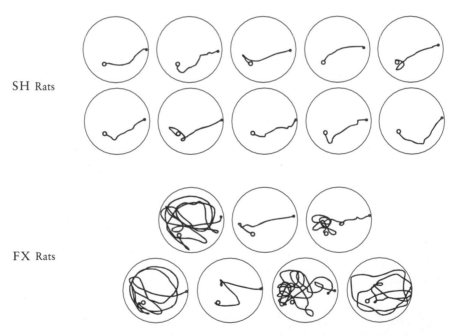

Figure 6.3 Tracking of swim paths in individual intact rats (SH) and rats with hippocampal damage (FX) on the probe trial that began from the "east" (rightmost start location). Intact rats almost always swam rather directly to the platform, but rats with hippocampal damage varied enormously, sometimes finding it directly and other times never locating the escape site. (From Eichenbaum et al., 1990.)

to be made. By contrast, rats with hippocampal damage were severely impaired when the same odor-discrimination problems were presented, but the procedures involved simultaneous presentation of the two odor cues and an explicit choice between them was required. Further investigations showed that rats with hippocampal damage could sometimes succeed in learning the simultaneous discriminations, and occasionally do as well as normal rats (Figure 6.4—compare to Figure 6.2). However, unlike normal rats, rats with hippocampal damage could not recognize the same stimuli when presented in novel pairings of familiar odor cues taken from different discrimination problems.

Similar to the findings on transitive inference and on water-maze learning, under conditions where learning occurs over many trial repetitions animals with hippocampal damage can succeed. Although they can repeat the learning event with the appropriately acquired biases, they cannot employ their memory to support judgments in novel challenges. This general finding, we argue, characterizes memory capacity without knowledge, that is, without the flexibility conferred by judgments made from a knowledge structure.

The Nature of Representations in Memory-without-Knowledge

A central issue in memory representation is how representations of stimuli become bound to one another in memory as new relations among these stimuli are learned. In his classic consideration of the "binding problem" in perception and memory, William James (1890/1918) suggested that stimuli may either be conceived as not distinct from one another and consequently may be bound by a conceptual *fusion* or, alternatively, may be discriminated as separate and then bound by *association* in memory. Our data indicate that animals with hippocampal damage are abnormally inclined to fuse rather than associate cues. For example, in the odor discrimination experiment just described we found that the pattern of behavior during the sampling was abnormal in rats with hippocampal damage. Normal rats sampled each of the cues independently, whereas rats with hippocampal damage sampled the two odors as if they were a single item, not hesitating to compare one odor with the other but responding to each stimulus configuration reflexively.

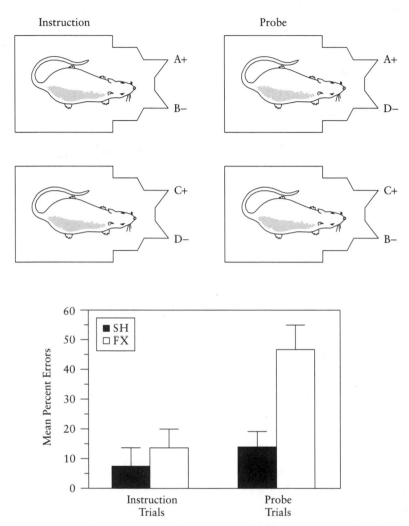

Figure 6.4   Performance of intact rats (SH) and rats with hippocampal damage (FX) on two simultaneous odor-discrimination tasks and on probe trials. In the first task, during instruction trials a rat was required to poke its nose into the port where odor A was presented in order to receive a reward, regardless of the left-right positions of odors A and B. In a subsequent task, rats were required similarly to select odor C over odor D. In the probe test the odors from both tasks were recombined in such a way that odor A had to be compared with odor D and odor B with odor D. Both groups of rats learned these problems and could perform equally well in repetitions of these instruction problems during the probe tests. In addition, intact rats readily recognized the correct odor selection when the odors were recombined, but rats with hippocampal damage were severely impaired, performing no better than chance at recognizing these highly familiar odors in new combinations. (From Eichenbaum et al., 1989.)

This finding led us to conclude that rats with hippocampal damage are abnormally inclined to fuse the representations of stimuli that are closely juxtaposed in space or time. And this abnormality in their representation could account for the inflexibility of memory expression. While the fusion of stimulus representations allowed them to succeed in repetitions of presented problems, it did not provide a form of representation that was useful when the animals were challenged to use their learning flexibly to solve new problems with separate stimulus elements.

Studies of human amnesia offer parallel insights into memory-without-knowledge. In the most compelling example of amnesia, the patient HM, it is now recognized that within his global and severe memory deficit is a broad set of distinctly preserved learning capacities. His acquisition of motor skills and perceptual priming were found intact. These findings were first viewed as exceptions to an otherwise global long-term memory impairment, but after further studies are viewed as merely examples of a large domain of preserved learning capacities observed in amnesic patients—including HM (see Cohen and Eichenbaum, 1993).

The range of intact learning capacities in amnesia includes motor, perceptual, and cognitive skills, and sensory adaptations and primings. Even learning that is severely impaired when subjects are asked to consciously recall or recognize items in the study phase, can be found fully spared in amnesic subjects when memory is assessed by more subtle measures (such as changes in response bias or speed after exposure to the test materials). These findings closely parallel the success of animals with hippocampal damage in acquiring biases in the selection of odor and spatial locations with appropriate reinforcement over many trial repetitions.

Yet, as in animals with hippocampal damage, spared learning in human amnesics has been characterized as "hyperspecific" in that successfully acquired memories can be expressed only in highly constrained conditions that imitate the conditions of original learning (Schacter, 1985). For example, several experiments have shown that the phenomenon of perceptual priming is intact in amnesia. Subjects are presented with words or pictures without any specific demand for remembering them. Both normal human subjects and amnesics reveal priming typically in one of two ways: by showing a bias toward completing an ambiguous word or picture fragment with the previously exposed item, or by identifying a repeated item more rapidly. However, priming effects such as these are seen only when the stimuli are presented in exactly the same format as during initial exposure, demonstrating an unusual specificity of access to this kind of memory. In studies specifically aimed at examining whether amnesics can acquire new associations, it has been found that indeed they can succeed, but only under conditions in which learning is revealed via implicit changes in speed or recognition, and the initial viewing conditions are replicated.

This hyperspecificity can be extended even to more everyday learning. For example, in one experiment that involved learning baseball facts in a question-and-answer format, a densely amnesic subject could correctly recall answers only if the test procedure included precise repetitions of the original questions used during learning (Schacter, 1985). In another study amnesics performed as well as normal subjects in learning a classification task that involved gradual acquisition of the capacity to predict the consequences of complex and probabilistic stimulus combinations (Reber, Knowlton, and Squire, 1996). Normal subjects could also answer questions about the predictive power of individual stimulus elements. These questions did not reinstantiate the test circumstances, and indeed were rated by subjects as assessing task knowledge indirectly and requiring flexible use of task knowledge. By contrast, despite their success in acquisition of the classification task, amnesic subjects failed the questions that relied on indirect and flexible use of memory.

Thus, as in the animal model, two forms of stimulus-binding can be distinguished in the performance of human amnesics. Amnesics are typically impaired in learning new associations, but with extra effort they do sometimes succeed. In these cases the associations appear to be *too* well bound; amnesic animals find it abnormally difficult to express memory for the original elements of a successfully acquired association when the elements are subsequently separated. In both human amnesics and animals with hippocampal damage, memory function can be surprisingly intact in certain respects, but is characterized by a loss of flexibility that is normally supported by a knowledge structure, the absence of which results in rigidity of access and expression of memory.

These experimental findings suggest that memory-without-knowledge can be characterized as capable of supporting a broad range of learning, but also as having two specific limitations. First, without a knowledge structure, information inordinately tends to become fused into large and complex chunks. Second, the expression of memory-without-knowledge is accordingly inflexible in that it can be accessed only within a limited scope that replicates the information-processing steps used to recover the chunks and associated biases obtained during original learning. In other words, memory is expressed only as a recompletion of the processing events that occurred during learning, typically with greater speed and a bias in perception or action that replicates the learning events. Such memory processing is comprehensive enough to guide complex behaviors that are high in motivation, emotion, and goal directedness. At the same time, this kind of learning occurs without introspection, investigation, or doubt. In precisely these ways memory-without-knowledge is the purest form of belief, an exaggeration or "caricature" of belief-driven behavior as we observe it in normal life.

Brain Systems that Support Memory-without-Knowledge

What brain systems support memory-without-knowledge, and how are the processing mechanisms of these systems characterized? Studies of these and related phenomena have led many students of memory to suggest that there are indeed multiple kinds of memory, each supported by different brain systems (Schacter and Tulving, 1994). Here we briefly consider some of the evidence that has been used to identify specific nonhippocampal systems that can mediate learning without knowledge, or acquisition of belief, and can do so surprisingly well under some circumstances. Before we review the functional roles of these systems, it will be useful to introduce them in terms of their anatomical pathways (Figure 6.5).

To the extent that most consider the cerebral cortex the main storehouse of memories, distinctions in access and expression of memories are determined by subcortical pathways with which the cortex interacts in supporting behavior. These considerations focus the attention of investigators on three main targets of cortical convergence onto subcortical structures, one involving cortical connections to the hippocampus, and the others involving cortical convergence onto the neostriatum and the amygdala. Evidence from several sources suggests that each of these pathways constitutes a distinct memory system.

Some of the strongest support for this view comes from studies by N. M. White and colleagues, who have directly compared the capacities of distinct brain systems in forms of spatial learning by rats. In their most recent and compelling investigations they accomplished a triple dissociation between memory functions supported by three different brain systems—one that involves the dorsal striatum, another that involves the amygdala, and the hippocampal system described above (McDonald and White, 1993). Distinctions among the ways these pathways support spatial learning were demonstrated in an experiment in which rats were trained on a radial maze (a maze having a central platform with eight arms radiating outward) to find food rewards. By carefully manipulating the task demands, McDonald and White created three different versions of the task for which performance on each required only one of these structures. The hippocam-

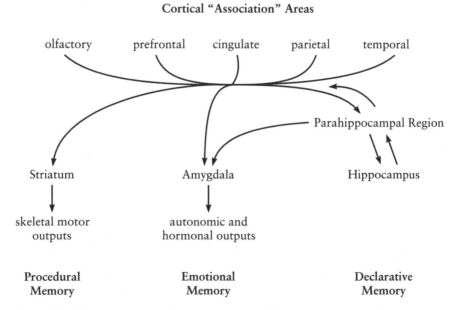

Figure 6.5 The anatomical pathways supporting different types of memory.

pal system predominated when the rats were encouraged to explore the maze and compare the experiences of entering each maze arm, as has been observed in several studies on hippocampal function in spatial learning and memory.

It was even more impressive that the other systems could support adequate spatial learning under some circumstances. A distinct system involving the neostriatum was enough to associate specific stimuli with an approach response when rats had to follow a cue to the locus of reward. And yet a third distinct system involving the amygdala could support the development of preferences and aversions to particular spatial locations when the rats were separately exposed to different sites that contained or did not contain rewards. Recent data on humans with brain damage and from brain imaging studies on normal humans have confirmed the distinct participation of a neostriatal pathway in response learning and the amygdala in emotional learning. So it appears there are at least two nonhippocampal pathways in animals and humans that can support unconscious forms of learning.

The characterizations formalized in these neuropsychological dissociations were in fact suggested much earlier by the philosopher Maine de Biran (1804/1929), who proposed the existence of three separate kinds of memory with different properties. Maine de Biran identified a specific system for the conscious recollection of ideas and events, what we have called the system for knowledge or declarative memory, as "representative memory." He distinguished this representative memory from two other unconscious mechanisms. First, he argued that "mechanical memory" supports the unconscious acquisition of motor and verbal habits. Second, he suggested that "sensitive memory" supports the unconscious acquisition of feelings associated with specific images and events.

Based on the above-described findings, Maine de Biran's propositions can now be interpreted as reflections of the different types of associations supported by separate anatomical pathways identified by White and colleagues: the convergence of sensory inputs and motor system connections in the neostriatum supporting mechanical memory (that is, *belief*), the convergence of sensory and affective inputs in the amygdala supporting sensitive memory (also *belief*), and the convergence of higher-order sensory inputs in the hippocampus mediating representative memory *(knowledge)*. Normal memory, we suggest, is characterized by a balance of the influences of these three parallel pathways and forms of memory. The consequences of imbalance among them is considered next.

Disorders of Belief and Knowledge

Our discussion so far has characterized belief as memory processes occurring in the relative absence of hippocampal function, and supported by pathways involving the neostriatum and amygdala. We have taken the position that damage to the hippocampal system results in an artificial imbalance in knowledge-driven behavior mediated by cortical-hippocampal pathways versus belief-driven behavior mediated by cortical-neostriatal or cortical-amygdala pathways. We now examine other instances of imbalance between belief and knowledge, as they occur in certain psychopathological syndromes. These are conditions in which the influence of knowledge (in the sense of hippocampally mediated representational flexibility) on behavior is abnormally attenuated or diminished.

Psychotic Disorders

Psychosis is characterized by drastic departure of an individual's system of interpretive schemata from that of the community. The influence of the pattern of reinforcement by experience on the structure of the interpretive schemata is also attenuated. In the terms used above, these changes can be characterized as functional defects of the knowledge structures of everyday life, with areas of prominent representational inflexibility. This inflexibility is most apparent in the symptom of delusionality, which involves a pervasive distortion of the use of memory in interpreting events in order to protect highly idiosyncratic beliefs. For example, a psychotic subject who suffers from the delusion that he is under surveillance by the Federal Bureau of Investigation will likely interpret a chance visit by a door-to-door salesman as incontrovertible evidence of the false belief, further strengthened by the salesman's shocked denial of any such undertaking. The psychotic individual's behavior in this situation is abnormally dominated by inflexible internal representations, which we hypothesize are mediated by nonhippocampal pathways.

The psychotic disorder most studied neurobiologically is schizophrenia. A repeated finding across several investigative techniques has been *hypofrontality* (Buchsbaum, 1991). Various prefrontal regions have been implicated, and a widely accepted model has invoked a resultant disinhibition and overactivation of nonhippocampal subcortical structures, including the neostriatum and amygdala, which are generally under tonic control of prefrontal inputs (Weinberger, 1987). This model is consistent with an abnormal prominence of nonhippocampal processes in mediating cognition, which might be expected to reduce representational flexibility.

Recent work has demonstrated that actively hallucinating schizophrenic subjects have reduced activation of the auditory cortex in response to external speech, suggesting saturation by internal (subcortical) inputs (David et al., 1995; Woodruff et al., 1996). Hallucinated perception is perhaps comparable to deluded belief in its lack of correctability by external reinforcement or lack of reinforcement. To date, no comparison has been made of brain activation in deluded versus nondeluded cognition (Yurgelun-Todd, personal communication, 1997).

Obsessive Compulsive Disorder (OCD)

In classic cases of OCD, afflicted subjects have diminished flexibility in the regulation of behavior, with full subjective awareness of the defect. This awareness suggests relative flexibility of cognition, with a defect at the level of the translation of intentions into behavior, including some aspects of subjective behavior (that is, intrusive "ego-alien" thoughts). Thus afflicted individuals may find themselves unable to resist vividly imagining terrible injuries befalling their child whenever that child is out of sight, despite realizing that the child is in no actual danger whatsoever; or they may be unable to resist repeatedly performing routine precautions (such as hand washing or lock checking), despite full awareness that these actions are completely unnecessary. Though knowledge structures are largely intact, their role in regulating behavior is significantly impaired.

On the basis of multiple functional imaging studies in humans, the pathophysiology of OCD has been hypothesized to relate to abnormal function of an orbitofrontal-neostriatal-thalamic circuit that may become inappropriately activated to the extent of overriding behaviors mediated by other pathways (Baxter et al., 1996). This suggests that the mediation of behavior in OCD is dominated by pathological response biases, although structures involved in cognitive appraisal (perhaps cortical-hippocampal circuits) may be unaffected, except in regard to their diminished influence on behavior. Thus, responses are dominated not by flexible knowledge structures but by inflexible beliefs.

Hysterical Disorders

Paradigmatic cases of hysteria include multiple personality disorder (recently renamed dissociative identity disorder); the conviction of having suffered unsubstantiable, apparently bizarre, traumatic life experiences, including alien abduction; satanic ritual abuse; and at least some cases of "retrieved memories" of extreme sexual and physical abuse of oneself, or groundless certainty that this has happened to one's children. In all these conditions the afflicted subject is typically responding to suggestions by psychotherapists or trusted peers that such apparently farfetched events are actually likely in their specific case, and the degree of social support is often quite intense (Merskey, 1995; Showalter, 1997). The high level of suggestibility of the typical affected subject, and the sense of high purpose lent to the subject by these psychological commitments, give their beliefs overriding durability even in the face of overwhelming counterevidence. The interpretations of the committed social supports are highly weighted, while more direct forms of evidence are dismissed.

Although there has been little systematic investigation of this patient population for evidence of specific brain abnormalities (Merskey, 1995), we hypothesize that the brain mechanisms underlying this condition may resemble those of the psychotic subject, except that here the restriction on representational flexibility is subject to social influence, rather than being rigidly autonomous as in the psychotic subject. Whatever neural processes underlie adherence to the accepted social group's norms seem to be highly active, and the frontal-hippocampal processes mediating representational flexibility appear to be impaired.

In all of these neuropsychiatric conditions, affected individuals are disposed to behave according to beliefs that are representationally inflexible and that do not permit full inferential use of memories in novel situations. Each condition presents clinically in a distinctly different way. In psychotic disorders there is extreme and inflexible idiosyncrasy in the interpretation of events, without a significant degree of susceptibility to social influence and without awareness of the impairment. OCD involves impairment in the capacity to behave in a manner consistent with intact representational flexibility, although there is typically vivid awareness of the defect, with cognitive appraisal being essentially unimpaired. In hysteria there is a usually shared idiosyncrasy of the interpretation of events, with extreme responsiveness to specific social influences, to the exclusion of other sources of reinforcement or lack of reinforcement of beliefs.

We hypothesize these conditions to reflect differing defects in the normal balance between belief and knowledge systems in the brain. All of them may involve defects of the cortical-hippocampal system, which our laboratory findings suggest underlies the representational flexibility we have termed *knowledge,* and consequent predominance of cortical-neostriatal and/or cortical-amygdalar systems that mediate rigid, habitual, and emotion-driven behavioral repertoires, which we have termed (pure) *belief.*

Putting the Memory Systems Back Together

So far our emphasis has been on unusual cases, both animal and human, in which the knowledge system has been compromised by ablation of specific structures or as a result of certain psychiatric disorders. These instances have served to identify the normal contribution of the knowledge system and demonstrate the characteristics of the belief system operating on its own. But none of these cases is normal. How do these systems operate under ordinary circumstances in animals and humans?

In this section we consider how these systems normally interrelate seamlessly to guide behavior. Our hypothesis is that they operate in parallel, but at any given time one predominates over the other in guiding behavior. Thus sometimes our behavior is "belief driven" and at other times it is "knowledge driven."

For example, one begins learning about a new topic area by a knowledge-driven approach. In this early phase, experiences are recorded along with the source of the information, and associations between learned items are made. This process iterates many times as new information is accumulated, leading to more elaborate associations and guiding their organization. Frequently some associations are broken so that new connections may intercede. Initially we may perceive a causal association between A and B. Later we find out that A causes B through a connection of A to X and X to B. Or A causes B only in context Y and not in context Z. These and many other associative elaborations add to, expand, and reorganize larger and larger networks of information. As the process continues, the specific source of each bit of information—the experience from which it was made—and many other dispensable aspects of the associations become lost. This occurs in part because the load of information otherwise becomes excessive, and in part because many incidental contiguities are not repeated or are contradicted. The end result of many iterations is the building of a knowledge structure that has all the properties we use to characterize cortical-hippocampal interactions. This base involves a large organized network of associations that can support flexible and inferential memory expression. It is constantly updated and modified through new experiences.

Eventually, however, as new experiences largely confirm the existing framework and add less and less new information, requiring less and less modification, the framework becomes more rigid and less amenable to major changes based on new or contradictory information. The processing strategy switches at some point to a belief-driven process, in which the presumption is that new information "must" fit the existing schema and provide further confirmation. When new information does not entirely fit, one of two things happens, as first characterized by Bartlett (1932). Either the disconcerting aspect of the new information is forgotten, or it is actually changed to fall in line with the current schema. This belief-driven process then can lead to memory loss, or to illusory or false memories. In most situations the belief-driven process can succeed only to a limited extent. As more and more new information is obtained that is disconfirming of the schema, eventually the strategy switches back to a knowledge-driven process. The inadequate schema is drastically altered or dropped for another schema.

Belief may survive a process in which specific details and episodes are lost to the overall knowledge structure. We *believe* something will happen even though we cannot recall a particular instance of its previous occurrence. And, because a belief can be strong, it may override the record of experiences on which it was built. Thus, belief can "drive" further knowledge processing. When recollections are required, the belief structure can dictate the contents and even modify them when constructing a memory that must fit the overall knowledge structure. Similarly, new information can be modified on input to fit a strong knowledge base.

The experimental findings presented above suggest that such processing may be rigid in the ways in which the knowledge structure is elaborated or modified. The stronger the structure and the more it has become a belief, the more limited the interpretation of new information, which is increasingly required to conform to the preexisting structure.

We like to think our conceptualizations are always subject to question, doubt, modification, and even disproof. To the extent that they are driven by cortical-hippocampal processing, this should be the case. But to the extent that the involvement of the system has become limited, other systems characterized by emotion and habit can largely replace this flexible processing.

Conclusion

In this review we have sought to understand belief though an analysis of memory processing. We have focused on a distinction between knowledge and belief and the different ways they operate in the service of memory. In our considerations of knowledge, we adopted characterizations proposed by James, Bartlett, Tolman, and Hebb, emphasizing the notion that knowledge is an organized network of information that can support flexible, inferential memory expression. Based on experiments that assess the flexibility of memory, we have seen that memory-with-knowledge and memory-without-knowledge can be distinguished by damage to the hippocampal region of the brain. Animals and humans with damage to the hippocampal region have robust learning and memory capacities, but lack the ability to express their memories flexibly and inferentially.

Studies on both animals with hippocampal damage and human amnesic patients have shown that successful memory-without-knowledge can be characterized as "hyperspecific" in that the nature of the memory representation involves fusion of stimuli and rigidity of the response paths available for memory expression, specifically limited to repetition of the circumstances of learning. We have discussed evidence that non-hippocampal systems involving cortical-striatal and cortical-amygdala pathways can support memory-without-knowledge. Finally, we have suggested that some psychiatric conditions parallel the consequences of loss of hippocampal-dependent memory processing and or exaggeration of corticostriatal or corticoamygdala memory processing, and so can be characterized in part as memory-without-knowledge.

In interpreting these experimental observations, we find it worth recalling the philosopher's distinction between belief and memory stated at the outset of this chapter, specifically that knowledge, unlike belief, must be "justified." Applying our experimental observations to this issue, we propose that a central feature of this required justification is the capacity to recover both direct and indirect associates of the known item, or have command of a body of facts and principles. Conversely, we propose that memory without this feature of knowledge is "pure" belief. In other words, we suggest that rats with hippocampal damage, for example, are able to solve a variety of complex olfactory and spatial tasks, but not make flexible inferences about them.

A few more analogies will summarize our main points. It may be simplest to think of knowledge-driven and belief-driven systems in a general way. Knowledge-driven memory processing is "bottom up," in that new experiences are paramount in forcing novel bits of information together to build or modify a memory scheme. It appears this processing is mediated by cortical-hippocampal interactions. By contrast, belief-driven memory processing is "top down," in that the general schema is paramount in guiding the interpretation of new experience to confirm convictions and to specify actions consistent with those convictions. We think this processing reflects less involvement of the cortical-hippocampal system and major roles for the cortical-neostriatal and cortical-amygdalar systems that are reflected in habits and emotionally driven beliefs.

This alternation of driving forces is interestingly analogous to Kuhn's (1970) characterization of scientific progress. Kuhn describes hypothesis generation as alternating with confirmation and elaboration processes. Initially a sketchy hypothesis is based upon and altered by new results of experiments and observations. Richer and richer, albeit continuously modified, hypotheses follow. Eventually, new data, sometimes seemingly inconsistent, are interpreted as consistent with the current framework, even if some aspects of the data must be ignored or modified by interpretation. If disconfirming evidence mounts beyond a critical point, a "revolution" occurs, whereby an old schema is dropped and another cycle of hypothesis building commences. We have suggested that analogous sequences characterize memory processing, supported by the parallel processing and interactions of distinct memory systems in the brain.

Some of the symptoms of psychosis, obsessive compulsive disorder, and hysteria present aberrations in which this normal alternation stops at a fixed belief-driven stage, potentially due to dysfunction of cortical-hippocampal interactions. For the unafflicted among us, the alternation of belief-driven and knowledge-driven processing facilitates the use of memory in daily life, allowing us to utilize memory effectively to guide responses in new situations, and to modify knowledge structures rapidly when circumstances warrant.

References

Bartlett, F. C. (1932). *Remembering: A study in experimental and social psychology.* London: Cambridge University Press.

Baxter, L. R., Saxena, S., Brody, A. L., Ackerman, R. F., Colgan, M., Schwartz, J. M., Allen-Martinez, Z., Fuster, J. M., and Phelps, M. E. (1996). Brain mediation of obsessive-compulsive disorder symptoms: Evidence from functional brain imaging studies in the human and nonhuman primate. *Seminars in Clinical Neuropsychiatry, 1,* 32–47.

Buchsbaum, M. S. (1991). Positron-emission tomography and regional brain metabolism in schizophrenia research. In N. D. Volkow and A. P. Wolf (Eds.), *Positron-emission tomography in schizophrenia research,* Progress in Psychiatry Series, 33. Washington, DC: American Psychological Association Press.

Chisholm, R. H. (1966). *Theory of knowledge*. Engelwood Cliffs, NJ: Prentice-Hall.

Cohen, N. J., and Eichenbaum, H. (1993). *Memory, amnesia, and the hippocampal system*. Cambridge, MA: MIT Press.

Cohen, N. J., and Squire, L. R. (1980). Preserved learning and retention of a pattern-analyzing skill in amnesia: Dissociation of knowing how and knowing that. *Science, 210*, 207–210.

David, A. S., Howard, R., Woodruff, P. W. R., Bullmore, E., Mellers, J. D., Whyte, M., Simmons, A., Williams, S. C. R., and Brammer, M. (1995). Schizophrenic hallucinations attenuate activation in the superior temporal lobes. *Proceedings of the Society of Magnetic Resonance and the European Society for Magnetic Resonance in Medicine and Biology, 1* (August 19–25).

Dusek, J. A., and Eichenbaum, H. (1997). The hippocampus and memory for orderly stimulus relations. *Proceedings of the National Academy of Sciences (USA), 94*, 7109–14.

Eichenbaum, H. (1997). Declarative memory: Insights from cognitive neurobiology. *Annual Review of Psychology, 48*, 547–572.

Eichenbaum, H., Fagan, A., Mathews, P., and Cohen, N. J. (1988). Hippocampal system dysfunction and odor discrimination learning in rats: Impairment or facilitation depending on representational demands. *Behavioral Neuroscience, 102*, 331–339.

Eichenbaum, H., Mathews, P., and Cohen, N. J. (1989). Further studies of hippocampal representation during odor discrimination learning. *Behavioral Neuroscience, 103*, 1207–16.

Eichenbaum, H., Otto, T., and Cohen, N. J. (1992). The hippocampus—what does it do? *Behavioral and Neural Biology, 57*, 2–36.

Eichenbaum, H., Otto, T., and Cohen, N. J. (1994). Two functional components of the hippocampal memory system. *Brain and Behavioral Sciences, 17*, 449–518.

Eichenbaum, H., Stewart, C., and Morris, R. G. M. (1990). Hippocampal representation in spatial learning. *Journal of Neuroscience, 10*, 331–339.

Hebb, D. O. (1949). *The organization of behavior*. New York: Wiley.

James, W. (1890/1918). *The principles of psychology*. New York: Holt.

Kuhn, T. S. (1970). *The structure of scientific revolutions* (2nd ed.). Chicago: University of Chicago Press.

Maine de Biran (1804/1929). *The influence of habit on the faculty of thinking*. Baltimore: Williams and Wilkins.

McDonald, R. J., and White, N. M. (1993). A triple dissociation of memory systems: Hippocampus, amygdala, and dorsal striatum. *Behavioral Neuroscience, 107*, 3–22.

Merskey, H. (1995). *The analysis of hysteria*. London: Gaskell.

Piaget, J. (1928). *Judgment and reasoning in the child*. London: Kegan, Paul, Trench, and Trubner.

Reber, P. J., Knowlton, B. J., and Squire, L. R. (1996). Dissociable properties of memory systems: Differences in the flexibility of declarative and non-declarative knowledge. *Behavioral Neuroscience, 110,* 861–871.

Schacter, D. L. (1985). Multiple forms of memory in humans and animals. In N. M. Weinberger, J. L. McGaugh, and G. Lynch (Eds.), *Memory systems of the brain* (pp. 351–380). New York: Guilford Press.

Schacter, D. L. (1987). Implicit memory: History and current status. *Journal of Experimental Psychology: Learning, Memory, and Cognition, 13,* 501–518.

Schacter, D. L., and Tulving, E. (1994). *Memory systems, 1994*. Cambridge, MA: MIT Press.

Scoville, W. B., and Milner, B. (1957). Loss of recent memory after bilateral hippocampal lesions. *Journal of Neurology, Neurosurgery and Psychiatry, 20,* 11–12.

Showalter, E. (1997). *Hystories: Hysterical epidemics and modern culture*. New York: Columbia University Press.

Squire, L. R., Knowlton, B., and Musen, G. (1993). The structure and organization of memory. *Annual Review of Psychology, 44,* 453–495.

Tolman, E. C. (1932/1951). *Purposive behavior in animals and men*. Berkeley: University of California Press.

Weinberger, D. (1987). The implications of normal brain development for the pathogenesis of schizophrenia. *Archives of General Psychiatry, 44,* 660–669.

Woodruff, P. R. W., Wright, I., Brammer, M., Howard, R., David, A. S., Bullmore, E., et al. (1996). Auditory hallucinations in schizophrenia alter cortical response to externally presented speech. *NeuroImage, 3* (3), S522.

Where in the Brain Is the Awareness of One's Past?

7

Endel Tulving

Martin Lepage

When a layperson ponders memory, what it is and what it does, that individual usually thinks that memory refers to the kind of mental capacity that makes possible learning or experiencing something now, then later remembering what it was that one learned or experienced. How it is accomplished usually does not concern the user of memory; it is a problem gladly left for the amusement of scientists. Indeed, for over a hundred years now, scientists in a variety of disciplines have tried to understand how memory works. Although they have made tremendous advances on many fronts, the main "discovery" to date has been that memory is extraordinarily complicated.

With the complications, however, have come some exciting prospects. One of these has to do with an aspect of memory that laypeople have always taken for granted and that scientists studying memory have managed to neglect—namely, the subjective element of the mental experience of remembering. To remember an event means to be consciously aware now of an experience that happened on an earlier occasion. It follows that remembering a past event as such is a conscious experience. For most of the long history of memory research, psychologists and others have assumed that the subjective and conscious recollective experience that accompanies memory performance was not amenable to scientific scrutiny. It was believed that there were no valid ways of directly getting at the subjective side of memory, at "remembering as conscious awareness." Brain imaging techniques, such as PET (positron emission tomography), fMRI (functional magnetic resonance imaging) and ERP (event-related potentials), have provided memory researchers with a new strategy to further the understanding of memory and awareness. With these recently developed techniques it has become possible to study the brain-mind correlates of remembering and to specifically examine the brain activity associated with different forms of memory and different types of subjective awareness that accompany recollection.

This chapter shares some of the excitement of memory research today with readers outside the field. The first part of the chapter stresses that there are many forms of memory, from habituation and simple classical conditioning to the loftiest thoughts that one can have based on what one has learned. Interestingly, most of these forms of memory, contrary to the public consensus, have nothing to do with the past. Instead, most forms of memory and learning studied in many areas of the life sciences have to do with the present and the future, not with the past. The single exception is episodic memory. It, and it alone, is very much concerned with the past.

The second part of the chapter describes episodic memory, which deals with a person's experienced past and makes possible "mental time travel" through subjective time. A special form of conscious awareness is required—otherwise we would not know whether we are just thinking about something or remembering. Evolution has seen fit to provide for that, too, with "autonoetic" awareness, which encompasses both the personal past and the personal future of an individual.

In the third portion of the chapter we present some material on subjective awareness and memory research using the techniques of brain imaging, research that is beginning to answer the question posed in the chapter's title: where in the brain is the awareness of one's past? Some of this research has been directed at distinguishing between the processes of encoding (getting information in) and retrieval (getting information out). A surprising finding is that the two hemispheres of the brain seem to be engaged in a kind of division of labor in which the left is doing more for encoding, whereas the right seems to be more interested in retrieval. Further exploration of this pattern, referred to as hemispheric encoding/retrieval asymmetry, or HERA, suggests that an important contribution of the right frontal lobe to episodic memory retrieval is the establishment and maintenance of a particular neurocognitive state, referred to as the episodic retrieval mode. It is this retrieval mode, supported by the prefrontal (especially right) cortex and its connectivity with other brain regions (especially in the medial temporal lobes), that we suggest gives rise to the highly subjective, autonoetic awareness of one's past. The hypothesis is supported by additional data, from both clinical cases of brain damage and studies of normal individuals' awareness of the past, that employ the technique of electrophysiological recording.

Our main theme is the subjective side of memory, the aspect that has to do with conscious awareness of not only space but time. This subjective side, specific to episodic memory and absent from all other forms of memory, has been difficult to pinpoint using the rules of science. New techniques of measuring and imaging the activity of the living brain have opened a window through which we are beginning to "see" the outlines of conscious awareness in memory in a way that was beyond the pale of science only a few years ago.

Memory and Time

Many organisms, including human beings, begin life with a host of biologically useful behavior patterns, or with the potential for postnatal maturation of such patterns that are released in appropriate situations. These instincts, effective ways of behaving in one's environment, have evolved over long periods and do not depend much on individual experience. For example, as shown by Eleanor Gibson many years ago, human infants, like the very young of other species, do not crawl off a "visual cliff" when given an opportunity to do so, but cling to the safe side of the divide, even during the very first test (Gibson, 1969).

Learning is another effective source of information that is useful for survival. It comes into play in situations that evolution does not know much about. Thus, the same young child, who knows without learning that mommies are to be approached and cliffs are to be avoided, must learn (through actual experience or vicariously) about the desirability of M&Ms and the danger of hot stoves. Despite the differences in origin, acquired knowledge can be as effective as innate knowledge in helping an organism to reach reproductive age and perhaps beyond.

All of the many different forms of memory, with a single exception, serve the same purpose as do the "instincts": they provide organisms with the means of behaving more effectively than would have been possible in the absence of the relevant acquired knowledge or skill. The experience at Time 1 allows the organism to respond more adaptively at Time 2, and this holds all the way from very simple forms of learning, such as habituation, to the most complex forms of acquired knowledge, such as the knowledge that all humans are mortal.

Another feature common to the vast majority of different forms of learning and memory is that none requires a conscious awareness of where or when or how the skill or knowledge used at the present moment was acquired. Remembering the particular occasion on which one learned about the mortality of living beings, or knowing how or why one knows something, is as irrelevant as the infant's lack of insight into the origin of her wisdom in refusing to crawl to mommy on the other side of what looks like empty space. Whether we think about a trout, a canary, our pet cat, or ourselves, survival clearly does not require conscious awareness of the past; it requires current skills and knowledge. This is why almost all evolved forms of learning and memory are oriented toward the present and the future, rather than the past. We designate these forms of memory collectively as "proscopic" (forward-looking) memory.[1]

Episodic Memory

The singular exception to the ubiquity and evolutionary significance of proscopic memory that serves the future without bothering about the past is episodic memory. It does exactly what the other forms of memory do not and cannot do; it enables the individual to mentally travel back into the personal past. A child remembers what happened at a friend's birthday party the day before, a young lover remembers the expression on his beloved's face in the moonlight, the scientist remembers the first time when a speaker at a conference mentioned her work, and so on. They all are happy possessors of this latest arrival on the evolutionary scene, episodic memory.

Figure 7.1 represents episodic and all other forms of memory as differences between the temporal relations among memory episodes. The

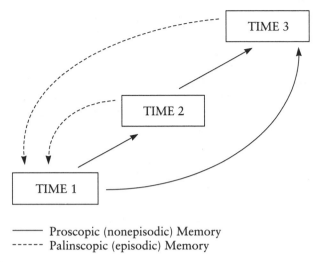

—— Proscopic (nonepisodic) Memory
----- Palinscopic (episodic) Memory

Figure 7.1   Schematic of time's arrows of proscopic (forward-looking) and palin-scopic (backward-looking) memory.

time's arrow of nonepisodic memory is straight and points to the future. Episodic memory's time is not an arrow, but rather a loop from Time 2 to Time 1. The influence of Time 1 at Time 2 expresses itself in a mental return to the past: the individual has a conscious awareness of reexperiencing here and now something of the experience of the earlier time. Because it allows us to mentally visit and "see" the past, we can refer to episodic memory as "palinscopic" (backward-looking) memory.[2] Thus, episodic memory makes possible one of the impossible dreams of the science fiction writer—time travel (see also Suddendorf and Corballis, 1997).

As with all familiar objects, we take our episodic memory for granted and do not spend even a minute marveling at the astounding evolutionary feat it represents. Nor do we marvel at what is an even more astounding feat of evolution: the looping arrow of episodic memory can loop once more at remembered Time 1 forward to imagined Time 3, which will follow Time 2. Episodic experiences of our personal past become a foundation for expectations about our personal future, and we can speak of individuals remembering the future. The time's arrow of proscopic (nonepisodic) memory becomes the time's circle of palinscopic (episodic) memory.

All this may sound a bit uninhibited. Scientists are people who say, "Don't tell me; show me!" It is easy to make all sorts of claims about all sorts of things in the universe, from superstrings and black holes to repressed memories and consciousness; but unless we can back these claims with empirical evidence, they remain what John Horgan, in his 1996 book entitled *The End of Science,* calls ironic science: commentary on the world, rather than a description of the world. When we talk about subjective time and autonoetic awareness, we do not mean to merely entertain the reader; we mean scientific business.

Our general approach is to relate concepts such as autonoetic awareness to happenings in the brain. When one simply describes how one remembers a past event and how it differs from reciting a learned fact, it is easy to remain uncertain about what it all means. But when such introspections are linked with objectively observable physiological changes in the brain, the story becomes a bit more interesting scientifically. And that is what we plan to do: link subjectively felt conscious awareness of past events to the activity of the living brain.

Before we look at the brain, however, we will find it useful to contrast episodic memory with its closest relative in the other (proscopic) family of memories. This exercise will not only give a better concept of episodic memory, but also prepare for appropriate comparisons when we focus on the brain.

Semantic Memory

This closest relative is called semantic memory. The name is somewhat misleading, but for historical reasons we are stuck with it (Tulving, 1983). Semantic memory is the kind of memory that makes it possible for organisms to acquire, store, and use information about the world in which they live, in the broadest possible sense. So whenever you see "semantic memory," think "knowledge of the world." The important thing is to remember that "semantic" here does not imply language in any sense. All kinds of animals who have no linguistic ability have excellent semantic memory—they know a lot about the kind of world in which they live. There is no evidence, however, that any species other than humans has episodic memory of the kind we have described.

Episodic and semantic memory have a large number of features in common, which is why they can be classified together as declarative, or cognitive, or propositional forms of memory. Table 7.1 gives a list of some of these commonalities: they are both large and complex and can hold immense amounts of information; they can handle a great variety of different kinds of information—visual, auditory, verbal, pictorial, spatial, and so on; the information they contain is representational and can be expressed in propositional and symbolic form; these propositions can be assessed for their truth value; the information they hold is flexibly accessible through a variety of retrieval routes, queries, prompts, and cues; both memory systems interact closely with other brain and behavior systems such as language, emotion, affect, and reasoning; finally, information in both is accessible to conscious contemplation: we can consciously reflect on what we know about the world and everything in it as well as we can think about what happened yesterday or what we did in summer camp at age ten.

If one focuses exclusively on all these commonalities, it is easy to conclude that the two kinds of memory are essentially the same, differing only with respect to the kind of material or kind of information with which they deal: (personally experienced) events versus (generally shared) facts. However, there are differences; and we believe they are crucial.

Some of these major differences between episodic and semantic memory are summarized in Table 7.1: they serve different functions; episodic memory is concerned with remembering past experiences as such, whereas semantic memory is concerned with the acquisition and use of knowledge; they differ with respect to evolutionary history, with episodic memory arguably representing the latest development; episodic memory lags behind semantic memory in human development (Perner and Ruffman, 1995); the underlying neuroanatomy differs, with episodic memory relying more on the frontal lobes (Schacter, 1987; Squire, 1987; Wheeler, Stuss, and Tulving, 1997); the time orientation is different, in that episodic memory is the only form of memory oriented toward the past. Finally, the conscious awareness that accompanies retrieval is also different: episodic memory is accompanied by a special kind of (autonoetic) conscious awareness, whereas semantic knowing is accompanied by another kind of (noetic)

Table 7.1   Commonalities and differences of episodic and semantic memory

Commonalities	Differences
Large and complex	Memory functions (remembering/knowing)
Support all kinds of information	Evolutionary
Representational	Developmental
Propositional	Neuroanatomical correlates
Truth value	Time orientation (past/future)
Flexibly accessible	Conscious awareness (autonoetic/noetic)
Interact with other systems	
Accessible to conscious contemplation	

conscious awareness (Tulving, 1993). Some of these differences are better established than others, and we could discuss all of them at length. One that is of particular significance for present purposes is the distinction between noetic and autonoetic awareness.

Memory and Consciousness

Although the terms "consciousness" and "awareness" are frequently used interchangeably, we draw a sharp distinction between them. In this chapter as elsewhere (Tulving, 1993), consciousness refers to the general capability of the brain that makes it possible for the individual to become aware of its world, whereas awareness refers to a particular expression or manifestation of that capability. Within any one kind of consciousness can be many kinds of awareness. Consciousness does not require an object; it is not about anything. Awareness does require objects and always is of something. One can be "in" a given state of consciousness, and within that state be aware of different things, depending on the object of awareness.

Most evolved forms of learning and memory in the animal kingdom have little to do with consciousness. The same is true of many of the forms of learning and memory on which human survival and happiness depend. Consciousness enters the picture only at the stage of higher forms of human memory, generically referred to as declarative or cognitive memory (Squire, 1987; Squire, Knowlton, and Musen, 1993; Tulving, 1983), composed of the two subtypes described above—semantic (knowledge of facts) and episodic (remembrance of events).

Awareness of one's past can occur through either of two forms of consciousness. The evolutionarily more recent and hence more sophisticated is autonoetic consciousness, the standard experiential mode of retrieval operations in the episodic memory system. It allows one to mentally travel back and forth in subjectively experienced time, a feat of the brain/mind that is probably unique in the animal kingdom. When we remember a particular past event, regardless of how vividly or accurately, we rely primarily on our autonoetic consciousness. When we are autonoetically aware of a past situation or past event, we focus our attention directly on our own past experience.

The evolutionarily older and more primitive form of consciousness that can provide access to the past is noetic consciousness. Noetic awareness accompanies an individual's interaction with aspects of his or her environment in the present. It is the standard experiential mode of retrieval operations in the semantic memory system. An individual thinking about the facts of the world is consciously aware of the relation between those thoughts and aspects of the world that are not perceptually present at the time. The experiential flavor of the noetic awareness of publicly sharable facts differs from that of autonoetic awareness of personally experienced past events.

A Patient with No Autonoetic Awareness

The story of a brain-damaged individual concretely illustrates the separability of noetic and autonoetic awareness. The case involves a man known as KC who has been extensively described elsewhere (Hayman, MacDonald, and Tulving, 1993; Tulving, Schacter, McLachlan, and Moscovitch, 1988). As a result of traumatic brain damage suffered in a motorcycle accident at age thirty, KC lost the ability to remember any personally experienced events, although in most other aspects his cognitive functions are reasonably intact and he remains indistinguishable from many other people who have suffered no brain damage. He knows much about the world and can even acquire new semantic information, although very slowly and laboriously. Thus, his noetic consciousness, his ability to become aware of aspects of the world not present to the senses, is entirely or largely intact. But he cannot consciously recollect any single or even repeated event from his entire life, regardless of how memorable the event by ordinary standards and regardless of how heavily he is cued or prompted. Thus, his autonoetic consciousness, his ability to become aware of past personal happenings, is totally dysfunctional.

Although they are rare, similar patients have been described by others (Calabrese et al., 1996; Hodges and McCarthy, 1993; Markowitsch et al., 1993). These patients do have mental access to their personal past, but the access is like that to any other aspect of the world with which they are familiar. Brain damage can produce individuals who are noetically aware of many autobiographical facts, but this kind of awareness is greatly impoverished in comparison with that afforded by autonoetic consciousness.

Studies on the effect of frontal lobe lesions on behavior implicate this brain region as an important neuroanatomical correlate of episodic memory and, consequently, of its associated state of autonoetic awareness (Wheeler et al., 1997). Functional neuroimaging studies have similarly revealed the contributions of the frontal lobes (among other regions) to episodic memory.

PET Studies of Episodic Memory

The relation between brain and mind has fascinated and frustrated scientists interested in memory for a long time. A popular way of posing the problem has been in terms of "localization of function," and a popular version of the question has been, Where are the memories in the brain?

Today we have many different kinds of memory, and multiple memory systems, and we think about them in terms of their constituent processes, such as encoding and retrieval. We also have substantial evidence suggesting that there are no specific memory centers in the brain, and probably not even specific storage sites. This is why we no longer ask, Where are the memories in the brain? Rather, we wonder about the neuroanatomical correlates of episodic encoding, or episodic memory retrieval.

We could ask this simple question: How similar and how different are the episodic encoding and retrieval circuits in the brain? A positron emission tomography (PET) experiment conducted by Shitij Kapur and Roberto Cabeza (Cabeza et al., 1997; Kapur et al., 1996) together with other members of the Toronto group suggests that the answer is: Surprisingly different. The subjects were twelve young men and women, university students. During different PET scans they were engaged in two different tasks. In the encoding task, they studied pairs of words, such as penguin–tuxedo, in preparation for the subsequent test. In the retrieval task, they saw previously studied pairs, one pair at a time, and had to decide whether the pair had appeared in the study list. This is an episodic-memory retrieval (recognition) condition. During the sixty-second scanning window, all the test pairs in fact were "old."

The brain maps of activation yielded by the subtraction of the retrieval activations from the encoding activations showed regions that were preferentially more active during encoding than during retrieval. These regions included the left prefrontal cortex, left anterior cingulate cortex, and left parahippocampal gyrus. The brain maps of activation yielded by the subtraction of encoding activations from the retrieval activations showed brain regions that were more active during retrieval than during encoding. The right prefrontal cortex, right anterior cingulate, and right inferior parietal cortex were the regions showing significant activation during the retrieval task.

Two observations are worth noting. First, there are striking differences between the brain regions activated during the encoding task and those activated during the retrieval task. We can assume that some common regions as well are activated during both encoding and retrieval, although they do not show in these analyses because they are "subtracted out" in the process. Nevertheless, the differences are surprisingly extensive. The two sets of activations are heavily lateralized in the two hemispheres: encoding activations are all in the left hemisphere, and retrieval activations are all in the right hemisphere. This stark dichotomy is not always observed, of course, but it does illustrate a kind of functional hemispheric laterality that seems to be real.

The second point is that, as almost always happens in these studies, the condition we call episodic encoding is also a condition of semantic-memory retrieval. The subjects use their knowledge of words, their meanings, and their relations when they impress the presented pairs of words on mind.

Hemispheric Encoding/Retrieval Asymmetry (HERA)

The data we have just described nicely complement the data yielded by many other PET studies, including the very first ones designed to investigate encoding and retrieval processes in episodic memory. These studies were done at the Hammersmith Hospital in London, England (Fletcher et al., 1995, 1996, 1997; Shallice et al., 1994); at Washington University in St. Louis (Buckner et al., 1995, 1996); and in Toronto (Kapur et al., 1994; Nyberg et al., 1996; Tulving et al., 1994b). Considered together, the data suggested a surprising empirical regularity: the left prefrontal cortex seemed to be differentially more involved than the right in retrieval of information from semantic memory, and in the simultaneous encoding information into episodic memory, whereas the right prefrontal cortex seemed to be differentially more involved than the left in episodic memory retrieval.

This pattern is referred to as HERA: hemispheric encoding/retrieval asymmetry in the frontal lobes (Tulving et al., 1994a). Although initially unexpected, and therefore greeted with some skepticism, the HERA pattern is now well established and indeed represents one of the most robust findings reported in the literature (Nyberg, Cabeza, and Tulving, 1996).

The overall HERA pattern can be economically described in terms of the interactions of three pairs of concepts: (a) encoding versus retrieval, (b) episodic versus semantic memory, and (c) left and right frontal lobes. This overall regularity is largely unaffected by specific conditions of the relevant experiments. Available evidence suggests that it holds equally for verbal and nonverbal materials. For instance, encoding of human faces has been shown to activate the left prefrontal cortex (Haxby et al., 1996) in the absence of comparable activation on the right, while recognition of previously studied faces has been shown to activate the right prefrontal cortex, in the absence of comparable activation on the left. Similar observations have been made with other nonverbal materials and line drawings of objects (for example, Owen, Milner, Petrides, and Evans, 1996). The encoding activations on the left have been observed under conditions of both intentional and incidental learning (Rugg, Fletcher, Frith, Frackowiak, and Dolan, 1997); the retrieval activations on the right have been observed in both recall and recognition tasks (Cabeza et al., 1997).

Although the general left/right encoding/retrieval pattern is remarkably consistent, within this general regularity exists considerable variability in localization of function, depending on the specific conditions of the various studies. This variability invites more detailed examination of the data. Analyses have begun, and the results are promising: it is possible to identify specific prefrontal regions that are involved in encoding and retrieval of particular aspects of the information (Buckner, 1996).

Analysis of the PET data from even a single experiment can rapidly become very taxing and complicated; analyses of data from many experiments are exceedingly so. One way of coping is to focus on specific aspects of the data, without forgetting that they are always part of a much larger and more comprehensive picture.

Retrieval Mode and the Frontal Lobes

In pursuing the implications of HERA, we focused on the episodic retrieval activation in the right frontal lobe, and asked the question, What does this right-frontal activation signify? Retrieval, like encoding, is not a single unitary process; it comprises many separate processes. When subjects are shown a group of words in an episodic recognition task and asked whether they have seen them previously in the experiment, several things happen: subjects go into what we call the episodic retrieval mode, trying to fit the present input into their mentally recovered past (Was this one of the words I saw while they were showing me all those words on the screen as I was lying here ten minutes ago?). They succeed incorrectly in recognizing many test items; they feel good about what they realize are successful "hits"; and they may also feel frustrated because of occasional felt uncertainties about their overall performance. All of this happens when subjects take a recognition test, and the right-frontal activation may signify any one thing or a combination of several.

We wondered initially, What will happen if we ask subjects to take a recognition test of previously studied words, but do not let them succeed in such recognition. We tested them, during the scanning window, with words that were all "new," that is, words they had not seen in the studied list. If the right frontal lobe "lit up," it signified the retrieval mode, the attempt to remember past happenings, and it meant that actual success or failure ("contacting the memory traces") did not matter. If the right frontal lobe did not light up in this situation, that meant that it had done so in previous studies because the subjects always succeeded in recognizing a substantial portion of test words.

We conducted two such studies and got identical results (Kapur et al., 1995; Nyberg et al., 1995). Right frontal activation was observed in a situation where subjects were tested with genuine "old" test words, and succeeded. With both retrieval attempt and retrieval success we achieve a nice confirmation of the HERA pattern: retrieval activation on the right, nothing showing on the left.

Our next question was, What happens when we test the subjects with new words, which they attempt to retrieve but fail by design? The pattern of brain activation was exactly the same: prominent activation on the right, nothing on the left. In the two conditions being directly compared here (one subtracted from the other), none of the words the subjects saw had been seen before in the experiment. But in this condition subjects were in retrieval mode; in the other condition they were not, they merely read the presented words. Thus, it seemed that right frontal activation was associated with the subject's being in episodic retrieval mode, rather than any success in the retrieval attempt.

A third comparison confirmed this picture: the subtraction of unsuccessful from successful retrieval. Subjects were in the retrieval mode in both conditions being compared, and the right-frontal retrieval-mode activation was subtracted out.[3]

Although it is far too early to begin formulating coherent stories of episodic memory in the brain, the available data do permit some speculations. One possible scenario is the following. The right frontal cortical regions, in concert with other parts of the retrieval network, are involved in the establishment and active maintenance of a specific neurocognitive state, or set, that is necessary but not sufficient for successful episodic retrieval. Probably many other such neurocognitive sets are actively maintained and in operation in the brain all the time. They determine the kind of processing that is performed on incoming and on-line information and presumably inhibit the many other kinds of processing that the brain is capable of performing on the same stimuli. The point is that the establishment, maintenance, and switching of these frontal sets require massive and presumably highly complex neuronal activity of a kind possible only for highly developed brains, such as those of humans and possibly other higher primates. This is where the story of episodic memory as a very recent evolutionary adaptation comes in.

One can imagine that, like other cognitive sets that psychologists have been studying since the days of the Würzburg School, episodic retrieval sets too represent a clever trick of nature that enables the brain to do a great deal of task-relevant processing of a stimulus before the stimulus occurs. In the case of episodic retrieval sets, it is possible to imagine that the processing done before successful ecphory occurs is that involved in suffusing the act of retrieval with the feeling of "warmth and intimacy" that William James ascribed to the recollection of personally experienced events. In more contemporary terms, we could say that the right frontal lobe plays a critical role in the creation of autonoetic awareness of the past, the kind of awareness that distinguishes episodic memory retrieval from semantic memory retrieval.

We are obviously treading on rather thin ice here; much more work is needed before we can tell how useful these kinds of speculations are. Indeed, before we can begin seriously wondering about the neuroanatomical correlates of autonoetic awareness—the awareness of self in one's subjective past—we should try to obtain evidence that autonoetic awareness can be distinguished from other kinds of awareness at the level of brain activity.

This is not an easy task. The major complication lies in the fact that conscious awareness is inextricably tied to preconscious and nonconscious processes that are always present in all cognitive activity. The difficulty caused by the tight coupling of conscious and nonconscious cognitive processes is well known to students of consciousness. The solution is logically simple: if we wish to capture something of the neural correlates of conscious awareness, we must be able, somehow, to pry apart the conscious and nonconscious processes in cognition.

Conscious Awareness and Electrophysiological Activity

We have recently completed an event-related potentials (ERP) study in which we took the first step toward such dissociation of different

kinds of conscious states and correlating them with the electrophysiological activity of the brain (Düzel, Yonelinas, Heinze, Mangun, and
Tulving, 1997). We adopted an experimental design that allowed us
to do two things. First, we separated autonoetic awareness of past
events from noetic awareness, and separated each of them from the
absence of any awareness of past events. Second, we separated the
electrophysiological signatures of the two different states of conscious
awareness from the electrophysiological signatures of those brain
processes that were present but did not contribute to these states. In
designing the experiment, we made use of two paradigms that have
been explored in cognitive psychology. One is the so-called R/K
(remember/know) paradigm that has been used in studies of episodic
recognition (Gardiner and Java, 1993). It is quite simple: When
the subject claims to recognize a test item as "old," she is asked to
reflect on the nature of her awareness of the past. Does she autonoetically remember the event of the target item's occurrence in the
study list, or does she noetically know the fact that the target
item was part of the list, without any autonoetic recollection of the
event?

The other paradigm—which we refer to as the DRM paradigm,
after the initials of its developers—was initially constructed by Deese
(1959) and further developed by Roediger and McDermott (1995).
This paradigm, in which close semantic associates of studied words
are used as "lures" in the yes/no recognition test, produces very high
rates of false alarms.

In brief, we adapted this paradigm to produce a large number of
true and false targets for recognition tests in which subjects made "remember" (autonoetic awareness) and "know" (noetic awareness)
judgments about all test items they called old. Subjects claimed both
autonoetic and noetic awareness for both true and false targets. Thus
we had four kinds of outcomes of the recognition test, and we examined the ERP waveforms associated with each. We assumed that the
components of the ERP waveform that were identical for true and
false targets reflected common features of retrieval, namely the subjects' judged state of conscious awareness. We also assumed that the
components of the waveform that differed for the true and false targets reflected processing differences of which the subjects were unaware. Those would be processes involved in the creation of the "en-

grams" that would be used in retrieval, and would necessarily be different for true and false engrams.

The study yielded two important findings. First, many components of the ERP waveforms were quite different for R and K judgments, that is, for autonoetic and noetic states of awareness of past events. Second, in the 600- to 1,000-millisecond recording window, the R and K judgments were essentially identical for true and false targets.

The scalp distribution associated with "remember" responses showed a widespread positivity, involving the anterior regions bilaterally and the left posterior regions more than the right posterior regions. In contrast, "know" responses were associated with a widespread negativity. The results are unambiguous: the brain's electrophysiological activity that is associated with autonoetic awareness of past events is rather strikingly different from the electrophysiological activity that is associated with noetic awareness.

Conclusion

We began this chapter by pointing to a fundamental distinction between different forms of memory in terms of how their operations are oriented in time. Contrary to traditional thinking, most forms of memory are future oriented. Conscious awareness of specific past happenings is irrelevant in these forms of memory. The single exception to the general picture is episodic memory. It is in many ways similar to semantic memory, but goes beyond it in that it is oriented to the past. It allows organisms that possess it to travel autonoetically through subjective time: from the present to the past, and through the past to the future. It is reasonable to assume that episodic memory is a recent evolutionary adaptation, possibly unique in humans. As such, it is subserved by special neural mechanisms. Indeed, early PET studies have pointed to specific neuroanatomical regions involved in episodic encoding and retrieval. An especially striking finding is hemispheric encoding/retrieval asymmetry (HERA) in the prefrontal cortex, possibly extending posteriorly: the left frontal lobes are differentially involved in semantic-memory retrieval and episodic-memory encoding, whereas the right frontal lobes are differentially involved in episodic-memory retrieval.

In the last part of the chapter we described data from an event-related potentials study that provided electrophysiological evidence for the distinction between autonoetic and autonoetic awareness as two modes of mental access to the past. Autonoetic awareness is identified with episodic memory and seems to depend critically on the frontal lobes. Noetic awareness, the evolutionary predecessor of autonoetic awareness, accompanies retrieval of information from semantic memory. Episodic retrieval mode is a neurocognitive set, maintained in the form of massively coherent neuronal activity in regions of the brain including the right prefrontal cortex. Autonoetic awareness of one's past, and one's future, is an emergent feature of such activity.

A general lesson to be drawn from this chapter is that episodic memory and autonoetic consciousness are true marvels of nature whose uniqueness has been frequently underestimated. With the advent of modern techniques for measuring and imaging the workings of the living brain, the prospects for a fuller appreciation of these wonders are much brighter.

References

Buckner, R. L. (1996). Beyond HERA: Contributions of specific prefrontal brain areas to long-term memory retrieval. *Psychonomic Bulletin and Review, 3,* 149–158.

Buckner, R. L., Petersen, S. E., Ojemann, J. G., Miezin, F. M., Squire, L. R., and Raichle, M. E. (1995). Functional anatomical studies of explicit and implicit memory retrieval tasks. *Journal of Neuroscience, 15,* 12–29.

Buckner, R. L., Raichle, M., Miezin, F. M., and Petersen, S. E. (1996). Functional anatomic studies of memory retrieval for auditory words and visual pictures. *Journal of Neuroscience, 16,* 6219–35.

Cabeza, R., Kapur, S., Craik, F. I. M., McIntosh, A. R., Houle, S., and Tulving, E. (1997). Functional neuroanatomy of recall and recognition: A PET study of episodic memory. *Journal of Cognitive Neuroscience, 9,* 254–265.

Calabrese, P., Markowitsch, H. J., Durwen, H. F., Widlitzek, H., Haupts, M., Holika, B., et al. (1996). Right temporofrontal cortex as critical locus for the ecphory of old episodic memories. *Journal of Neurology, Neurosurgery, and Psychiatry, 61,* 304–310.

Deese, J. (1959). On the prediction of occurrence of particular verbal intrusions in immediate recall. *Journal of Experimental Psychology, 58,* 17–22.

Düzel, E., Yonelinas, A. P., Heinze, H. J., Mangun, G. R., and Tulving, E. (1997). Event-related brain potential correlates of two states of conscious awareness in memory. *Proceedings of the National Academy of Sciences (USA), 94,* 5973–78.

Fletcher, P. C., Frith, C. D., and Rugg, M. D. (1997). The functional neuroanatomy of episodic memory. *Trends in the Neurosciences, 20,* 213–218.

Fletcher, P. C., Frith, C. D., Grasby, P. M., Shallice, T., Frackowiak, R. S. J., and Dolan, R. J. (1995). Brain systems for encoding and retrieval of auditory-verbal memory: An in vivo study in humans. *Brain, 118,* 401–416.

Fletcher, P. C., Shallice, T., Frith, C. D., Frackowiak, R. S. J., and Dolan, R. J. (1996). Brain activity during memory retrieval: The influence of imagery and semantic cueing. *Brain, 119,* 1587–96.

Gardiner, J. M., and Java, R. I. (1993). Recognizing and remembering. In A. F. Collins, S. E. Gathercole, M. A. Conway, and P. E. Morris (Eds.), *Theories of memory* (pp. 163–188). Hillsdale, NJ: Lawrence Erlbaum.

Gibson, E. I. (1969). *Principles of perceptual learning and development.* New York: Appleton-Century-Crofts.

Haxby, J. V., Ungerleider, L. G., Horwitz, B., Maisog, J. M., Rapoport, S. L., and Grady, C. L. (1996). Face encoding and recognition in the human brain. *Proceedings of the National Academy of Sciences (USA), 93,* 922–927.

Hayman, C. A. G., MacDonald, C. A., and Tulving, E. (1993). The role of repetition and associative interference in new semantic learning in amnesia. *Journal of Cognitive Neuroscience, 5,* 375–389.

Hodges, J. R., and McCarthy, R. A. (1993). Autobiographical amnesia resulting from bilateral paramedian thalamic infarction. *Brain, 116,* 921–940.

Horgan, J. (1996). *The end of science.* New York: Addison-Wesley.

Kapur, S., Craik, F. I. M., Jones, C., Brown, G. M., Houle, S., and Tulving, E. (1995). Functional role of the prefrontal cortex in retrieval of memories: A PET study. *Neuroreport, 6,* 1880–84.

Kapur, S., Craik, F. I. M., Tulving, E., Wilson, A. A., Houle, S., and Brown, G. M. (1994). Neuroanatomical correlates of encoding in episodic memory: Levels of processing effect. *Proceedings of the National Academy of Sciences (USA), 91,* 2008–11.

Kapur, S., Tulving, E., Cabeza, R., McIntosh, A. R., Houle, S., and Craik, F. I. M. (1996). The neural correlates of intentional learning of verbal materials: A PET study in humans. *Cognitive Brain Research, 4,* 243–249.

Markowitsch, H. J., Calabrese, P., Liess, J., Haupts, M., Durwen, H. F., and Gehlen, W. (1993). Retrograde amnesia after traumatic injury of the fronto-temporal cortex. *Journal of Neurology, Neurosurgery, and Psychiatry, 56,* 988–992.

Nyberg, L., Cabeza, R., and Tulving, E. (1996). PET studies of encoding and retrieval: The HERA model. *Psychonomic Bulletin and Review, 3,* 135–148.

Nyberg, L., McIntosh, A. R., Cabeza, R., Habib, R., Houle, S., and Tulving, E. (1996). General and specific brain regions involved in encoding and retrieval of events: What, where, and when. *Proceedings of the National Academy of Sciences (USA), 93,* 11280–85.

Nyberg, L., Tulving, E., Habib, R., Nilsson, L.-G., Kapur, S., Houle, S., Cabeza, R., and McIntosh, A. R. (1995). Functional brain maps of retrieval mode and recovery of episodic information. *Neuroreport, 7,* 249–252.

Owen, A. M., Milner, B., Petrides, M., and Evans, A. C. (1996). A specific role for the right parahippocampal gyrus in the retrieval of object-location: A positron emission tomography study. *Journal of Cognitive Neuroscience, 8,* 588–602.

Perner, J., and Ruffman, T. (1995). Episodic memory and autonoetic consciousness: Developmental evidence and a theory of childhood amnesia. *Journal of Experimental Child Psychology, 59,* 516–548.

Roediger, H. L. III, and McDermott, K. B. (1995). Creating false memories: Remembering words not presented in lists. *Journal of Experimental Psychology: Learning, Memory, and Cognition, 21,* 803–814.

Rugg, M. D., Fletcher, P. C., Frith, C. D., Frackowiak, R. S. J., and Dolan, R. J. (1997). Brain regions supporting intentional and incidental memory: A PET study. *Neuroreport, 8,* 1283–87.

Schacter, D. L. (1987). Memory, amnesia and frontal lobe dysfunction. *Psychobiology, 15,* 21–36.

Schacter, D. L., and Tulving, E. (1994). *Memory systems 1994.* Cambridge, MA: MIT Press.

Shallice, T., Fletcher, P., Frith, C. D., Grasby, P., Frackowiak, R. S. J., and Dolan, R. J. (1994). Brain regions associated with acquisition and retrieval of verbal episodic memory. *Nature, 368,* 633–635.

Squire, L. R. (1987). *Memory and brain.* New York: Oxford University Press.

Squire, L. R., Knowlton, B., and Musen, G. (1993). The structure and organization of memory. *Annual Review of Psychology, 44,* 453–495.

Suddendorf, T., and Corballis, M. C. (1997). Mental time travel and the evolution of the human mind. *Genetic, Social, and General Psychology Monographs, 123,* 133–167.

Tulving, E. (1983). *Elements of episodic memory*. New York: Oxford University Press.

Tulving, E. (1993). Varieties of consciousness and levels of awareness in memory. In A. Baddeley and L. Weiskrantz (Eds.), *Attention: Selection, awareness, and control. A tribute to Donald Broadbent* (pp. 283–299). Oxford: Clarendon Press.

Tulving, E., Kapur, S., Craik, F. I. M., Moscovitch, M., and Houle, S. (1994a). Hemispheric encoding/retrieval asymmetry in episodic memory: Positron emission tomography findings. *Proceedings of the National Academy of Sciences (USA), 91,* 2016–20.

Tulving, E., Kapur, S., Markowitsch, H. J., Craik, F. I. M., Habib, R., and Houle, S. (1994b). Neuroanatomical correlates of retrieval in episodic memory: Auditory sentence recognition. *Proceedings of the National Academy of Sciences (USA), 91,* 2012–15.

Tulving, E., Schacter, D. L., McLachlan, D. R., and Moscovitch, M. (1988). Priming of semantic autobiographical knowledge: A case study of retrograde amnesia. *Brain and Cognition, 8,* 3–20.

Wheeler, M. A., Stuss, D. T., and Tulving, E. (1997). Toward a theory of episodic memory: The frontal lobes and autonoetic consciousness. *Psychological Bulletin, 121,* 331–354.

Notes

1. We are grateful to Professor Jaan Puhvel for adapting this term for us from the classical Greek.
2. Again, our thanks to Professor Puhvel for adapting this term.
3. There are, of course, other activations in post-Rolandic cortical regions that do reflect the differences between successful and unsuccessful retrieval, reflecting other retrieval processes and perhaps including sites at which previously stored traces are activated. But that is another story, and much more work is needed before we can have much confidence in what the data seem to be telling us.

Memory and Belief in Autobiographical Recall and Autobiography

Constructing and Appraising Past Selves 8

Michael Ross
Anne E. Wilson

One of us (MR) was recently invited to complete a survey on diet, lifestyle, and health conducted on middle-aged alumni of the University of Toronto. Having burdened many others with research questionnaires, MR felt obliged to respond as best he could. Respondents were asked how many hours per week, on average, they had spent on various activities in the past year (sitting at home, standing or walking around at home); how frequently, on average, they had consumed various beverages and foods (per day, per week, per month); and how often each year during different decades of their life they had engaged in recreational pursuits (swam at an outdoor pool, sunbathed, hiked, played baseball, soccer, and football, or climbed a glacier). Respondents were also asked to describe themselves now and in the past on specific dimensions (current weight versus weight at age 20).

MR did not find these questions easy to answer, although he was fairly certain of some of his responses. Growing up in Toronto, he had seen lots of ice and snow, but no glaciers. The first time he could remember encountering a glacier was in the early 1970s, at the Columbia Ice Fields in the Canadian Rockies. He recalled walking a little on the glacier and riding over it in a tourist vehicle, so he decided to give himself credit for climbing a glacier.

One difficulty with most of the questions was that they could not be answered simply by retrieving stored memories. Few people have stored how many hours per week they sit at home, or how frequently

231

per year they sunbathed between the ages of 20 and 29. Answers to such questions have to be constructed from memories (number of hours remembered as sitting at home yesterday), arithmetic calculations (to construct averages), and people's beliefs about how they have changed or remained the same over time. For example, MR was certain that, like most people, he was skinnier at age 20 than in middle age, but how much so?

Also, MR was concerned that his preferences might have colored his answers. Some of the questions probed for healthy and unhealthy behavior. Respondents were asked how often they ate regular-fat ground beef versus medium-fat and lean ground beef. A health-conscious person, MR would like to believe that he favors the leaner cuts of meat. Yet he recalled that he occasionally buys regular-fat ground beef in the belief that it yields tastier hamburgers than its leaner counterparts. How often does he consume each type of beef? MR also engaged in an internal debate when answering questions about smoking. How frequently did he smoke pipes and cigars, and at what age did he give them up? In sum, MR's answers were constructions, reflecting his beliefs, preferences, and guesses, as well as his retrieval of stored memories.

Constructing the Past

Clearly, one is not often asked such detailed questions about personal behaviors over the life span. Nonetheless, the process of trying to answer these questions is probably fairly representative of autobiographical recall in general. Autobiographical memory is a constructive process: evidence for its creative nature comes from a variety of sources. First, different people sometimes report contrasting recollections of the same episodes (Ross, 1981, 1997; Ross and Sicoly, 1979). One of our favorite conflicting memories involves Sir Fredric Bartlett, an advocate of the constructive approach to memory. In the preface to a book published in 1932, Bartlett wrote that the Laboratory of Experimental Psychology at Cambridge was formally opened on "a brilliant afternoon in May 1913." Bartlett offered no indication that he felt a need to verify the veracity of this memory. Instead, this noted constructivist evidently accepted the accuracy of his own recall. Interestingly, another person present at the opening of the laboratory, Sir

Godfrey Thompson, remembered that it poured rain (Zangwill, 1972). Although some memory conflicts no doubt reflect differences in how people originally perceived and stored events, others may be attributable to people's differing beliefs and goals at the time of retrieval (Ross, 1997).

There is more direct evidence that people's current goals and knowledge influence recollections. Research on nonliterate societies indicates that social groups alter their histories to make them consistent with their present knowledge (Goody and Watt, 1968; Henige, 1980; Ong, 1982; Packard, 1980). For example, at the time the British arrived in Ghana in the early part of this century, the state of Gonja was divided into seven territories, each ruled by its own chief (Goody and Watt, 1968). When British authorities asked them to explain their territorial arrangement, the Gonja reported that the founder of their state, Ndewura Jakpa, had divided the land so that each of his seven sons ruled one territory. Shortly after the British arrived, two of the seven states in Gonja disappeared as a result of changes in boundaries. Sixty years later, historians again recorded the myths of state. In the updated version, Ndewura Jakpa had only five sons and the Gonja failed to mention the founders of the two territories that had ceased to exist.

Efforts to alter inconvenient aspects of the past also occur in literate societies (Goody and Watt, 1968; Ross and Buehler, 1994). In his autobiography Natan Sharansky (1988) described modifications to the *Great Soviet Encyclopedia*. The first target of revision was Lavrenty Beria, a chief of the secret police who was executed for being a British spy. Subscribers to the encyclopedia were instructed to destroy the article on Beria and were provided additional information on the Bering Strait to fill the gap in the pages. According to Sharansky, subscribers frequently received such missives.

Less dramatically perhaps, people also revise their own personal histories. Long-term recollections are often constructions that reflect the impact of people's beliefs, knowledge, and goals at the time of retrieval, in addition to stored memories (Bartlett, 1932; Fischhoff and Beyth, 1975; Greenwald, 1980; Mead, 1929/1964; Ross, 1989; Ross and Buehler, 1994; Singer and Salovey, 1993). A number of experimental studies demonstrate the impact of current beliefs on autobiographical recall. Ross, McFarland, and Fletcher (1981) provided some university students with arguments that frequent brushing of teeth helps the teeth and gums; others received information that it was harmful. Participants subsequently recalled how often they had brushed their teeth in the past few weeks. The group persuaded that brushing was harmful reported a lower frequency than those given the opposite communication. In another study Santioso, Kunda, and Fong (1990) induced individuals to believe that extroversion is superior to introversion, or the reverse. Later, those who favored extroversion more readily recalled engaging in extroverted behaviors than did those who preferred introversion. Feldman Barrett (1997) studied the relation of people's enduring self-concepts to their recollections. Respondents kept diary ratings of their emotional experiences and subsequently recalled the emotions they had reported. Those who scored high on a neuroticism scale remembered experiencing more negative emotion than they had reported; conversely, respondents who scored high on extroversion remembered feeling more positive emotion than they had reported earlier.

The Impact of Implicit Theories on Recall

Ross (1989) examined the impact of a particular type of current knowledge on people's autobiographical recall. He proposed that individuals possess implicit theories about the stability of attributes and that they use these theories to construct their past standing on a personal attribute when memories fade or are difficult to access. Implicit theories incorporate specific beliefs regarding the inherent stability of an attribute, as well as general principles concerning the conditions likely to promote change. Within a culture, individuals share many implicit theories. For example, people in our culture seem to suppose that an adult's attitude toward an ethnic group will normally remain stable over time, but might change under certain circumstances, such as increased exposure to that group (Ross, 1989). A theory of this sort is implicit, in that people typically do not learn it through formal education and may rarely discuss it.

To demonstrate the role of implicit theories in recall, we invite the reader to answer the following question: What was your attitude toward capital punishment five years ago? Most people find it difficult to retrieve a past attitude directly from memory. Ross suggested that people often answer such questions by means of a two-step process. Because present beliefs are generally more salient and available than earlier beliefs, individuals begin by considering their current attitude. They then construct their earlier attitude by inferring whether it would have been different from, or similar to, their present position. To determine their attitude toward capital punishment five years ago, people might ask themselves, "Is there any reason to suppose that I felt differently than I do now?" Because adults normally assume that their beliefs are consistent over time (Ross, 1989), most people should infer that their prior attitude was similar to their current belief. They may then corroborate their judgment by selectively recalling instances of past behavior that are congruent with the presumed earlier belief.

Implicit theories often are quite accurate and yield recollections that correspond well with the person's original views. At other times, people's theories may lead them astray. Even valid theories of human behavior do not apply to all contexts and individuals. Ross (1989) reported numerous examples of biases in recall that he attributed to misleading assumptions of personal stability. For example, several researchers demonstrated that people who had recently experienced a change in attitudes exaggerated the consistency between their earlier and their new opinions. In one of these studies, participants described how they had recalled their earlier attitudes: many reported that they assumed their beliefs to be stable over time and that they inferred their previous opinions from their current attitudes.

More recently, Levine (1997) asked supporters of Ross Perot to report their emotional reaction to his abrupt withdrawal from the U.S. presidential race in July 1992. Perot reentered the race the following October and eventually received nearly a fifth of the popular vote. After the elections in November, Levine asked supporters to recall their earlier emotional reaction to Perot's withdrawal and to describe their current feeling toward him. People's memories of their earlier emotion were biased in the direction of their current appraisal of Perot.

McFarland and Ross (1987) found a similar effect in people's recollection of their earlier evaluation of dating partners. People who fell more in love after their initial evaluations exaggerated, and those who fell less in love underestimated, the degree to which they had previously reported caring for their partner. The findings from these two studies suggest that people suppose that their emotional reactions to individuals are fairly stable over time and that they use their current assessments as a basis for inferring their earlier feelings.

Just as individuals sometimes exaggerate their stability, they may also overestimate the degree to which they have changed. Retrospective overestimation of change is likely when people experience a circumstance that they expect to produce change, but that in reality has minimal impact. Self-help programs are a context in which people's expectancies and hopes of change are likely to be disappointed. Although such programs often have considerable face validity, they tend to be remarkably unsuccessful (Ross and Conway, 1986). Another study explored the relation between memory and expectations for change in the context of a study-skills program. After asking university students to evaluate their study skills, researchers randomly assigned half of them to a study-skills program that lasted several weeks and the remaining half to a control condition. Although participants in the treatment program expected to improve their skills (and grades), their program, like most other study-skills courses, was ineffective. At the conclusion of the course, participants in the treatment and control conditions were asked to recall their original rating of their study skills. They were reminded that the researcher had the initial ratings and would assess the accuracy of their recall. Participants who took the course remembered their preprogram rating as being worse than they had initially reported. In contrast, control participants exhibited no systematic bias in recall. The biased recollections of the participants would support their theory that the program had improved their skills. More generally, a tendency to revise the past in order to claim personal improvement may explain why many individuals report that they benefit from ineffective pop therapies and self-improvement programs (Conway and Ross, 1984).

Individuals revise their memories in other contexts on the basis of apparently erroneous theories of change. After reviewing the research literature on the menstrual cycle, McFarland, Ross, and DeCourville (1989) concluded that many women hold theories that exaggerate the effects of menstruation on their physical and psychological well-being.

Why do women fail to alter their beliefs on the basis of their personal experiences? McFarland and her colleagues suggested a possible answer to this question: Perhaps women inadvertently bias their recall in a way that corroborates their theories of menstrual distress. McFarland and her associates conducted a diary study that offered support for their hypothesis. When not menstruating, women engaged in theory-guided retrieval that led them to overestimate the difference between their present level of well-being and their status during their last period. For example, although their levels of depression did not vary systematically across the menstrual cycle, women recalled being more depressed during their last period than they had reported at the time.

The research on autobiographical recall does not indicate that biased recollections are more common than accurate recollections, or that people's implicit theories are generally false. Indeed, in some of the studies described above, researchers reported impressive degrees of accuracy as well as evidence of biased recall (Feldman Barrett, 1997; Levine, 1997). Also, research conducted on autobiographical memory in other contexts has revealed that people's recollections can be fairly accurate, at least for the gist of past experiences (Neisser, 1982). The studies we have described do suggest, however, that individuals' self-concepts, beliefs, and implicit theories influence their recollections.

Appraising Past Selves

To this juncture, we have focused on the content of recall. Recollections often have evaluative aspects as well. People remember events as being happy or sad, and judge their past actions favorably or harshly. Moreover, individuals are sometimes motivated to recall the past in ways that enhance their current views of themselves. In the remainder of the chapter, we present a theory of motivated temporal self-appraisal and preliminary research that supports it.

The theory concerns people's retrospective evaluations of themselves through time. Our interest in this topic was sparked by both psychological research and everyday observation. Research indicates that individuals in our culture tend to view themselves as superior to their peers on a wide range of personality traits and abilities (Taylor and Brown, 1988). Observation of everyday behavior suggests, however, that people typically are far more humble about their earlier attributes and achievements. Here, for example, is actor Mary Tyler Moore's appraisal of her life at the age of 60: "Of all the lives that I have lived, I would have to say that this one is my favorite. I am proud that I have developed into a kinder person than I ever thought I would be. I am less critical than I ever was, and as a result, I'm less critical of myself" (Gerosa, 1997, p. 83). Such derogation of past selves is intriguing because today becomes yesterday; in retrospect, today's superior self seems unremarkable.

Examples of this tendency to criticize past selves are common in published autobiographies. Consider the novelist James Salter's (1997) description of how he reevaluated his prowess as a fighter pilot during the Korean War:

> When I returned to domestic life I kept something to myself, a deep attachment—deeper than anything I had known—to all that had happened. I had come very close to achieving the self that is based on risking everything, going where others would not go, giving what they would not give. Later, I felt I had not done enough, had been too reliant, too unskilled. I had not done what I set out to do and might have done. I felt contempt for myself, not at first but as time passed, and I ceased talking about those days, as if I had never known them. (p. 159)

Ruth Jacobs (1987) captured the inclination to feel contempt for past selves in her poem "Bag Ladies": "Bags of memories/tell us who we were/before we were wise" (p. 167). People's views of their life sometimes seem to mirror the Bildungsroman, a form of novel in which the heroic features of the leading character emerge slowly over time (Buckley, 1974).

People's recollections of improvement may at times reflect their theories of development. A generally shared conception within our culture is that people improve with age on a host of traits, at least until quite late in their life span (Heckhausen and Krueger, 1993). If Tyler Moore's recall is influenced by her theories of aging, she may not view her own improvement as unique, but rather a common occurrence for people in her culture, age group, and social class.

We must also emphasize that people's perceptions of improvement over time are sometimes accurate. Individuals learn from experience. They may judge the present self to be superior to previous versions because it is.

Finally, although modesty about the past may be widespread, it is not inevitable. People tell stories about former achievements as well as about the times that they were "young and foolish." In formulating a theory of temporal self-appraisal, we attempt to describe the *psychological* factors that lead people to revise their evaluation of past selves upward or downward. Furthermore, we examine whether people perceive such shifts to be specific to themselves or more general.

A Theory of Temporal Self-Appraisal

Beginning with the well-validated premise that people in our culture are motivated to think highly of themselves (Baumeister, 1998; Higgins, 1996; Sedikides, 1993), we infer that people are disposed to evaluate the past in a manner that makes them feel content with themselves now. We suggest that people maintain or augment their typically positive views of themselves sometimes by derogating, and other times by enhancing, their former selves. We describe additional ways in which individuals vary their recall to preserve favorable views of themselves.

What psychological factors determine the direction of people's evaluations of past selves? The theorizing of Tesser and his colleagues on social comparison provides some clues (Tesser, 1980, 1988; Tesser and Campbell, 1982; Tesser and Paulhus, 1983). Analyzing how individuals maintain their self-esteem in light of another person's success, these researchers emphasized two variables: the importance of the comparison dimension, and the individual's closeness to the other person. When the achievement occurs on a dimension that is unimportant to self, increased closeness to a successful individual enhances people's self-worth. When the dimension is insignificant, people can bask in the reflected glory of the successful individual (Cialdini et al., 1976). In contrast, people's self-esteem can suffer a blow when a close friend succeeds on a personally important dimension. One's own performance may seem inferior by comparison. Tesser (1988) suggests that people employ several psychological mechanisms to avoid feeling inferior: downplaying their closeness to a successful individual, deemphasizing the significance of the dimension on which the success occurred, or minimizing the magnitude of the other person's achievement.

We propose, metaphorically, to consider past selves as other individuals who range in closeness to current self, and have achievements or failures on attributes that vary in importance to the present self. We suggest that people can maintain their favorable view of current self by shifting their evaluation of past selves, by modifying the significance they attach to the attributes in question, or by altering their judgments of the temporal distance between present and past selves. Like Albert (1977), we consider the relevance to intraindividual (temporal) comparisons of dimensions that have been shown to influence social comparisons. Next, we specify the meaning of each of the key constructs in the model: attribute importance, temporal distance, and retrospective evaluation. We then describe their interrelationships in the context of temporal appraisals.

Attribute Importance

We define an attribute as important if people believe that it helps them to attain significant goals. The importance people accord to attributes can change over time. Characteristics that were important to former selves may seem less important to current selves, and vice versa. Attribute importance can vary with time for a number of reasons. People's goals may change; consequently, attributes that help them to attain specific goals may rise or fall in significance. Also, individuals may maintain the same goals over time, but their means of achieving these goals may shift. For example, as a teenager, Ilana valued dancing because it helped her to obtain the admiration of her peers. In middle age, dancing may seem less important. If her goals have changed, she may no longer seek the approval of her peers. If social approval is still a goal, she may have different ways of achieving it than starring on the dance floor.

Changes in attribute importance can be general as well as idiosyncratic. The importance of some attributes changes with age for most people. Dancing and test-taking ability are likely to have a larger impact on the self-evaluation of teenagers than of 50-year-olds. Because

attribute importance can shift over time, we need to differentiate between current and past importance when considering their impact on
temporal self-appraisal.

Temporal Distance

Temporal distance is partly captured by the passage of time. People
should typically feel closer to recent former selves than to distant past
selves. Their experience of time, however, can differ from actual duration. Previous research reveals that the more detailed one's memory of
an episode, the more recent it seems (Brown, Ripps, and Shevell,
1985). In contrast, the greater the number and novelty of events recalled in the period since the target episode, the more distant it seems
(Block, 1989). Although "time flies" when a person is busy and engaged in interesting activities, that period may feel longer in retrospect
than a similar amount of time in which the person either does very little or performs only routine activities.

   People's experience of temporal distance may also reflect their feelings of similarity to, and empathy for, earlier selves. Because similarity
between selves normally decreases with temporal distance, perceived
similarity may be used as a cue for inferring temporal distance. Selves
that people perceive to be similar should seem close together in time.
William James (1890/1950) emphasized the importance of feelings of
empathy to judgments of distance from past selves. According to
James's reasoning, if Ilana continues to feel discomfort on remembering an event that embarrassed her, then she should feel close to the
self that experienced the event. In contrast, if she can now laugh at
her earlier reactions, then she should feel more distant from her
former self.

   In sum, we associate temporal distance with the psychological experience of closeness between former and current selves. We suggest
that the experience of closeness varies with time, but also with a number of other factors relating to the vividness, nature, and affective
quality of the memories.

Retrospective Evaluation

In considering whether people enhance or deprecate past selves, we
need to specify relative to what. For example, people may evaluate

past selves less favorably than present selves, evaluate past selves less well in retrospect than they did originally, and finally, evaluate past selves as mediocre compared to their peers, but judge present selves to be superior to their peers. The first two forms of disparagement could reflect the reality that people often learn from experience, as well as implicit theories regarding how attributes change over the life span in most people. The last contrast is significant because it cannot be readily interpreted in these ways. Improvement with age does not directly imply improvement relative to one's peers. If Ilana presumes that social skills improve with age, then she could view herself as in the 50th percentile on social skills at both age 16 and age 20, even though she sees personal improvement. In contrast, if she perceives her improvement to be relatively special, then she should perceive herself to be more superior to her peers in the present than in the past. When temporal self-appraisal is motivated by a desire to think highly of the current self, people tend to view their improvement as quite unique. A perception of distinctive improvement is presumably more self-enhancing than a belief that one is simply developing at the same rate as everyone else. Logically, of course, *most* people cannot change from ordinary to exceptional, relative to their peers.

Relationships among Attribute Importance, Temporal Distance, and Retrospective Evaluation

Each of the variables in our model—attribute importance, temporal distance, and retrospective evaluation—can serve as both cause and effect and is associated interactively with the remaining two. Tesser (1988) made a similar claim for social comparisons. The psychological implications of the dimensions may be quite different, however, when the comparisons are temporal rather than interpersonal. Next, we suggest how each of the variables is determined by the other two.

Predicting Retrospective Evaluation
We propose that perceived temporal distance interacts with attribute importance to influence people's evaluations of their earlier selves. People should generally evaluate a temporally close past self favor-

ably, especially on currently important attributes. Because people experience close selves similarly to current selves (Albert, 1977), individuals may maintain or enhance their current self-worth by inflating the successes of recent selves and discounting their failures, especially on major dimensions.

In contrast, people may be more inclined to deprecate far-off selves. As perceived temporal distance increases, a negative evaluation of a former self should be less likely to tarnish the current self. Furthermore, derogation of distant selves has psychological advantages. An unfavorable past can serve as a downward comparison that helps people to appreciate their current achievements (Wills, 1981). Also, by derogating past selves relative to current selves, individuals can see improvement. People feel good about themselves when they see themselves as moving toward their goals (Baumeister, 1998; Carver and Scheier, 1990; Jones, Rock, Shaver, Goethals, and Ward, 1968). Individuals may be especially motivated to derogate past selves on important attributes, because they can then see themselves as improving on these crucial dimensions.

In sum, we predict that temporal distance and attribute importance combine to influence temporal retrospective evaluations. Close selves will be evaluated more favorably than distant selves; close selves will be evaluated more favorably on currently important than on unimportant attributes; and distant selves will be evaluated more favorably on currently unimportant than on important attributes.

When do people hesitate to derogate even distant selves? We have suggested that people deprecate former selves when doing so enhances their judgment of present selves. From this perspective, individuals should be reluctant to criticize a remote self if they see its defects as tainting the present self. If, for example, people's past behavior could be construed as immoral, then even exemplary conduct in the more recent past may not fully counteract the evaluative implications of their earlier actions ("once a thief, always a thief"). As a result, individuals may seek to justify such actions to themselves or minimize their negative connotations.

More generally, people have implicit theories concerning the mutability of traits (Dweck and Leggett, 1988). They view some personal characteristics as readily changeable and others as invariable. People should be particularly interested in denying that their past behavior reveals evidence of unchangeable negative traits.

We propose, as well, that people may enhance distant selves on attributes that have decreased in importance over time. Suppose, for example, that a middle-aged man played sports when he was younger because it earned him the admiration of his peers. Presume, also, that his athletic prowess has declined with age, but that he now has other ways of earning social approval. He may then celebrate and even embellish his former athletic achievements. By dwelling on earlier achievements, he is reminded of successful goal attainment. This type of enhancement of the past can be likened to "basking in reflected glory" (Cialdini et al., 1976) and have a positive effect on present self-regard.

In contrast, enhancing the past on currently important attributes should be detrimental to self-views. If a middle-aged man still wanted to be a star athlete at his present age, then glorifying his past achievements would highlight his subsequent decline. Interestingly, people may often be able to avoid seeing themselves as declining on *important* attributes. People generally view their positive qualities as more meaningful than their negative qualities (Baumeister, 1998; Pelham, 1991). Therefore, perceptions of dwindling achievement may tend to be associated with reductions in the significance of an attribute.

A decrease in the importance of an attribute should depend on a shift in goals or the means of attaining them. When such alterations do not occur, a comparison to better-off former selves should be discouraging. For example, unemployed individuals who focus on their earlier periods of employment experience depression and lowered self-esteem rather than elation (Sheeran, Abrams, and Orbell, 1995). Presumably they are unable to bask in the reflected glory of their former selves, because the attribute on which they declined remains meaningful to them.

Predicting Temporal Distance
We propose that people's evaluations of past selves combine with the current importance of the attributes to influence people's perceptions of temporal distance. People should generally judge unfavorably evaluated past selves to be temporally remote, especially when the attrib-

utes assessed are important. By distancing negatively evaluated past selves, people can avoid deprecating their present selves. In contrast, people can enhance the present self by perceiving successful past selves to be close, especially when the success occurs on critical dimensions. By narrowing the temporal distance, individuals can continue to take credit for their earlier achievements. We predict, then, that negatively evaluated former selves are seen as more temporally distant than favorably evaluated past selves, that negatively evaluated former selves are seen as more temporally distant when the dimensions of evaluation are important rather than unimportant, and that favorably evaluated former selves are seen as temporally closer when the dimensions are important rather than unimportant.

Predicting Attribute Importance

Finally, people's evaluations of former selves should interact with perceived temporal distance to influence estimates of the importance of an attribute. Previous research indicates that people view their positive qualities as more important than their negative qualities (Baumeister, 1998; Pelham, 1991), and Tesser (1988) reasoned that people can reduce the perceived importance of an attribute to alleviate the pain of an unfavorable *social* comparison. We predict that individuals should typically consider unfavorably evaluated attributes to be unimportant, especially in close selves; in contrast, they should regard favorably evaluated attributes to be important, especially in close selves.

Alternative Explanations for Derogating Past Selves

According to the theory of temporal self-appraisal, people deprecate their past if it makes them feel better in the present. There are factors beyond those described in the theory, however, that can contribute to disparagement of former selves. People may work particularly hard to better themselves on important attributes and therefore may actually improve more on these dimensions. Also, the passage of time often allows people to adopt a more dispassionate view of the past. For example, when reviewing a conflict after anger has subsided, individuals may conclude that they were not as blameless as they had thought earlier (Wilson, Celnar, and Ross, 1997). Furthermore, individuals may obtain information over time that leads them to reassess downward their past actions or qualities. Perhaps they learn that the outcomes of their actions were not as favorable as they had anticipated. Disillusionment of this sort is probably common, because people are often too optimistic about their futures (Armor and Taylor, forthcoming). And mistakes may seem more obvious in hindsight than they appeared at the time (Fischhoff and Beyth, 1975). In retrospect, people may view errors of judgment as foolish blunders, even though their original decisions were appropriate in light of the then-available information.

We suggest that such interpretations explain only some of the variance in temporal appraisals, and that our model yields predictions and data not accounted for by the competing explanations. The model differs from the alternative interpretations in predicting that people vary their assessments of importance and closeness, as well as their evaluations of past selves. The predictions involving distance and importance help differentiate temporal self-appraisal theory from other plausible interpretations of a tendency to denigrate past selves (for example, hindsight bias). Moreover, although such a long list of plausible mechanisms may make it seem inevitable that people will derogate their pasts, the model of temporal self-appraisal predicts that people will sometimes instead glorify former selves.

Finally, although we focus on *self*-perceptions, the temporal self-appraisal model can be extended to individuals' views of other people, relationships, surroundings, and possessions through time. The theory is relevant whenever people feel strongly about an entity, whenever their association with it has extended over time, and whenever it helps them to accomplish important goals. The theory predicts that if a marriage (or automobile) is currently going well and is important to people, then they may view past problems in the relationship (with the automobile) as psychologically more distant than they would if the relationship (or automobile) currently needed repair. Also, if the quality of a relationship (automobile) has declined, then people may reduce its importance to their goals.

Research Questions and Supporting Evidence

Derogation of Past Selves

As discussed earlier, Conway and Ross (1984) found that individuals who took an ineffective study-skills course remembered their preprogram ratings as being worse than they had reported initially. One interpretation of this finding is that participants deprecated their earlier attainments to see improvement on a dimension that mattered to them. However, another conceivable interpretation suggested by Conway and Ross is that participants simply believed in the efficacy of the program; overestimating their improvement, they exaggerated the discrepancy between their current and their earlier skill levels. There is no need to assume that participants' bias in recall is motivated by a desire for self-enhancement.

We have conducted several studies to examine whether people disparage their past selves more generally, and to provide a preliminary assessment of our temporal self-appraisal model. To minimize self-presentational concerns in all studies, we assured respondents that their answers would remain confidential and anonymous.

In an initial study, we asked university students to list adjectives that described what they were like at age 16 and what they are like now. We coded the adjectives into three categories: positive, negative, and neutral. Participants used more negative traits (for instance, moody, mean, snobby) and fewer positive traits (for example, friendly, confident, dedicated) to describe their 16-year-old selves than to describe their current selves. Yet participants viewed even their former selves fairly favorably. On average, 59 percent of the adjectives used to describe 16-year-old selves were positive and 25 percent were negative; the comparable figures for present selves were 77 percent and 14 percent.

Next, we asked another group of university students to talk into a tape recorder, describing what they are generally like now, relative to their peers, and what they were like at age 16. Participants spontaneously offered more positive and fewer negative comments about current than about past selves. They praised their 16-year-old selves in 45 percent of their statements and criticized them 35 percent of the time. Sixty-six percent of participants' descriptions of present selves were favorable and only 18 percent were derogatory.

People's perception of improvement over time in the above research may reflect reality and/or their implicit theories of how attributes change with age. If deprecation of the past is motivated by a desire to regard the present self favorably, then individuals should view themselves as improving more than their peers over a similar period of development. We examined this hypothesis in several different ways.

In one study, pairs of adult siblings evaluated themselves and their sibs on a variety of relationship behaviors and attributes (such as problem-solving skills). At least one member of each pair was a university student and the other was a maximum of four years older or younger. They rated themselves and their sibs in the past year and when they were growing up (defined as under 12 years old). Participants generally reported themselves to be superior to their sibs in the recent past and inferior or equal in the more remote past. Although they march together through time, individuals see themselves as exhibiting greater improvement than their brothers or sisters.

In another study, we asked university students to evaluate their standing relative to their same-age peers on seven positive attributes, including social skills, willingness to stand up for own beliefs, and consideration. Participants assessed themselves on these characteristics as they are now, relative to others of their current age, and as they recalled being at the age of 16, relative to their same-aged peers. On each dimension participants compared themselves to others on a seven-point scale, with the midpoint labeled "same as most." Seventy-one percent of participants rated themselves as better than most of their peers at their current age. Only 53 percent rated themselves as better than most at age 16.

These studies suggest that young adults view their earlier selves as relatively ordinary and their current selves as superior, compared to same-aged peers. Do older participants show the same tendencies? We asked the parents of one of our university samples to evaluate themselves on the identical seven attributes as their children had. Parents assessed themselves relative to their same-aged peers in the present, and at the ages of 19 and 16. Parents in this sample, ranging in age from 44 to 55, evaluated themselves much more favorably than their peers at the present time. They were significantly less in awe of themselves at the ages of 19 or 16. Parents rated their past 19-year-old selves less favorably than their 19-year-old children evaluated current selves. Parents also did not differentiate between their 19-year-old and 16-year-old selves (they were equally undistinguished), whereas their children were far more impressed with their current 19-year-old selves than with their 16-year-old selves. Like young adults, middle-aged people view their present selves much more favorably than past selves.

Next, we greatly expanded the number of attributes on which university students evaluated themselves. We included ten positive (for example, resourceful, pleasant), ten negative (for instance, bigoted, dull), and ten more neutral or descriptive (reserved, impulsive) attributes as assessed by Saucier (1994). We also used a different scale of relative standing, asking people to estimate their percentile rank relative to their age group. On the positive and negative traits, we replicated the tendency to rate the current self as superior to one's peers and the past self as less exceptional. On the neutral traits, participants assessed themselves as ordinary now and in the past. Neutral traits presumably have few implications for self-worth.

Across different measures and samples, then, we found that people view themselves as relatively superior in the present and more ordinary in the past. The finding that participants see greater improvement in themselves than in their peers is not readily interpreted as reflecting either implicit theories or reality. This finding is consistent with the idea that participants deprecate past selves in order to enhance current selves. We next examine whether derogation of past selves does indeed serve to boost people's ratings of their present selves.

Derogation of Past Selves Enhances Ratings of Present Selves

We have suggested that criticizing temporally remote past selves allows people to see improvement and therefore feel better about their current selves. A study by Strack, Schwarz and Gschneidinger (1985) provides indirect support for this hypothesis. These researchers examined the impact of recalling positive or negative events on current life satisfaction. Remembering recent positive events enhanced, and recalling recent negative experiences lowered, current satisfaction. A more complex pattern emerged when participants recalled events from the more distant past. If the participant reexperienced the positive or negative affect associated with the event, then satisfaction was influenced in the same direction as it was for recent events. In contrast, if the event was remembered without the original emotion, then recalling positive events lowered current satisfaction, and negative events enhanced it. These results suggest that if a past is experienced as distant (defined by the lack of reexperienced emotion), then focusing on negative aspects can enhance people's current life satisfaction.

In our own research, we have found that providing individuals with the opportunity to deprecate past selves leads them to further enhance their current selves. In several of the studies described earlier, the order of the ratings was counterbalanced. Some participants evaluated remote past selves before they appraised current selves; others completed the evaluations in the reverse order. Although participants evaluated current selves more favorably than past selves regardless of order, they assessed current selves even more favorably after appraising (and derogating) their former selves. This finding is compatible with our notion that denigration of distant former selves can serve to enhance people's views of their current selves.

Derogation of Past Selves Increases with Distance

Our theory predicts that deprecation of past selves increases with temporal distance. As a preliminary test of the hypothesis that people are more likely to derogate remote pasts, we examined the relation between the current age of university students and evaluations of earlier selves in our various studies. Although the undergraduate population is predominantly composed of young adults, some of the studies were conducted with participants from night classes that included more older students. Participants' current ages ranged from 18 to 76 years, and they all rated a past self of 16 years of age. Thus, some participants were relatively close to the past self, whereas others were very distant. As predicted, the older individuals currently are, the more unfavorable their assessment of their 16-year-old selves (r ranged between $-.21$ and $-.50$).

Derogation of Past Selves Increases with Importance of Characteristics

Finally, we examined participants' self-evaluations on traits that varied in importance. In several studies participants evaluated the current importance of the target attributes, after reporting their past and present self-evaluations. About 50 percent of the individual traits revealed significant effects for current importance. As predicted, individuals exhibited greater derogation of past selves relative to current selves on currently important traits. Many of the traits for which this effect was not obtained evidenced little variance in importance ratings (for instance, almost everyone thought it was important to be reliable). Thus no distinction could be made among the self-evaluations of people who valued the trait to differing extents.

We have suggested that people may enhance past selves on attributes that they see as declining in importance with age. Because the attribute is relatively unimportant to them now, they are not threatened by attributing superior performance to a former self. Our analyses of the importance ratings provide some evidence to support this hypothesis. In one study we asked participants to evaluate both how important attributes were to them in the past and how important the attributes were now. We examined sixteen characteristics individually, by comparing the self-ratings of people who reported an increase, a decrease, or no change in the importance of the attribute over time. Thirteen of the traits yielded the expected pattern of results. People who reported that an attribute declined in importance (for example, it was more important for them to be athletic at age 16 than now) enhanced their past relative to their present self-ratings (they reported being better athletes at age 16 than they are now). People who reported that traits increased in importance showed the greatest depreciation of their past standing on those characteristics.

Future Directions

We have focused on evaluations of distant and present selves. Some of the more interesting predictions concern the closeness and importance dimensions, and evaluations of recent past selves. We are currently conducting studies to examine additional predictions from the temporal self-appraisal model. We intend to extend the model also to examine perceptions of objects and relationships through time.

In our current theorizing, we have focused on people's personal reasons for derogating or enhancing the past. Recollections are often public, however, and people's evaluations of past selves may also reflect self-presentational concerns. Individuals are best liked when they strike a balance between humility and self-enhancement (Jones, 1990; Schlenker, 1980; Schlenker and Leary, 1982). By criticizing their past and enhancing their present qualities, people can make use of previous selves to provide humility and of present selves to provide self-enhancement. In addition, criticism of the past may lend credibility to individuals' favorable evaluations of their present attainments.

There are risks, however, to flagellating even past selves. Research on impression formation suggests that observers may sometimes average evaluations across time, weighting unfavorable and earlier information more heavily than favorable and later information (Anderson, 1981; Asch, 1946; Kanouse and Hanson, 1971). These effects appear in studies in which people are typically presented with a list of different trait adjectives (for example, intelligent, shy, lazy, kind) and asked to form overall impressions of a target person. It is unclear whether similar findings would be obtained if targets described themselves as improving over time on a specific trait such as social skills.

Derogating the past will be an effective self-presentational technique only if audiences' unfavorable judgments of a rememberer's past selves do not diminish their assessments of his or her current self. To discourage audiences from fusing the two selves, rememberers may emphasize the distance between their present superior and former inferior selves. Also according to our model, rememberers should publicly attribute unfavorable attributes to past selves only if they perceive the stain as erasable, as when an extremely positive portrayal of the present self more than compensates for one's earlier failings. Rememberers should be less likely to dwell on deficiencies that are seen as immutable.

Finally, we are intrigued by the possibility of cultural differences in temporal self-appraisal. There is evidence that people from collectivist cultures are less likely to enhance current selves than are Europeans and North Americans (Markus, Kitayama, and Heiman, 1996). We wonder whether people in our individualistic culture typically see themselves as superior to their peers because they use temporal comparisons when evaluating themselves, and social comparisons when evaluating other people. Temporal comparisons would be more likely for self because people are more aware of their own histories. Social comparisons may be more likely for others because one lacks temporal information and because oneself is a salient social comparison for others.

The nature of the comparison (social versus temporal) may matter because, on average, social comparisons should yield less favorable evaluations of a target individual than temporal comparisons. Presumably one can almost always identify other people who are better than a target individual on any specific attribute. In contrast, when people look backward in time they may see their current self as superior to any of its predecessors on that same attribute.

Why do people from collectivist cultures not self-enhance? Perhaps they use different standards of comparison for self-assessments than Europeans and North Americans. Because group membership is salient to them, individuals from collectivist cultures may use the same social comparisons when evaluating themselves or other people. As a consequence, their judgments of themselves would parallel their evaluations of other people.

Conclusion

We began by describing how people's knowledge and beliefs at the time of retrieval can influence the content of their recall. We observed that people often judge the past while remembering it; they recall their actions as wise or foolish. We suggested that people seem very willing to criticize their past actions and attributes. Such derogation seems surprising; people in our culture generally have high opinions of themselves. We proposed, however, that deprecation of past selves is not inconsistent with favorable evaluations of present selves. By derogating past actions, people are able to perceive themselves as improving over time.

More generally, we suggested that people are motivated to view their pasts in ways that enhance their current self-view. We proposed a model in which people can maintain their favorable views of themselves by shifting their evaluations of past selves, by modifying the importance they attach to the attributes in question, or by altering their judgments of the temporal distance between present and past selves.

Earlier discussions of autobiographical recall (such as Ross, 1989) depicted rememberers as earnestly trying to recall the past as accurately as possible, using the available information. From this perspective, biased recall is an inadvertent result of misleading personal theories or of changes in knowledge or beliefs. In contrast, the temporal self-appraisal model presents rememberers as motivated to recall the past in a way that enhances their current views of themselves. According to this model, rememberers are sometimes more interested in self-enhancement and self-presentation than in discovering and reporting the facts of their pasts. Of course, these alternatives do not exhaust the possible goals of an autobiographer. When recall is public, for example, another aim of the rememberer may be to tell a story that an audience would find comprehensible and enjoyable (Ross and Buehler, 1994; Ross and Holmberg, 1990).

We will resist the temptation to conclude that our current perspective is superior to our former analysis (and thereby provide additional support for the temporal appraisal model). Instead, we note that the approaches complement each other. Both analyses emphasize the reciprocal relation between autobiographical memory and people's private and social concerns. Autobiographical memory affects how people see themselves and how others view them. At the same time, people's personal and social concerns influence how and what they remember. This reciprocal relation between recall and personal and social interests makes autobiographical memory a fascinatingly complex subject, of interest to a broad cross-section of humanists and scientists. We mine a rich vein, and we expect that it will keep us engaged for many years to come.

References

Albert, S. (1977). Temporal comparison theory. *Psychological Review, 84,* 485–503.

Anderson, N. H. (1981). *Foundations of information integration theory.* New York: Academic Press.

Armor, D. A., and Taylor, S. E. (Forthcoming). Situated optimism: Specific outcome expectancies and self-regulation. In M. P. Zanna (Ed.), *Advances in experimental social psychology,* Vol. 30. New York: Academic Press.

Asch, S. E. (1946). Forming impressions of personality. *Journal of Abnormal and Social Psychology, 41,* 1230–40.

Bartlett, F. C. (1932). *Remembering: A study in experimental and social psychology.* London: Cambridge University Press.

Baumeister, R. (1998). The self. In D. T. Gilbert, S. T. Fiske, and G. Lindzey (Eds.), *Handbook of social psychology* (4th ed.), Vol. 2, pp. 680–740. New York: McGraw Hill.

Block, R. A. (1989). Experiencing and remembering time: Affordances, context, and cognition. In I. Levin and D. Zakay (Eds.), *Time and human cognition: A life-span perspective* (pp. 333–364). Amsterdam: Elsevier.

Brown, N. R., Ripps, L. J., and Shevell, S. K. (1985). Subjective dates of natural events in very long-term memory. *Cognitive Psychology, 17,* 139–177.

Buckley, J. H. (1974). *Season of youth: The Bildungsroman from Dickens to Golding.* Cambridge, MA: Harvard University Press.

Carver, C. S., and Scheier, M. F. (1990). Origins and functions of positive and negative affect: A control process view. *Psychological Review, 97,* 19–35.

Cialdini, R. B., Borden, R. J., Thorne, A., Walker, M. R., Freeman, S., and Sloan, L. R. (1976). Basking in reflected glory: Three (football) field studies. *Journal of Personality and Social Psychology, 39,* 406–415.

Conway, M., and Ross, M. (1984). Getting what you want by revising what you had. *Journal of Personality and Social Psychology, 47,* 738–748.

Dweck, C. S., and Leggett, E. L. (1988). A social-cognitive approach to motivation and personality. *Psychological Review, 95,* 256–273.

Feldman Barrett, L. (1997). The relationship among momentary emotional experiences, personality descriptions, and retrospective ratings of emotion. *Personality and Social Psychology Bulletin, 23,* 1100–10.

Fischhoff, B., and Beyth, R. (1975). "I knew it would happen": Remembered probabilities of once-future things. *Organizational and Human Performance, 13,* 1–16.

Gerosa, M. (1997, Fall). Moore than ever. *Ladies' Home Journal,* pp. 79–83.

Goody, J., and Watt, I. (1968). The consequences of literacy. In J. Goody (Ed.), *Literacy in traditional societies* (pp. 27–68). London: Cambridge University Press.

Greenwald, A. G. (1980). The totalitarian ego: Fabrication and revision of personal history. *American Psychologist, 35,* 603–618.

Heckhausen, J., and Krueger, J. (1993). Developmental expectations for the self and most other people: Age grading in three functions of social comparison. *Developmental Psychology, 29,* 539–548.

Henige, D. (1980). The disease of writing: Ganda and Nyoro kinglists in a newly literate world. In J. C. Miller (Ed.), *The African past speaks: Essays on oral tradition and history* (pp. 240–261). Kent, England: Wm Dawson.

Higgins, E. T. (1996). Self digest: Self-knowledge serving self-regulatory functions. *Journal of Personality and Social Psychology, 71,* 1062–83.

Jacobs, R. H. (1987). Bag ladies. In S. H. Martz (Ed.), *When I am an old woman I shall wear purple*. Watsonville, CA: Papier-Mache Press.

James, W. (1890/1950). *Principles of psychology*. New York: Dover.

Jones, E. E. (1990). *Interpersonal perception*. New York: Freeman.

Jones, E. E., Rock, L., Shaver, K. G., Goethals, G. R., and Ward, L. M. (1968). Pattern of performance and ability attribution: An unexpected primacy effect. *Journal of Personality and Social Psychology, 39*, 496–502.

Kanouse, D. E., and Hanson, R. (1971). Negativity in evaluations. In E. E. Jones, D. E. Kanouse, H. H. Kelley, R. E. Nisbett, S. Valins, and B. Weiner (Eds.), *Attribution: Perceiving the causes of behavior* (pp. 47–62). Morristown, NJ: General Learning Press.

Levine, L. J. (1997). Reconstructing memory for emotion. *Journal of Experimental Psychology: General, 126*, 165–177.

Markus, H., Kitayama, S., and Heiman, R. J. (1996). Culture and basic psychological principles. In E. T. Higgins and A. W. Kruglanski (Eds.), *Social psychology handbook of basic principles*. New York: Guilford Press.

McFarland, C., and Ross, M. (1987). The relation between current impressions and memories of self and dating partners. *Personality and Social Psychology Bulletin, 13*, 228–238.

McFarland, C., Ross, M., and DeCourville, N. (1989). Women's theories of menstruation and biases in recall of menstrual symptoms. *Journal of Personality and Social Psychology, 57*, 522–531.

Mead, G. H. (1929/1964). The nature of the past. In A. J. Reck (Ed.), *Selective writings: George Herbert Mead* (pp. 345–354). Chicago: University of Chicago Press.

Neisser, U. (1982). John Dean's memory: A case study. In U. Neisser (Ed.), *Memory observed: Remembering in natural contexts*. San Francisco: W. H. Freeman.

Ong, W. J. (1982). *Orality and literacy*. New York: Methuen.

Packard, R. M. (1980). The study of historical process in African traditions of genesis: The Bashu myth of Muhiyi. In J. C. Miller (Ed.), *The African past speaks: Essays on oral tradition and history* (pp. 157–177). Kent, England: Wm Dawson.

Pelham, B. W. (1991). On confidence and consequence: The certainty and importance of self-knowledge. *Journal of Personality and Social Psychology, 60*, 518–530.

Ross, M. (1981). Egocentric biases in attributions of responsibility: Antecedents and consequences. In E. T. Higgins, C. P. Herman, and M. P. Zanna (Eds.), *Social cognition*. Hillsdale, NJ: Lawrence Erlbaum.

Ross, M. (1989). The relation of implicit theories to the construction of personal histories. *Psychological Review, 96*, 341–357.

Ross, M. (1997). Validating memories. In N. L. Stein, P. A. Ornstein, B. Tversky, and C. Brainerd (Eds.), *Memory for everyday and emotional events* (pp. 49–82). Hillsdale, NJ: Lawrence Erlbaum.

Ross, M., and Buehler, R. (1994). Creative remembering. In U. Neisser and R. Fivush (Eds.), *The remembering self* (pp. 205–235). New York: Cambridge University Press.

Ross, M., and Conway, M. (1986). Remembering one's own past: The construction of personal histories. In R. M. Sorrentino and E. T. Higgins (Eds.), *The handbook of motivation and cognition: Foundations of social behavior*. New York: Guilford Press.

Ross, M., and Holmberg, D. (1990). Recounting the past: Gender differences in the recall of events in the history of a close relationship. In J. M. Olson and M. P. Zanna (Eds.), *Self-inference processes: The Ontario Symposium on personality and social psychology*, Vol. 6 (pp. 135–152). Hillsdale, NJ: Lawrence Erlbaum.

Ross, M., McFarland, C., and Fletcher, G. J. O. (1981). The effect of attitude on the recall of personal histories. *Journal of Personality and Social Psychology, 40,* 627–634.

Ross, M., and Sicoly, F. (1979). Egocentric biases in availability and attribution. *Journal of Personality and Social Psychology, 37,* 322–336.

Salter, J. (1997). *Burning the days.* New York: Random House.

Santioso, R., Kunda, Z., and Fong, G. T. (1990). Motivated recruitment of autobiographical memories. *Journal of Personality and Social Psychology, 59,* 229–241.

Saucier, G. (1994). Separating description and evaluation in the structure of personality attributes. *Journal of Personality and Social Psychology, 66,* 141–154.

Schlenker, B. R. (1980). *Impression management: The self concept, social identity, and interpersonal relations.* Monterey, CA: Basic Books.

Schlenker, B. R., and Leary, M. R. (1982). Audiences' reactions to self-enhancing, self-denigrating, and accurate self-presentations. *Journal of Experimental Social Psychology, 18,* 89–104.

Sedikides, C. (1993). Assessment, enhancement, and verification determinants of the self-evaluation process. *Journal of Personality and Social Psychology, 65,* 317–338.

Sharansky, N. (1988). *Fear no evil.* New York: Random House.

Sheeran, P., Abrams, D., and Orbell, S. (1995). Unemployment, self-esteem, and depression: A social comparison theory approach. *Basic and Applied Social Psychology, 17,* 65–82.

Singer, J. A., and Salovey, P. (1993). *The remembered self: Emotion and memory in personality.* Toronto: Maxwell Macmillan International.

Strack, F., Schwarz, N., and Gschneidinger, E. (1985). Happiness and reminiscing: The role of time perspective, affect, and mode of thinking. *Journal of Personality and Social Psychology, 49,* 1460–69.

Taylor, S. E., and Brown, J. D. (1988). Illusion and well-being: A social psychological perspective on mental health. *Psychological Bulletin, 103,* 193–210.

Tesser, A. (1980). Self-esteem maintenance in family dynamics. *Journal of Personality and Social Psychology, 39,* 77–91.

Tesser, A. (1988). Toward a self-evaluation maintenance model of social behavior. In L. Berkowitz (Ed.), *Advances in experimental social psychology,* Vol. 21 (pp. 181–227). New York: Academic Press.

Tesser, A., and Campbell, J. (1982). Self-evaluation maintenance and the perception of friends and strangers. *Journal of Personality, 59,* 261–279.

Tesser, A., and Paulhus, D. (1983). The definition of self: Private and public self-evaluation maintenance strategies. *Journal of Personality and Social Psychology, 44,* 672–682.

Wills, T. A. (1981). Downward comparison principles in social psychology. *Psychological Bulletin, 90,* 245–271.

Wilson, A. E., Celnar, C., and Ross, M. (1997). Siblings' self and other perceptions of past and present conflict. Poster presented at American Psychological Association conference, Chicago.

Zangwill, O. L. (1972). Remembering revisited. *Quarterly Journal of Experimental Psychology, 24,* 123–138.

Memory and Belief in Development　　9

Katherine Nelson

Do infants have memory? What kind? For how long? Do young children remember specific events—do they have episodic memories? If they do, why don't we as adults remember those events too? (After all, we recall a great deal from later in childhood—from our school days, for example, which, relatively speaking, is not much longer ago than early childhood.) This is the "infantile amnesia" problem identified by Freud, which has been receiving renewed attention among developmental psychologists after a long period of benign neglect in psychology circles. And if we do remember events from early childhood, how do we know that they really happened rather than being something that someone told us or that we just imagined? How can we believe what children tell us about things that happened to them? Are they making it up?

These questions are among those that have driven research in the developmental psychology of memory for the past twenty years. Before then there was little interest in and less investigation of these topics or others that might bear on these issues. In addition, for the last decade or so interest has burgeoned in what seems to be a different topic: when and how do young children achieve a "theory of mind" (or a psychological understanding) such that they can entertain the possibility that someone has a false belief, or that they themselves believed something in the past that turns out not to be true in the present?

In this chapter I present the case that these two seemingly divergent streams of research converge on the same developmental process, in-

259

volving a potential for entertaining simultaneously two (or more) different representations of reality. The child's emerging capacity at about 4 to 5 years of age to use language as a medium of mental representation is seen as the key to unlocking that potential. This emerging language capacity in turn begins to challenge the young child's initially firm conviction that immediate experience yields enduring and irrefutable knowledge.

Briefly, the claim is that initially the young child's mind and world agree perfectly: for the child the world is as the mind delivers. As a result, the mind itself is transparent and not accessible to reflection by the child. Of course, the child recognizes that other people, such as parents, might know about aspects of the world that are unknown by the child. Because for the child there is perfect agreement between mind and world, there is no need and no place for a separate *concept* of mind, or of belief, true or false, beyond the observed states of the real world in the present. As states of the world change over time, the record is simply overwritten—updated to accord with present perceived reality. Development of mind and memory then involves radical changes in the potentials for knowledge, belief, and self-understanding.

In the following sections I review the basis for these claims about the child's mind, and about what happens to bring about an understanding that mind and world may differ, that beliefs are not necessarily true, that the past need not and should not be overwritten by the present. I begin with the evidence from studies of children's personal memories, and proceed with an overview of the pertinent research on theory of mind and a look at related domains of development. Finally, I gather these strands together to reveal relationships characteristic of the more complex mind-view that emerges by the middle childhood years.

Event Schemas, Episodes, and Narratives in Early Development

An extensive body of research by C. Rovee-Collier and her students, examining memory in infants and toddlers, demonstrates memory for contingent action-event relations over weeks and even months (Rovee-Collier and Shyi, 1992). In addition, research shows that toddlers

(1- to 2-year-olds) may observe, with or without immediate imitation, brief sequences of actions that are causally related to a goal state and recall them when cued after a delay of six months or more (Bauer, Hertsgaard, and Dow, 1994; Hudson and Sheffield, 1993; Mandler, 1990; Meltzoff, 1995). Further, the effect of a "reminder" in the form of one part of the sequence, presented at a critical time lag, may serve as a reinstatement of the originally remembered sequence and result in an extension of the retention interval—often for twice as long as it might otherwise have been (Rovee-Collier, 1995).

However, it is clear from common observation as well as from scientific research (Nelson, 1986, 1989b; Perlmutter, 1980) that by age 1 the infant "knows" about routine events, locations, people, and sets of objects. This kind of memory or knowledge goes beyond the perceptual/motor schemas focused on by Piaget (1952); or by Glenberg (1997), which represent the child's or person's direct interactions with the world. In addition, it includes situational and social specifications; it is reasonable to think of the infant at this age as having schemas or scripts that guide participation in familiar routine events. We have called these general event representations (Nelson, 1986; Nelson and Gruendel, 1981) and consider them to be a kind of or precursor to semantic memory or generalized knowledge base.[1] By 2 years of age, children demonstrate this kind of knowledge not only through symbolic play but also through anticipation of events and engagement in manipulating minor changes in routines, while insisting on the exact maintenance of important rituals such as a bedtime routine (Nelson, 1989b). By 3 years, many young children can articulate a whole scripted event, although in skeletal form. For example, one 3-year-old reported a restaurant script in response to a prompt: "We eat and then we go home" (Nelson, 1978, 1986). That is, the child can externalize the script in language, although there is no evidence that at this age language is effective in establishing a script.

Also during the third and fourth years, many children begin to participate actively with parents in recalling specific episodes that they have experienced in the form of verbal narratives. Children may then use language to indicate some memory that we might be tempted to call episodic, about something that happened one time in the recent past—pointing to a picture and naming the participants, for example.

But the child's ability to articulate this memory is largely dependent on the parent for providing scaffolding cues and elaborations. The child's contributions tend to be in the form of fragments, suggestive of parts of scenes rather than narratives. An example from Engel's (1986) study of mother-child talk about the past illustrates the point:

C: Mommy, the Chrysler Building.

M: The Chrysler Building?

C: The Chrysler Building?

M: Yeah, who works in the Chrysler Building?

C: Daddy.

M: Do you ever go there?

C: Yes, I see the Chrysler Building\picture of the Chrysler Building.

M: I don't know if we have a picture of the Chrysler Building. Do we?

C: We went to . . . my Daddy went to work.

M: Remember when we went to visit daddy? Went in the elevator, way way up in the building so we could look down from the big window?

C: Big window.

M: Mmhm.

C: When . . . we did go on the big building?

M: Mmhm, the big building. Was that fun? Would you like to do it again? Sometime.

C: I want to go on the big building.

In this excerpt the child contributes the topic (the Chrysler Building) and the fragments about Daddy and work, but Mother provides the narrative about the experience that ties the memory into a story with an evaluative component ("Was that fun?") and a suggestion of a repeat visit in the future.

Much research on this process of parent-child memory talk has been documented, and there is considerable evidence that indicates that elaborative scaffolding of the child's contribution to the verbalization of the memory contributes to the retention of both that specific memory and episodic memories in general (Fivush, 1991). Additionally, narrative style of talk during an experience, in contrast to a focus on categories and attributes of objects, contributes to the child's retention of information about the experience over a subsequent period (Tessler and Nelson, 1994). Moreover, a toddler's own use of language during recall of an action sequence at one session is associated with greater retention of the memory after a six-month delay (Bauer and Wewerka, 1997). Future talk may also influence what is remembered, although this effect is less well studied and the evidence is equivocal (Nelson, 1989a).

What kind of memory the studies of early memory in infancy and the toddler years demonstrate is debated—whether recall or recognition, implicit or explicit, procedural or episodic. Perhaps we should not worry too much about the exact category; we may need to describe these early-memory phenomena in different terms than those applicable later in development. I hesitate to term them episodic because of the lack of evidence that the infant or toddler consciously remembers that the sequence of actions that go with a particular object were experienced at a singular time and place in the past; the alternative is that the infant or toddler is reminded of the sequence by the sight of the associated object but does not place the remembering as having been experienced (*autonoetic,* to use Tulving's term), only as a recallable sequence of actions (Nelson, 1994). This phenomenological distinction is of course difficult if not impossible to make for a nonverbal organism, which the 1- to 2-year-old primarily is. (The same difficulty holds for other nonverbal creatures such as the clever chimpanzee.) In light of evidence from later developments, the distinction of episodic versus nonspecific knowledge is nonetheless important.

The challenge for developmentalists is to trace the development of a capacity or skill from a point where it is not in place to its mature form, while remaining neutral with respect to the fit of the analytic categories applied to the mature system. For the memory researcher this implies that the categories of *episodic* and *semantic* may not be appropriate to this early beginning point. Pillemer and White (1989) argue that adults' very early memories tend to be fragments of visual scenes, sometimes including bits from other perceptual modalities. This is consistent with the type of contributions that 2- and 3-year-olds make to memory talk with adults, like that of the 2-year-old child quoted. The implication is that the child's memory, like the adult's for the same early event recalled in later years, is different from later memories. It is not truly episodic, although it retains fragments of episodes recognizable to the adult listener (or later to the adult re-memberer) as based on a personal experience.

Arguing that the memory that we observe in later infancy and early childhood subsequently develops into the categories that Tulving (1983) defined as episodic and semantic, we can think of some types of early memory as protoepisodic and other types as protosemantic. Then we might speculate that young children's protosemantic memory is realized in action, whereas their protoepisodic memory is realized in images. Is the implication that semantic memory grows out of proce-dural? Perhaps; at least it appears to be supported by procedures that are acquired and known implicitly. But the child's scripts—caretaking routines, for example—include more than the sequence of actions. They invoke the roles of other people in the routine, and the use of objects as well as their characteristics and locations, appropriate lan-guage, and other modes of communication. In other words, they are multimodal though organized around action.

To summarize briefly, protoepisodic fragments and scripts may turn into full memories when elaborated into narratives through talk with parents. Effects of these different processes can be seen in memo-ries from childhood recalled later by adults, resulting in some cases in false beliefs about events from early life that are held with strong con-viction. Two examples are telling. The first is a report by Jean Piaget of his earliest "memory," quoted in his own words:

One of my first memories would date, if it were true, from my second year. I can still see, most clearly, the following scene, in which I believed until I was about fifteen. I was sitting in my pram, which my nurse was pushing in the Champs Elysées, when a man tried to kidnap me. I was held in by the strap fastened around me while my nurse bravely tried to stand between me and the thief. She received various scratches, and I can still see vaguely those on her face. Then a crowd gathered, a policeman with a short cloak and a white baton came up, and the man took to his heels. I can still see the whole scene, and can even place it near the tube station. When I was about fifteen, my parents re-ceived a letter from my former nurse saying that she had been converted to the Salvation Army. She wanted to confess her past faults and in particular to return the watch she had been given as a reward on this occasion. She had made up the whole story, faking the scratches. I therefore must have heard, as a child, an account of this story, which my parents believed, and projected it into the past in the form of a visual memory. (Piaget, 1962, pp. 187–188)

This "memory" must have been implanted in Piaget's mind through family conversations about the dramatic event, but instead of retaining the source knowledge—verbal report—the young Piaget incorporated it into his then-emerging personal memory. No doubt the details of the visual scene were based on other experiences that he had with his nursemaid on walks along the Champs Elysées, providing script knowledge on which to draw. This making up of a memory wholly on the basis of verbal representation is rather unusual. But it and similar reports have led to the conclusion—on the part of laypeople as well as many experts—that early memories, especially those retrieved in adulthood, are very unreliable.

More usual than the incorporation of a full account of a past experience such as Piaget's is the construction of an early-self story from bits and pieces of visual imagery fragments and family conversations that fit with them. These may be valid reports of what really happened, or they may be distorted. Comparisons of memories by different family members may provide insight into this process; typically, each sibling has a different point of view reflecting a different developmental stage and relation within the group (Bruner, 1990; Sebris, 1992).

Sebris compared childhood memories by sibling pairs of a dramatic episode: leaving their childhood homes in Latvia toward the end of World War II. She found substantial differences in accounts, in terms of both action sequences and emotions. In one case she was able to document, through comparison of narratives as well as through historical record, that a younger child had assimilated two or three different events shared by all the family members and had projected them backward in time to provide a dramatic rendering of the central scene of leaving their homeland. This memory, like Piaget's, remained vivid and was held with conviction throughout forty years of adult life until finally challenged by the accounts of her two siblings.

Reluctantly this woman began to accept, in light of historical records as well as the siblings' claims, that her account must be wrong; but she reported that it continued to seem right. This strong but inaccurate memory was a construction by a person who at 4 years of age when the trip from Latvia took place was the youngest studied by Sebris. Unlike Piaget, each fragment of her "memory" could be traced to an actual occurrence. No doubt these had been talked about at the time they were experienced, and also during subsequent years as the family waited to emigrate to the United States. The weaving into a coherent whole that made sense to the child was an individual construction that nicely fits Bartlett's (1932) conception of how memory operates.

These false memory constructions reported by adults raise important issues about how language enters into and changes memory during early childhood. In addition, research findings on the effects of memory talk on children's subsequent recall have provoked the question of the mechanism behind the relation between language as used in talk about past, present, and future experiences, and the establishment and retention of memory for these experiences. What does language do for memory in the development of the child? Of course, what language does for the child it may also do for the adult.

Function of Scripts, Episodes, and Narratives

The evident relation of memory talk to later retention of episodic memories in childhood and into adult life provide the background for a theory of memory function and the social origins of autobiographical memory (Nelson, 1993c, 1993d). I briefly review this proposal and our more recent work on verbal reinstatement, before turning to work on false belief and theory of mind in early childhood in order to trace connections between them.

An assumption of the social origins theory is that the basic function of memory for any organism, including humans, is to support and direct action in the present ecological environment and to anticipate future outcomes. Memory has value for the present and future because it predicts on the basis of past probabilities (Nelson, 1988, 1989b, 1993b, 1993c; see Glenberg, 1997, for a similar conception). Memory for recurrent conditions and routine actions (as in scripts) is most useful for this pragmatic purpose. Memory for a one-time occurrence of some event (if the event is not life threatening) is not especially useful, given its low probability of recurrence. It is suggested that the basic memory system is designed to retain information about frequent and recurrent events, to discard or overwrite information about unrepeated events, and to integrate new information about variations in recurrent events into a general knowledge system based on schemas and scripts.

As noted earlier, script-type knowledge of routines is evident very early in development. In the basic system a new experience alerts the person to set up a new schema, which at first may be similar to an episodic memory; but with further experience with events of the same kind it comes more and more to have the function and characteristics of a script. Such a process has been observed for adults as well as for children (Fivush, 1984; Hudson and Nelson, 1986; Linton, 1982; Thompson, Skowronski, Larsen, and Betz, 1996).

A further proposal is that memories for novel events may be retained for a time in a temporary, episodic memory space. If a similar event recurs during that time, it becomes part of the generic system. If a similar event does not recur during that period, the episode as a whole may be eliminated from memory and component bits may be distributed to other schemas (Schank and Abelson, 1995). In this functionally based system, assumed to be in place from at least late infancy, all event memory is either generic knowledge—scriptlike—or *temporarily* episodic. Thus the basic episodic system is hypothesized to be a holding pattern, not a semipermanent memory system.

What then is the function of autobiographical memory, in which single-occurrence events are often retained for decades? The hypothesis is that sharing memory with others is the catalyst that establishes autobiographical memory. By age 4 years children enjoy and actively participate in talking with others about their lives. Sharing memories provides an important context for social participation as well as self-reflection. However, identifying this social function does not in itself explain why personal autobiographical memories continue to persist.

We might want to share some experiences with others, but some personal memories—vivid as they may be—are not generally viewed as appropriate for sharing.

The hypothesis that social interaction is the basis for autobiographical memory has been put forth by a number of developmentalists, most within a Vygotskian framework (Fivush, 1991; Hudson, 1990; Nelson, 1992; Pillemer, Picariello, and Pruett, 1994; Pillemer and White, 1989). Vygotsky, the Soviet developmental theorist of the 1920s and 1930s, proposed a general principle of "higher mental functioning" based on the premise that all higher-level functions appear first on the intermental plane and second on the intramental plane (Vygotsky, 1978). According to this principle, after overt recounting becomes established, covert recounting or conscious reexperiencing to oneself may take place. This principle may explain the function of memory talk in evoking long-term personal and socially shared memory narratives.

Beyond social and personal value, what is the mechanism that enables episodic memories to persist over time, often for decades? How does either talking with others about an experience or talking to oneself about it result in retention of an autobiographical memory? The hypothesis behind our current work is that reinstatement through verbal means is the mechanism that becomes activated in early to middle childhood and makes enduring personal memories possible.

Reinstatement

Reinstatement through partial reenactment or contextual cues can act on the basic memory system theorized here by raising the probability that the experienced event will recur. A learned response on the verge of forgetting may be reinstated if a part of the context of the original learning is re-presented prior to test. The response may thus be reactivated and preserved over a longer time than would otherwise be expected. Reinstatement appears to be a basic characteristic of memory across species and developmental stages, originally identified in animals (Campbell and Jaynes, 1966) and extensively studied in infants, as noted previously (Rovee-Collier and Hayne, 1987; Rovee-Collier and Shyi, 1992).

Reactivation, rehearsal, and reinstatement are related but not identical processes. *Reactivation* involves experiencing some part of the activity or the context on a second occasion sufficient to bring the previous experience into active memory. *Rehearsal* involves an active strategy of repeating to oneself parts of the experience to be remembered, usually more than once. *Reinstatement* may result from reactivation or rehearsal, or from reexposure through talk or observation to another episode of the event. In addition, *repeated recall* may result in rehearsal effects, reinstatement effects, or confusion of one's memory by suggestions from interviewers (as documented in many child testimony cases). Moreover, as noted previously, *repeated experience* of an event has the well-documented effect of establishing a script or schema, leading to the confusion of details of different occasions. The original memory of the event may be distorted through any one of these processes, resulting in some cases in suggestibility effects, where the suggestion of an interviewer or other person, or inserted text or pictures, enters into one's memory and is either confused with, suppresses, or supplements part of the original (Ceci and Bruck, 1993). *Suggestibility* should be seen as one possible variation of the normal effects of repetition in a social and variable environment.

Our current research is based on the hypothesis that language comes to serve a reinstating function during the preschool years. Effects of reactivation through reenactment or through partial re-presentation on children's long-term retention of memories have been demonstrated in late infancy and early childhood (Fivush and Hamond, 1989; Hudson, 1991). Reinstatement in these studies has been accomplished through reactivating a behavioral response—an action in response to a stimulus. The assumption that we are working with is that an important effect of verbally sharing an experience with others is to reinstate and thus to preserve the memory. Reinstatement through verbal means is therefore hypothesized to be the mechanism that makes possible the onset of autobiographical memory in early childhood.

Language could not be an effective means of reinstatement unless a child can use language as a medium for the representation of a complex event. As previously discussed, children begin conversing with parents (and others) about past experiences around age 2. However, the child's mastery of language is not sufficient at that age to support the representation of an event presented solely through linguistic means (Nelson, 1996). It is not until about age 3 that children are minimally competent conversational partners (Bloom, 1991), and it is not until the school years that they demonstrate competence in constructing complex discourse narratives (Karmiloff-Smith, 1986; Nelson, 1996). In the early preschool years, children are gaining grammatical competence but they are not yet able to represent and interpret connected discourse.

According to Schank and Abelson (1995), social knowledge is basically story understanding. They see the process as follows: "understanding [someone else's story] boils down to finding a story of your own that is similar to the story you are hearing. If there is a very close match, then telling your story in response signals that you have understood . . . If there is not a close match, you will have to work hard to come up with a more remote response . . . by constructing one from scene by scene details" (p. 82).

This sketch implies a complex process of comprehension suggesting that a preschool child who lacks much experience with stories of self or other, and is relatively unpracticed in the skills of story construction, will have significant problems in relating her own memories to those of others. Whether or not one buys this model, the fact is that young children do not yet have either the knowledge or the skills required to do the "hard work" that the model requires. For very young children some part of a conversation about the past may evoke memory of an event, in essence acting as a verbal label to access the memory. However, understanding that another person's memory for an event is the same as, or differs from, one's own requires more than evocation through a verbal cue.

As children gain experience with language over the preschool years, they begin to use language to represent events in memory in more elaborate ways that may be effective in both comprehension and production of remembered episodes. Reconstructing an event verbally with another person could be expected to have a much stronger reinstating effect than simple evocation through verbal cues, but this possibility depends on the further development of language as a potential representational medium. By this reasoning, verbal recounts might result in weak effects of reactivation through labeling for younger children, and stronger effects through reconstruction and comparison of narrative representations, the latter becoming possible toward the end of the preschool period. Our research is currently concerned with these issues, focused on the effects of different types of reactivation and verbal reinstatement of an event with children of different ages during the preschool years.

The consequences of narrating personal experiences with others may have a profound effect on the child's understanding of his or her own self-history as well as the subjectivities of others. Dennett has commented on similar effects of human discourse in the following terms: "The advent of language was . . . [a] boon for human beings, a technology that created a whole new class of objects-to-contemplate, verbally embodied surrogates that could be reviewed in any order at any pace. And this opened up a new dimension of self-improvement—all one had to do was to learn to savour one's own mistakes" (Dennett, 1994, p. 177). He goes on to note that chimpanzees and other primates "never dispute over attributions, and ask for the grounds for each others' conclusions. No wonder their comprehension is so limited. Ours would be, too, if we had to generate it all on our own." In particular, if we had to generate a self-history through autobiographical memory, as well as an account of others' knowledge and beliefs, without the advantage of language, how would we do it? This is the state of the 3-year-old, who appears to be linguistically competent but who uses language primarily for pragmatic, not for representational, purposes.

The Age-4 Transition
Stage theories in developmental psychology often are formulated in such a way that it appears that a child leaps suddenly from one stage to the next, that the light dawns one day and the child comes into Knowledge like Adam and Eve in the Garden. Although ours is a kind of stage theory, based on the attainment of a critical level of language competence, it posits a long period of hearing and using language in exchanging views about those invisible states of memory, knowing, thinking, and anticipating future activities between self and other, eventuating in a new capacity to entertain two different possible states

of reality—what is and what was, or what will be; or what I did and what someone else did and thought. The child is enabled thereby to make a transition from an *experiencer* to a *narrativisor* state. Through the sharing of unique as well as similar accounts of shared and un-shared events and thoughts, the child's knowledge system is extended beyond its dependence on direct experience and becomes reorganized in more complex and abstract ways (Nelson, 1993a, 1996). An important part of that reorganization is the acquisition of other people's stories and the formulating of one's own memories in narrative formats, including the "landscape of consciousness" as well as the "landscape of action" (Bruner, 1990).

These developments imply a transition period between $2^1/_2$ and 5 years—often termed the age-4 transition—during which this system undergoes significant change and within which related changes in other domains of cognitive functions are observed. The transition period includes many indications, beyond the move from experiencer in the present to narrativisor of past and future states, that some fundamentally important function is developing or failing to develop.

Theory of Mind and False Belief.   Best known from a multitude of studies of transitional phenomena in the 3- to 5-year-old age range is the younger child's ignorance of or denial of the possibility of false-belief states on his or her own part as well as that of another (Astington, 1993; Astington, Harris, and Olson, 1988; Lewis and Mitchell, 1994). Several classic tasks (such as the Maxi task and the Sally Ann task) involve a character's placing an item in a distinctive spot (a cupboard, a basket), then leaving the area; while that character is away, another character moves the item to a different distinctive spot (a drawer, a box). The child's task is to report where the first character will look for the item when he or she returns to get it (Wimmer and Perner, 1983). Children younger than 4 years typically fail this change-of-location task, stating that the uninformed child will look for the desired item in the place where it is now, rather than in the place where he (or she) left it.

This response has led to the conclusion that young children are incapable of attributing false belief, on the grounds that if they understood that the protagonist entertained a false belief about the location of the desired object, they would predict that that is where he would look for it. The actual response implies that the child attributes to the other only a true belief, one that corresponds to the true state of the world. In addition, the child's understanding of possible sources of belief is brought into serious question in this response pattern. From whence, in the child's mind, comes Maxi's belief that the candy is in the drawer (the reality state) rather then where he left it? Too little attention has been directed to this issue.

The larger conclusion generally drawn from this line of research is that children younger than about 4 years have not achieved the equivalent of the folk psychological theory of mind, attributing or predicting actions on the basis of epistemic states. By 5 years, almost all Anglo-American children do pass the false-belief tests; they are said then to have acquired a theory of mind. These results have been replicated many times and are not contested.[2] What is in dispute is how to account for these achievements. (See Carrithers and Smith, 1996, for a discussion of the many alternative theoretical accounts, both developmental and from a more general philosophical perspective.)

Related Developments. Perhaps even more provocative than the standard theory-of-mind results, in a task where the child of 3 or even 4 years is either told or shown where a toy is hidden, she will fail to acknowledge the source of her knowledge, especially when the source is language. When asked "Did I tell you or did you see?" the young child tends to answer randomly. Surprisingly, children have difficulty with this type of task up to the age of 5 years (Gopnik and Graf, 1988; Perner, Leekam, and Wimmer, 1987).

One phenomenon that has been observed in several different experimental tasks is that children of 3 years or younger seem to be unaware of former states of the self. Theory-of-mind studies brought out this surprising finding provocatively in what is called the deceptive box task. In this task the child is shown a box that usually holds candies and then discovers on opening it that it contains pencils. When asked what he or she thought the box contained before it was opened, 3-year-old children do not accept that they first thought it contained candies. They fail to acknowledge this as vociferously as they fail to predict that someone else will think it contains candies.[3] This finding suggests that children have no insight into their own mental functioning, although they clearly have awareness of their physical and active selves—as demonstrated among other ways by the mirror recognition test, which children tend to pass between 18 and 24 months.

Strangest of all along these lines is the evidence showing that 3-year-old children will fail to connect a video of themselves taken during a game played just minutes previously with their present state (Povinelli, Landau, and Perilloux, 1996). A sticker surreptitiously placed on a child's head during the game and clearly visible to the child watching the video elicits no response from the young child viewing its replay a few minutes later, whereas by 4 years most children will reach up to remove the sticker. In this case, as in the deceptive box task, it is as though the child sees no connection between present reality and past physical or mental state.

The puzzle evoked by this body of evidence is how children can have episodic memories of experiences, as demonstrated in their talk with parents (Fivush and Hamond, 1990) and in their daily activities at home (Dunn, 1988), yet fail to connect past and present selves in terms of knowledge or even physical states. The evidence suggests that there must be an important difference between personal memories in early childhood and those of older children or adults. It is not just that memories are forgotten unless reinstated; they must have a different character. They are not truly episodic, as already argued, and they come and go under different conditions. At the least the younger child's memory of immediately prior experience does not seem to be accessible to recall *as a memory* of personal experience.

Another less well documented aspect of the transition period around 3 to 4 years of age is the assimilation of other people's experience to oneself. Miller has documented several cases of this kind (Miller, Hoogstra, Mintz, Fung, and Williams, 1993; Miller, Potts, Fung, Hoogstra, and Mintz, 1990). In the account of her son's use of the story of Peter Rabbit in different retellings, she points out how he uses the story to deal with his own experience and fears of a garden. In other cases the child seems to be assimilating story characters and experiences to herself (Wolf and Heath, 1992), as well as other children's and adults' experiences that become reformulated as her own.

The vulnerability to suggestions from interviewers, which is at its height in the years between 3 and 5, may be another manifestation of the same transition state. It is as though misleading suggestions, whether verbal or nonverbal, creep into the child's memory and become part of it. Also, source errors in memory (for example, between thinking, acting, and saying) have been found to be particularly vulnerable in the preschool years (Johnson and Hirst, 1993).

Much work on perspective taking in the early years suggests a gradual move from an egocentric position that others will see what the child sees, to taking account of the other's perceptual access to the same scene (Flavell, 1992). This research suggests that a good understanding of what others can know from what they can see is a late achievement of the preschool years, similar to the understanding of knowledge sources previously noted.

Summary and Implications

Under the presumption that all of the cognitive phenomena cited here as characteristic of children in the transitional 2- to 5-year age range may reflect the same or a similar cause or set of causal factors, it seems reasonable to reach for an explanation beyond the phenomena of the false-belief tests and beyond the attribution of a lack of or defective kind of theory of mind. To that end, Table 9.1 summarizes the related developments of this period, including but not confined to memory and false belief, that suggest developmental commonalities (see Flavell and Miller, 1997, for a review of many of these developments). The developmental achievements summarized in Table 9.1 do not of course fully cover even the cognitive domains of interest during this period (for example, advances in mathematical, spatial, and temporal knowledge). What they do suggest is that in domains pertaining to psychological understanding of self and other, as well as in memory and language, there are striking commonalities in the developmental sequence.

In particular, at 2 years of age there is little or no awareness of different perspectives or belief states, and although there is mirror self-recognition and differentiation of activity roles, there is no concept of an enduring self. Grammar is developing, but language use is primar-

Table 9.1 Summary of related developments at ages 2 to 5 years

Age	Language	Perspective / source	Theory of mind	Self-other knowledge	Memory
2 years	Beginning grammar Brief conversations No narrative	Level 1 perspective/no knowledge source awareness	Beginning use of mental state terms for perception and emotion	Activity roles Self-awareness/ self-recognition	Scripts Nonspecific fragments
3 years	Complex sentences Brief conversations Script reports	Level 1 perspective taking/no knowledge source awareness	Mind reading in familiar settings	No delayed recognition of self / limited awareness of past self mental states	Flexible scripts Some specific episodes Suggestible
4 years	Basic grammar Longer conversations Personal narratives, action only Story comprehension	Beginnings of Level 2 perspective taking and knowledge source awareness	False belief emerging	Delayed self-recognition Attribution of past epistemic states	Enduring specific episodes Suggestible
5 years	Conversations Narratives and stories with intentionality	Percept, knowledge source awareness Level 2 perspective	False belief	Personal past and future Self-concept	Episodic / autobiographical Less suggestible

Notes: Language—grammatical competence, conversational competence, narrative understanding.
Perspective/source—perspective taking, knowledge source awareness.
Theory of mind—performance on standard theory-of-mind tasks.
Self-other knowledge—self-recognition standard and delayed self and other knowledge attribution in theory-of-mind tasks, self in narratives, self-concept.
Memory—generic script/schema, nonspecific episodic fragments, specific episodes, suggestibility—from cumulated memory.
(See text for reference citations.)

ily pragmatic; conversations are primitive (in Piaget's terms, talk is egocentric). Memory is articulated only in fragments and is most evident in the child's action scripts.

At age 3, we find emerging awareness in virtually all of these domains, including perspective taking, conversational ability, episodic memory reports, and some limited success on theory-of-mind tasks in familiar situations. At age 4 years, children understand stories, produce personal narratives, solve theory-of-mind and more complex perspective-taking tasks; by age 5 years, all of these achievements, including source knowledge, are more firmly established, and the ability to articulate knowledge in language is strikingly more evident.

The question raised by such summaries is whether the apparent coincidences are a consequence simply of greater experience, of general cognitive growth, or of some specific factor that underlies all—or whether the apparent concurrence is an artifact, and each domain is explainable in terms of its own specific developmental sequence. These are indeed difficult relations to unravel. It may be that future investigations of neural development will provide new insights, or that further probing of specific temporal contingencies among the competencies in question may imply different possible developmental patterns. But given our current understanding, the convergence pattern appears compelling and can be best explained in terms of the dramatic impact of language in human life and thought, as noted by Dennett in the quotation cited previously. Dennett is not of course the first person to suggest that language must make a difference in how we understand other people's intentionality (see Smith, 1996, and Whiten, 1996, for other examples directed specifically at theory-of-mind questions). Moreover, researchers increasingly recognize that language skills are more closely related to success on theory-of-mind tasks than is the child's age (Dunn, 1994; Lewis, 1994; Nelson, 1996; Siegal and Peterson, 1994), supporting the idea that the ability to exchange perspectives on the world with others is critical to the development of understanding mental states.[4]

In this view, success on theory-of-mind tests reflects precisely the same kind of understanding of self and other and of past, present, and future that is achieved through shared verbal representations of experience with other people, and that is reflected in the establishment of an autobiographical memory system toward the end of the preschool period (Nelson, 1997). Moreover, the basis for this achievement is not simply a transition from experiencer to narrativisor, but from a *single-minded representation* of reality to a *multiple-level representational* memory system, in which the language mode represents intramentally as well as intermentally.

This proposal is consistent with the hypothesis advanced by Donald (1991) regarding the evolutionary origins of the modern mind conceived of as a hybrid representational system. Nelson (1996) spells out the connections between Donald's theory and mine. Donald described four levels of memory represented in different modes: events, mimesis, language or narrative, and external memory systems, the last enabling the development of logic and scientific theory. Information may be retained at any of these levels of memory available to the modern adult mind. In his theory, each succeeding level was an advance over the preceding one in evolution or (for external memory systems) in human history. But all are simultaneously available in the hybrid mind of literate humans today.

Donald emphasizes the enormous cognitive changes that resulted with each successive level. What I have suggested is that equally enormous changes in cognitive functioning are made possible in early childhood as children move from the more restricted modes of event representations and mimesis to the social-exchange potential of language and narrative, which makes possible the maintenance of conflicting simultaneous representations of reality.[5]

The implications of the transition from one reality to dual or multiple representations are provocative. It is important to acknowledge some of the more startling effects of the one-reality view characteristic of the child age 3 and younger, not all of which are understood at present. Some implications that can be tentatively drawn, based on the research reviewed here, are the following.

One reality means living in the present. Past states that conflict with present states are overridden in memory. Past states that do not conflict may be "remembered" in a nonspecific way and "recalled" in contexts suggestive of the original experience, including verbal context cues. Such recall is not remembering a prior experience per se, but

calling on prior experience to guide present action and interpret interactions, assumed to be the basic memory function (see Nelson, 1993a,
1993b for details). The idea of a specific past in which previous experiences took place is, in contrast, a construction of language users.
Similarly, the idea of a specific future beyond the immediate present is
not conceivable in the state of one reality. The single-mind view of reality also projects one's own view onto all others who share one's current environment. Research on children's perspective taking has documented this state in young children, and it is underscored by the
research on own and other's theory of mind.

The suggestibility literature (Ceci and Bruck, 1993) implies that the
transition from a single-mind status to a multimind status may contain its own pitfalls. When the developing representational system begins to open a pathway through which representations in language
can find their way into the mental representation spaces, it appears
that such representations may at first be not just as powerful as actual
experience, but even more powerful. Thus verbal suggestions may become vivid states of reality for the 3- or 4-year-old. Or the new verbal
information may be treated simply as updating of a prior knowledge
state, old and new not kept separate. In this case the verbal representation will overwrite the memory of the experience itself. The child
who has lived a life without consciousness of a false-knowledge state
may not be able to acknowledge the conflict between the experience
and the verbal message.

We are presently investigating this possibility in our laboratory
(Nelson, Plesa, and Henseler, 1998). Some of the 3-year-olds we have
tested are capable of accepting a verbal message that conflicts with
knowledge based on their own prior action (say, of where they left a
picture) and use the message to locate the picture but do not then recall the original location. Others appear to be merely confused by the
conflicting information. Only one child in this study recalled and
acted on the original action-based knowledge but did not recall the
verbal message, implying a general priority of verbal input at this age.
By age 4 years, most children both remember the original location and
use the verbal message to locate the picture in the new location.

The transition in cognitive function taking place between 3 and 5
years of age must involve two critical parts, which may emerge in se-

quence. First, mental representations must accept verbal messages about the states of the world. Next, verbal representations must be kept separate from "own" direct experience of states of the world based on perception and action. The different representations may then be compared, and both may be retained as true—but true of different times and places. Without this latter capacity, source confusions (own experience as opposed to other's information) will be unconstrained. Indeed, an important aspect of this development must be a new awareness of source information.

This transition phase leads to new realizations that there may be two (or more) representations of reality; that one may be true and another false; that one may have been true in the past and is no longer; that another person may hold a belief that is not the same as one's own, but that one of these may be more valid—more true of the world—than another. A mature view of course holds that there may be different beliefs about the same reality, but this is a later achievement.

During the transition phase the child may go to great lengths to reconcile conflicting representations. One child in an earlier study (Plesa, Goldman, and Edmondson, 1995), given a deceptive box test in which a raisin box with a clear raisin picture on the front was opened to reveal crayons and then closed again, explained it this way: "It's magic . . . there's raisins when it's closed and crayons when it's opened." Seemingly bizarre beliefs of this kind on the part of young children are not merely reflections of the failure to construct a folk theory of mind or to simulate others' mental states, and they clearly are not the simple result of maturation of a theory-of-mind mechanism module (three competing accounts of theory-of-mind understanding). Rather, they reflect something basic about human cognitive structure and function—in particular about how the acquisition of a capacity for representation in language, first between self and other and then for self alone, may radically change how memory and cognition work, at the same time introducing a new and deeper understanding of self and other.

The idea that representation potential changes during the early childhood years is hardly novel. It was one of Bruner's contributions to understanding cognitive growth (Bruner, Olver, and Greenfield,

1966), an idea that was given less credit than it deserved in the heyday of Piagetian enthusiasms. More recently, Karmiloff-Smith (1985, 1991) outlined a theory based on the idea that representations that were initially implicit could be redescribed at an explicit level. This theory is not age dependent as the present one is, and although it incorporates language it does not depend on it in the same way. Similarly, Perner (1991) has developed a theory of levels of representation that is age dependent but not language dependent. His theory addresses the problems of theory-of-mind studies, and he relates success in those tasks to an emerging capacity for episodic memory, basing his ideas quite explicitly on Tulving's theory of episodic and semantic memory systems. Perner suggests that children younger than 3 years are incapable of autonoetic functions because they lack experiential awareness (Perner and Ruffman, 1995).

Perner's theory, applied to the problem of infantile amnesia, has many points in common with the thesis presented here. However, I believe that the problem of experiential awareness is a symptom of a wider restriction on understanding that is reflected in the many related developments summarized in Table 9.1. Remembering as such, as Perner and Ruffman (1995) put it, emerges in concert with many other developments in self-understanding, understanding of sources of knowledge, others' perspectives, the specific past and future. These are all matters made manifest in talk. The potential for understanding may be implicit in the child's experiential representations, but their emergence as specific understandings remains to be evoked through conversations with others, both adults and children.

For these reasons I believe that emergence of language as a representational mode is much more dramatic in its impact than many contemporary developmentalists do, and that it is much more instrumental in bringing about a change in both memory and understanding of belief states in self and other. I believe language representational capacities can account for developmental phenomena and can make sense of otherwise puzzling and unconnected research findings.

Beyond these claims about development, by accepting the metaphor of the hybrid mind that Donald put forth we may be able to understand (if not to explain) why adults as well as children are simultaneously susceptible to suggestion, vulnerable to source errors, and convinced of the validity of their own memories even in the face of challenge and documentation.

Return then to the assumption that the mind begins—phylogenetically and ontogenetically—as single-minded, convinced of its own true view of reality. Other views presented to the child through visual or symbolic media may be all too easily assimilated to this true view. It may take effort to keep them distinct; what "really happened" may be lost in the effort. Young children may be more vulnerable to this sort of integration than adults, but after the age of 4 or 5 years it is a matter of degree, not kind. There is a difference between assimilating a view that does not conflict with one's own, supplementing one's own view of reality through the acquisition of new information, and accepting a view that conflicts with one's own. In earliest childhood, conflicting views cannot be maintained; later, two conflicting views—past and present, mine and yours—can be recognized, kept separate, and reflected on. This is an essential achievement of human development.

As seen in developmental research, as well as in accounts of adults' memories from their early childhood, confusions of knowledge source account for many inaccuracies in memory that are unrecognized or unacknowledged by the rememberer. Whereas we as adults know and remember with hybrid minds, it seems that phenomenologically we continue to "know" with one mind. Thus we remain vulnerable to the illusion of certainty that what we remember must have happened. Reports that conflict with memory are not in danger of being accepted as "ours," but vigilance is required to prevent the assimilation of others' accounts, as well as of fantasies or dreams, that are consistent with our own experience from becoming part of our singular personal past and subsequently being defended as such.

How then can we discriminate false memory from true? The lesson I draw from developmental research is that the process must be the same as discriminating false belief from true belief, whether in childhood or in adulthood. We search for evidence in our own experiences related to the memory, look for evidence of sources of knowledge and belief, and compare notes with others who may have information relating to the memory or belief—and who may view it from a perspective different from our own. Without taking advantage of this specifically human capacity to compare notes, we are left within the boundaries of our single-mind limits on truth finding, the limitations of which children aged 3 to 5 years are just beginning to escape. Thereafter, children are able to reflect on their own and others' mental states, and to form narratives of their own self-histories—even as they recognize that others' constructions of experience may differ from their own.

References

Astington, J. W. (1993). *The child's discovery of the mind.* Cambridge, MA: Harvard University Press.

Astington, J. W., Harris, P. L., and Olson, D. (Eds.). (1988). *Developing theories of mind.* Cambridge: Cambridge University Press.

Baron-Cohen, S., Tager-Flusberg, H., and Cohen, D. (Eds.). (1993). *Understanding other minds: Perspectives from autism.* Oxford: Oxford University Press.

Bartlett, F. C. (1932). *Remembering: A study in experimental and social psychology.* Cambridge: Cambridge University Press.

Bauer, P. J., Hertsgaard, L. A., and Dow, G. A. (1994). After 8 months have passed: Long-term recall of events by 1- to 2-year-old children. *Memory, 2,* 353–382.

Bauer, P. J., and Wewerka, S. S. (1997). Saying is revealing: Verbal expression of event memory in the transition from infancy to early childhood. In P. W. van den Broek, P. J. Bauer, and T. Bourg (Eds.), *Developmental spans in event comprehension and representation* (pp. 139–169). Mahway, NJ: Lawrence Erlbaum.

Bloom, L. (1991). *Language development from two to three.* New York: Cambridge University Press.

Bruner, J. S. (1990). *Acts of meaning.* Cambridge, MA: Harvard University Press.

Bruner, J. S., Olver, R. R., and Greenfield, P. M. (1966). *Studies in cognitive growth.* New York: Wiley.

Campbell, B. A., and Jaynes, J. (1966). Reinstatement. *Psychological Review, 73,* 478–480.

Carrithers, P., and Smith, P. K. (1996). *Theories of theories of mind.* New York: Cambridge University Press.

Ceci, S. J., and Bruck, M. (1993). Suggestibility of the child witness: A historical review and synthesis. *Psychological Bulletin, 113,* 403–439.

Dennett, D. (1994). Language and intelligence. In J. Khalfa (Ed.), *What is intelligence?* (pp. 161–179). New York: Cambridge University Press.

Donald, M. (1991). *Origins of the modern mind*. Cambridge, MA: Harvard University Press.

Dunn, J. (1988). *The beginnings of social understanding*. Cambridge, MA: Harvard University Press.

Dunn, J. (1994). Changing minds and changing relationships. In C. Lewis and P. Mitchell (Eds.), *Children's early understanding of mind: Origins and development* (pp. 297–310). Hillsdale, NJ: Lawrence Erlbaum.

Engel, S. (1986). Learning to reminisce: A developmental study of how young children talk about the past. Doctoral dissertation, City University of New York Graduate Center.

Fivush, R. (1984). Learning about school: The development of kindergartners' school scripts. *Child Development, 55,* 1697–1709.

Fivush, R. (1991). The social construction of personal narratives. *Merrill-Palmer Quarterly, 37,* 59–82.

Fivush, R., and Hamond, N. R. (1989). Time and again: Effects of repetition and retention interval on two year olds' event recall. *Journal of Experimental Child Psychology, 47,* 259–273.

Fivush, R., and Hamond, N. R. (1990). Autobiographical memory across the preschool years: Toward reconceptualizing childhood amnesia. In R. Fivush and J. A. Hudson (Eds.), *Knowing and remembering in young children* (pp. 223–248). New York: Cambridge University Press.

Flavell, J. H. (1992). Perspectives on perspective taking. In H. Beilin and P. Pufall (Eds.), *Piaget's theory: Prospects and possibilities* (pp. 107–139). Hillsdale, NJ: Lawrence Erlbaum.

Flavell, J. H., and Miller, P. H. (1997). Social cognition. *Handbook of child psychology* (5th ed.), Vol. 2. New York: Wiley.

Glenberg, A. M. (1997). What memory is for. *Behavioral and Brain Sciences, 20,* 1–56.

Gopnik, A. (1993). How we know our minds: The illusion of first-person knowledge of intentionality, *Behavioral and Brain Sciences, 16,* 1–14.

Gopnik, A., and Graf, P. (1988). Knowing how you know: Young children's ability to identify and remember the sources of their beliefs. *Child Development, 59,* 1366–71.

Gopnik, A., and Wellman, H. (1994). The theory theory. In L. A. Hirschfeld and S. A. Gelman (Eds.), *Mapping the mind* (pp. 257–293). New York: Cambridge University Press.

Hudson, J. (1991). Effects of re-enactment on toddlers' memory for a novel event. Poster presented at the biennial meeting of the Society for Research on Child Development, Seattle.

Hudson, J., and Nelson, K. (1986). Repeated encounters of a similar kind: Effects of familiarity on children's autobiographical memory. *Cognitive Development, 1,* 253–271.

Hudson, J., and Sheffield, E. (1993). Effects of re-enactment on toddlers' memory after 2, 8, and 12 months. Poster presented at the biennial meeting of the Society for Research on Child Development, New Orleans.

Hudson, J. A. (1990). The emergence of autobiographic memory in mother-child conversation. In R. Fivush and J. A. Hudson (Eds.), *Knowing and remembering in young children* (pp. 166–196). New York: Cambridge University Press.

Johnson, M. K., and Hirst, W. (1993). MEM: Memory subsystems as processes. In A. F. Collins, S. E. Gathercole, M. A. Conway, and P. E. Morris (Eds.), *Theories of memory* (pp. 103–139). Hillsdale, NJ: Lawrence Erlbaum.

Karmiloff-Smith, A. (1985). Language and cognitive processes from a developmental perspective. *Mind and Language, 1,* 61–85.

Karmiloff-Smith, A. (1986). Language development beyond age five. In P. Fletcher and M. Garman (Eds.), *Language acquisition* (2nd ed.) (pp. 455–474). Cambridge: Cambridge University Press.

Karmiloff-Smith, A. (1991). Beyond modularity: Innate constraints and developmental change. In S. Carey and R. Gelman (Eds.), *The epigenesis of mind: Essays on biology and cognition* (pp. 171–197). Hillsdale, NJ: Lawrence Erlbaum.

Lewis, C. (1994). Episodes, events, and narratives in the child's understanding of mind. In C. Lewis and P. Mitchell (Eds.), *Children's early understanding of mind: Origins and development* (pp. 457–480). Hillsdale, NJ: Lawrence Erlbaum.

Lewis, C., and Mitchell, P. (Eds.). (1994). *Children's early understanding of mind: Origins and development.* Hillsdale, NJ: Lawrence Erlbaum.

Lillard, A. S. (1997). Other folks' theories of mind and behavior. *Psychological Science, 14,* 96–107.

Lillard, A. S. (1998). Ethnopsychologies: Cultural variations in theories of mind. *Psychological Bulletin, 123,* 3–32.

Linton, M. (1982). Transformations of memory in everyday life. In U. Neisser (Ed.), *Memory observed: Remembering in natural contexts.* San Francisco: W. H. Freeman.

Mandler, J. M. (1990). Recall of events by preverbal children. *Annals of the New York Academy of Sciences, 608,* 365–393.

Meltzoff, A. N. (1995). Infantile amnesia? New data from infancy. Paper presented at the biennial meeting of the Society for Research in Child Development, Indianapolis.

Miller, P. J., Hoogstra, L., Mintz, J., Fung, H., and Williams, K. (1993). Troubles in the garden and how they get resolved: A young child's transformation of his favorite story. In C. A. Nelson (Ed.), *Memory and affect in development,* Vol. 26 (pp. 87–114). Hillsdale, NJ: Lawrence Erlbaum.

Miller, P. J., Potts, R., Fung, H., Hoogstra, L., and Mintz, J. (1990). Narrative practices and the social construction of self in childhood. *American Ethnologist, 17,* 292–311.

Nelson, K. (1978). How young children represent knowledge of their world in and out of language. In R. S. Siegler (Ed.), *Children's thinking: What develops?* (pp. 225–273). Hillsdale, NJ: Lawrence Erlbaum.

Nelson, K. (1986). *Event knowledge: Structure and function in development.* Hillsdale, NJ: Lawrence Erlbaum.

Nelson, K. (1988). The ontogeny of memory for real events. In U. Neisser and E. Winograd (Eds.), *Remembering reconsidered: Ecological and traditional approaches to the study of memory* (pp. 244–276). New York: Cambridge University Press.

Nelson, K. (Ed.). (1989a). *Narratives from the crib.* Cambridge, MA: Harvard University Press.

Nelson, K. (1989b). Remembering: A functional developmental perspective. In P. R. Solomon, G. R. Goethals, C. M. Kelley, and B. R. Stephens (Eds.), *Memory: Interdisciplinary approaches* (pp. 127–150). New York: Springer-Verlag.

Nelson, K. (1992). Emergence of autobiographical memory at age 4. *Human Development, 35,* 172–177.

Nelson, K. (1993a). Developing self-knowledge from autobiographical memory. In T. K. Srull and R. Wyer (Eds.), *The mental representation of trait and autobiographical knowledge about the self,* Vol. 5 (pp. 111–120). Hillsdale, NJ: Lawrence Erlbaum.

Nelson, K. (1993b). Events, narratives, memories: What develops? In C. Nelson (Ed.), *Memory and affect in development: Minnesota symposium on child psychology,* Vol. 26 (pp. 1–24). Hillsdale, NJ: Lawrence Erlbaum.

Nelson, K. (1993c). Explaining the emergence of autobiographical memory in early childhood. In A. Collins, M. Conway, S. Gathercole, and P. Morris (Eds.), *Theories of memory* (pp. 355–385). Hillsdale, NJ: Lawrence Erlbaum.

Nelson, K. (1993d). The psychological and social origins of autobiographical memory. *Psychological Science, 4,* 1–8.

Nelson, K. (1994). Long-term retention of memory for preverbal experience: Evidence and implications. *Memory, 2,* 467–475.

Nelson, K. (1996). *Language in cognitive development: The emergence of the mediated mind.* New York: Cambridge University Press.

Nelson, K. (1997). Finding oneself in time. In J. G. Snodgrass and R. L. Thompson (Eds.), *Annals of the New York Academy of Sciences.* New York: New York Academy of Sciences.

Nelson, K., and Gruendel, J. (1981). Generalized event representations: Basic building blocks of cognitive development. In M. Lamb and A. Brown

(Eds.), *Advances in developmental psychology,* Vol. 1 (pp. 131–158). Hillsdale, NJ: Lawrence Erlbaum.

Nelson, K., Plesa, D., and Henseler, S. (1998). Children's theory of mind: An experiential interpretation. *Human Development, 41,* 7–29.

Perlmutter, M. (Ed.). (1980). *Children's memory,* Vol. 10. San Francisco: Jossey-Bass.

Perner, J. (1991). *Understanding the representational mind.* Cambridge, MA: MIT Press.

Perner, J., Leekam, S. R., and Wimmer, H. (1987). Three year-olds' difficulty with false belief. The case for a conceptual deficit. *British Journal of Developmental Psychology, 5,* 125–137.

Perner, J., and Ruffman, T. (1995). Episodic memory and autonoetic consciousness: Developmental evidence and a theory of childhood amnesia. *Journal of Experimental Child Psychology, 59,* 516–548.

Piaget, J. (1952). *The origins of intelligence in children.* New York: Norton Library.

Piaget, J. (1962). *Play, dreams, and imitation in childhood.* New York: W. W. Norton.

Pillemer, D. B., Picariello, M. L., and Pruett, J. C. (1994). Very long-term memories of a salient preschool event. *Applied Cognitive Psychology, 8,* 85–106.

Pillemer, D. B., and White, S. H. (1989). Childhood events recalled by children and adults. In H. W. Reese (Ed.), *Advances in child development and behavior,* Vol. 21 (pp. 297–340). New York: Academic Press.

Plesa, D. N., Goldman, S., and Edmondson, D. (1995). Negotiation of meaning in a false belief task. Poster presented at the biennial meeting of the Society for Research in Child Development, Indianapolis.

Povinelli, D. J., Landau, K. R., and Perilloux, H. K. (1996). Self-recognition in young children using delayed versus live feedback: Evidence of a developmental asynchrony. *Child Development, 67,* 1540–54.

Rovee-Collier, C. (1995). Time windows in cognitive development. *Developmental Psychology, 31,* 147–169.

Rovee-Collier, C., and Hayne, H. (1987). Reactivation of infant memory: Implications for cognitive development. In H. W. Reese (Ed.), *Advances in child development and behavior,* Vol. 20 (pp. 185–283). New York: Academic Press.

Rovee-Collier, C., and Shyi, G. (1992). A functional and cognitive analysis of infant long-term retention. In M. L. Howe, C. J. Brainerd, and V. F. Reyna (Eds.), *Development of long-term retention* (pp. 3–55). New York: Springer-Verlag.

Schank, R. C., and Abelson, R. P. (1977). *Scripts, plans, goals, and understanding.* Hillsdale, NJ: Lawrence Erlbaum.

Schank, R. C., and Abelson, R. P. (1995). Knowledge and memory: The real story. In R. S. Wyer, Jr. (Ed.), *Knowledge and memory: The real story*, Vol. 8 (pp. 1–86). Hillsdale, NJ: Lawrence Erlbaum.

Sebris, S. B. (1992). Autobiographical childhood narratives: Processes of remembering and reconstructing. Doctoral dissertation, City University of New York Graduate School.

Siegal, M., and Peterson, C. C. (1994). Children's theory of mind and the conversational territory of cognitive development. In C. Lewis and P. Mitchell (Eds.), *Children's early understanding of mind: Origins and development* (pp. 427–456). Hillsdale, NJ: Lawrence Erlbaum.

Smith, P. K. (1996). Language and the evolution of mind-reading. In P. Carruthers and P. K. Smith (Eds.), *Theories of theory of mind* (pp. 344–354). Cambridge: Cambridge University Press.

Tessler, M., and Nelson, K. (1994). Making memories: The influence of joint encoding on later recall. *Consciousness and Cognition, 3*, 307–326.

Thompson, C. P., Skowronski, J. J., Larsen, S. F., and Betz, A. L. (1996). *Autobiographical memory: Remembering what and remembering when*. Mahwah, NJ: Lawrence Erlbaum.

Tulving, E. (1983). *Elements of episodic memory*. New York: Oxford University Press.

Vygotsky, L. S. (1978). *Mind in society: The development of higher psychological processes*. Cambridge, MA: Harvard University Press.

Whiten, A. (1996). When does smart behaviour-reading become mind-reading? In P. Carruthers and P. K. Smith (Eds.), *Theories of theory of mind* (pp. 277–292). Cambridge: Cambridge University Press.

Wimmer, H., and Perner, J. (1983). Beliefs about beliefs: Representation and constraining function of wrong beliefs in young children's understanding of deception. *Cognition, 13*, 103–128.

Wolf, S. A., and Heath, S. B. (1992). *The braid of literature: Children's worlds of reading*. Cambridge, MA: Harvard University Press.

Notes

1. The term "generalized event representations" was chosen (Nelson and Gruendel, 1981) to avoid the implication of a propositional script format. However, the predictive implications of script theory (Schank and Abelson, 1977) have proved to fit the young child's knowledge base of everyday routine events very well (Nelson, 1986). This fit of course does not imply that the child's memory format is propositional.

2. Although earlier cross-cultural studies suggested that theory-of-mind achievements would be found universally, independent of culture or language, more recent reviews (Lillard, 1997, 1998) have emphasized differences in cultural theories and achievements.

3. In a study carried out in my laboratory we have found that 3-year-olds are more willing to admit to a different knowledge state if we ask what they said was in the box rather than what they thought. Nonetheless, the pattern of results remains striking and puzzling.

4. Additional support for this view may come from the specific difficulty that autistic persons have with theory-of-mind tasks, given their problems with the communicative functions of language. However, the interpretation of autism in relation to theory of mind is controversial. A prominent theory runs the causal relation in the other direction: that a theory-of-mind deficit is a critical causal factor underlying autism (Baron-Cohen, Tager-Flusberg, and Cohen, 1993).

5. Theories in the scientific sense are not attained until after the third transition. The developmental implication is that the attribution of theories to young children should be cautiously made and only in a loose metaphorical sense, the sense in which most writers use the term. Some theorists of theory of mind, however, adhere to a much stronger sense of theory and view very young children as "little scientists" (Gopnik, 1993; Gopnik and Wellman, 1994).

Autobiography, Identity, and the Fictions of Memory

10

Paul John Eakin

Memory's mythmaking is necessary to life.
Philippe Lejeune, 1991

Looking back, I suspect that I have always regarded memory as autobiography's anchor, the source of that core of factual truth that enables us to distinguish autobiography's fiction from the other kind we more commonly call fiction.[1] Recent research on memory, however, has radically destabilized such a notion; memory, whether we like it or not, is one more source of fiction, and I want to reckon with that fact as I explore in this chapter the relation between autobiography and identity.

One More Fiction

I need first to clarify my use of the term "fiction." Steering clear of any pejorative connotations, any sense of untruths or lies, I will be speaking of fiction in its root meanings: that which is formed, shaped, molded, fashioned, invented.[2] Autobiographies are not only fictions in this sense, albeit fictions of a special, memory-based kind, they are fictions about what is itself in turn a fiction, the self. The self is properly understood as a metaphor for the subjective reality of consciousness. Although recognition of the self as a kind of fiction is a commonplace of our skeptical postmodern age, it in no way attenuates the psychological reality of the experience to which concepts of self or identity refer.[3] The psychologist John Shotter (1989) captures the perennial appeal of this experiential notion of selfhood as follows: "Central . . . is the apparently self-evident *experience* that one's own *self* (one's 'I,' or ego, or whatever else it may be called) exists somewhere 'inside' one, as something unique and distinct from all else that there is—and it is *that,* its substantial existence, which guarantees one's personal identity" (p. 137).

If this experientialist view of the self seems to guarantee personal identity, it is memory that guarantees the guarantee. Yet memory is no more immune to fiction than the autobiographical text or the psychological experience of selfhood. The latest developments in brain science confirm the extent to which memory, the would-be anchor of selves and lives, constructs the materials from the past that an earlier, more innocent view would have us believe it merely stored. Israel Rosenfield (1988) argues that memories share the constructed nature of all brain events: "recollection is a kind of perception, . . . *and every context will alter the nature of what is recalled*" (p. 89; emphasis added).[4] If memory indeed is the anchor of autobiographical truth, of texts and selves, if autobiography really is in some fundamental way an art of memory, then any shift in our conception of memory is bound to have important consequences for our thinking about autobiography and identity.

The discussion of memory and belief in the remainder of this chapter unfolds, then, against a constructivist backdrop, a sense that our representations of the real—literary, psychological, neurological—are dynamic and constructed rather than static and mimetic in nature. I begin by examining the ways in which memory and belief are configured in autobiography, focusing on the concept of continuous identity. Then I place this concept in a developmental perspective, examining the emergence in early childhood of what Ulric Neisser has termed the extended self. In the final section I show how one introspective autobiographer, the German novelist Christa Wolf, grapples with continuous identity, contesting its apparent self-evidence and deepening, as she does so, our insight into the existential purpose of memory's fictions.

Continuous Identity

If it is a commonplace to conceive of autobiography as an art of memory, it may seem curious that autobiographies rarely dramatize the working of memory itself as process. As Philippe Lejeune observes, with few exceptions, most autobiographers proceed to tell their stories with only the most perfunctory and conventional acknowledgment of the memory problems they inevitably encounter.[5] Life writers find it reassuring to subscribe to a comparatively simple notion of memory as a storehouse in which the past is preserved intact, conveniently awaiting autobiographical recall in any present. As Michael Sheringham (1993) astutely comments, this "secular myth, deeply rooted in the Western tradition, . . . involves a sublimation whose most striking feature, in the context of autobiography, is perhaps the way it elides the subject's active participation in the work of memory" (p. 289).[6]

Following Lejeune and Sheringham, we can divide autobiographers into two unequal camps: the overwhelming majority, who place their trust in the concept of an invariant memory that preserves the past intact, allowing the original experience to be repeated in present consciousness; and a small group of dissenters, who argue against such a possibility. For students of memory, the issue can be formulated as follows: Can past experience be repeated, or is it necessarily—psychologically and neurologically—*constructed* anew in each memory event or act of recall?

In the celebrated episode of the *petite madeleine* dipped in tea, Marcel Proust gives the dream version of invariant memory: "Eat, drink, and the past shall be yours," the passage seems to say. And who can resist the appeal of the Proustian sacrament of memory? The eating of the cake and the drinking of the tea trigger an ecstasy of recall in which the very "souls" of past things, all the "residue" of Combray, "overcome death and return to share our life."[7] Vladimir Nabokov (1966) defines this ecstasy precisely as the "enjoyment of timelessness" (p. 139), and his autobiographical art evokes again and again moments of total and perfect recall, as in this stunning passage: "*I see again* my schoolroom in Vyra, the blue roses of the wallpaper, the open window . . . The mirror brims with brightness; a bumblebee has entered the room and bumps against the ceiling. Everything is as it should be, nothing will ever change, nobody will ever die" (pp. 76–77; emphasis added). Invariant memory permits the triumph over time.

Summarizing recent research on memory, Larry R. Squire (1995) reminds us that "memory is not a single faculty but consists of different systems that depend on different brain structures and connections" (p. 198). The traditional notion of memory, however, as a single mental faculty varying only in strength and accessibility (p. 208), dies hard. Epiphanies of recall on the order of Nabokov's "I see again" abound in autobiographies.[8] It is as though we believe that our consciousness provides an unchanging, transparent, colorless medium in which—in Proust's famous figure—the exquisite Japanese paper flowers of the past can open, expand, and bloom once more (p. 36). In a probing sketch of his childhood in Brisbane, however, the Australian novelist David Malouf (1986) gives the lie to this faith in invariant memory. The startling climax of his compelling sketch of his childhood home, the essay "12 Edmondstone Street," is his recognition that memory does not preserve the past; instead, it interferes with its recovery:

> Here we come to a limit . . . a threshhold we cannot cross, since even if we could find the door to that room, we cannot now find in ourselves the body, the experiencing mind-in-the-body, to go through. That body is out of reach . . . What moving back into it would demand is an act of *un*-remembering, a dismantling of the body's experience that would be a kind of dying, a casting off, one by one, of all the tissues of perception, conscious and not, through which our very notion of body has been remade. (p. 64)

Because the body changes and consciousness alters, the recovery of the past—autobiography's project—is, in a deep psychological and neurological sense, impossible.

The dynamic conception of memory espoused by Malouf, which seems to bar our reentry into the lost world of the past, carries with it nonetheless profound compensation in enabling us to maintain a sense of continuous identity over time. If the self is continuously evolving, becoming "different," then memory's task is to allow for the possibility of identity, of being the "same," that would otherwise be lacking. Thus memory's fallibility, its proclivity for revisionist history, may prove, paradoxically, to be redemptive. In this view, memory would be not only literally essential to the constitution of identity, but also crucial in the sense that it is constantly revising and editing the remembered past to square with the needs and requirements of the self we have become in any present.[9]

Jerome Bruner and other "narrative psychologists" have made a very persuasive case for the decisive role played by narrative in identity formation.[10] The neurologist Oliver Sacks (1987) formulates this link between narrative and identity memorably as follows: "It might be said that each of us constructs and lives, a 'narrative,' and that this narrative *is* us, our identities" (p. 110). Following William James (1890/1981), I trace the germ of this self-narration that provides identity's core to the individual's recognition of consciousness both as continuous and as his or her own. Defining "the stream of thought," James writes: "But in . . . the sense of the parts [of consciousness] being inwardly connected and belonging together because they are parts of a common whole, the consciousness remains sensibly continuous and one. What now is the common whole? The natural name for it is *myself, I,* or *me*" (Vol. 1, p. 232). What we call the self emerges, then, in James's reasoning, as the "name" for consciousness which we "own" or acknowledge as belonging to us continuously over time.[11] And it is narrative, as the supremely temporal form, that permits us to articulate precisely this memory-dependent experience of continuous identity.[12]

Whether or not the capacity for making narrative should be regarded as the sine qua non of identity, however, should give us pause.[13] Complementing Daniel L. Schacter's (1996) findings on the implicit memories of amnesics (pp. 163–176), William Hirst (1994) argues that an individual "can have a dynamic changing self-concept even without personal narratives," for "memories may be implicit or stored in the social setting around us" (p. 255). Nevertheless, for both Hirst (p. 271) and Schacter (pp. 149–150, 160), there is no question that the self of the amnesic is radically altered by the loss of explicit memory.[14]

The identity that is impaired by the failure of explicit memory is what Ulric Neisser terms the extended self. Neisser (1988) distinguishes usefully "among several kinds of self-specifying information, each establishing a different aspect of the self" (p. 35). I draw particular attention to his concept of the extended self, for this is the self of memory and anticipation, the self existing outside the present moment. It is the extended self whose history is recorded in autobiography, and I want now to examine the origins of this self and its practice of self-narration in early childhood.

The Narrative Culture of Memory

The notion that autobiographical memory is socially and culturally constructed may at first seem counterintuitive. From Rousseau's *Confessions* on down, readers have been conditioned by the ideology of individualism to think of autobiography as a theater in which the self's uniqueness, privacy, and interiority are on display. Instead, Kenneth J. Gergen (1994) argues aggressively for "social constructivism" as the most appropriate perspective through which to approach the phenomena of autobiographical memory: "To report on one's memories is not so much a matter of consulting mental images as it is engaging in a sanctioned form of telling" (p. 90).

Other developmental psychologists working on autobiographical memory in the last decade—I am thinking of Katherine Nelson, Robyn Fivush, Peggy J. Miller, Catherine E. Snow, and Dennie Palmer Wolf—support Gergen's social constructivist assumptions. Analyzing parent-child conversations about the past, they stress the interpersonal context in which the extended self emerges, they highlight the role of rules and conventions in the formation of autobiographical memories, and they show how the young child gradually assimilates these narrative practices.[15] A study by Robyn Fivush and Elaine Reese (1992), "The Social Construction of Autobiographical Memory," is characteristic of the drift of this research. Tracing the process through which the child "internalizes . . . the culturally available narrative forms for recounting and for representing past experiences" (p. 115), they conclude, "In this way, children begin forming a more overarching, narratively organized life story" (p. 117).

Fivush (1988) identifies the primary function of autobiographical memory as that of "organizing our knowledge about ourselves, a self-defining function" (p. 277). She articulates, moreover, the complex interrelationship between the extended self (the self in time) and its store of autobiographical memories, and the difficulty of sorting out the ways in which language and narrative, interpersonal exchange and cultural formations, contribute to its unfolding:

> The self-concept and memories of past experiences develop dialectically and begin to form a life history. The life history, in turn, helps organize both memories of past experiences and the self-concept. The life history is essentially what Barsalou calls the extended time lines, or the person's "story line." It is only with the construction of the life history that we have true autobiographical memory. (pp. 280–281)

As the dialectical cast of this formulation suggests, Fivush and Reese (1992) eschew any notion of determinism in their account of the parent-child conversations in which "children learn the conventionalized narrative forms which eventually provide a structure for internally represented memories" (p. 115): they view "both the child and the adult as playing active roles in the construction of autobiography" (p. 118).

Turning to the work of Catherine E. Snow and Dennie Palmer Wolf, I want to suggest that the development of autobiographical memory in early childhood prepares for the writing of autobiography—when it occurs—in adult life. The distance between little Emily's "narratives from the crib," studied by Nelson (1989) and her colleagues, and literary autobiography of the kind I am about to discuss is not so great as it might seem: both belong to a single, continuous, lifelong trajectory of self-narration. Analyzing transcripts of parent-child conversations recorded over a period of several years, Snow (1990) distinguishes between "memories located in the parental mind, which are transferred to the child but not actually shared by the child before transferal, and memories which children have some access to, though they are undeniably enriched and structured by parental intervention" (p. 227). "Ultimately," she concludes, "children become the authors of their own autobiographies and the repository of their own memories" (p. 232).

The child's growth toward what Snow terms "autonomous remembrances" (p. 232) is investigated in fascinating detail by Wolf (1990), who traces the emergence of what she terms "an *authorial self*" (p. 185) between the ages of two and four years. She documents the child's progressive ability to manipulate memories in a proto-literary fashion, rendering "the 'same' experience in a variety of formats" (p. 185), playing with voices and versions of an event, and becoming increasingly attracted to "fiction, with all of its selections, transformations, and distortions" (p. 197). Of special note, as an anticipation of the autobiographer's stance, is the child's mastery in "memory talk" of the double point of view that governs retrospect: "the person who identifies with the younger, distant person (the object of the memory) and the person who engages in recollection (the subject who currently has the memory)" (p. 192). The child who has learned through memory talk "to speak as subject and object, author and critic, character and narrator" (p. 208) is a budding autobiographer. Fivush, Snow, and Wolf link autobiographical memory to narrative forms, to the making of fiction, to the exercise of authorship, and Nelson (1988) has emphasized the dawning sense of audience, the pleasure-producing sociality, of these promptings: children learn that "sharing memories with others is in fact a prime social activity" (pp. 266–267).[16]

Central to the binding of autobiographical memories in all self-narrations, early and late, is the "I" of autobiographical discourse, which bridges the gap between the present and the past. It is the linchpin of autobiography's fictions of memory.

Constructing and Deconstructing Identity in Christa Wolf's *Patterns of Childhood*

In what sense can the extended self be said to maintain a continuous identity? That is, in what sense can we say that we are what we were? What connection—if any—is there between self-narrations early and late? Is the child really father of the man? Only the functioning of memory permits such a notion of the extended self in the first place; memory underwrites it. Yet if we now accept a dynamic, constructivist view of memory, we must recognize the extended self as necessarily a fiction in the sense I have been using the term; it is a fiction of memory, and its story, its autobiography, is also a fiction of memory.

Most autobiographers, however, embrace the fiction of the extended self as fact, proclaiming the continuous identity of selves early and late, and they do so through the use of the first person, autobiography's most distinctive, if problematic, generic marker: the "I" speaking in the present—the utterer—is somehow continuous with the "I" acting in the past—the subject of the utterance. This simultaneous double reference of first-person autobiographical discourse to the present and the past masks the disruptions of identity produced by passing time and memory's limitations.

I have chosen Christa Wolf's *Patterns of Childhood* (1976) to illustrate the problems involved in an autobiographer's use of the memory-based concept of continuous identity precisely because her text rejects any easy acceptance of this fiction as fact. Wolf's narrative deconstructs the notion that who we were and who we are now can be said in any simple sense to be the same person: as Malouf reminds us, the body changes, consciousness changes, memories change, and identity changes too, whether we like it or not. Thus Wolf's text does not employ the first person, signaling to the reader that the genre's conventional assumption of continuous identity is not operating in her self-narration in the familiar way. Here the narrator speaks not as "I" but as "you," and she addresses her earlier self not as "I" or Christa but as "she"—her earlier self even has a different name: Nelly.[17] Yet *Patterns of Childhood* is indeed Wolf's self-narration, one that works steadily, as we shall see, to reforge the link between selves past and present. Wolf recognizes the extended self not only as a fiction of memory but also as an existential fact, necessary for our psychological survival amid the flux of experience.

Looking back some twenty-five years after the end of World War II, the German novelist seeks to understand her own participation in the pernicious ideology of the Third Reich: as a teenager, she had been an ardent member of a Hitler youth group. But how, the narrator asks, can she connect with an earlier self she has repudiated and repressed? How to begin, when at least three distinct stories claim her attention? In this intricately layered narrative, Wolf tracks all three chronologies of her inquiry into the past simultaneously: Nelly's childhood in the 1930s through World War II up to 1946, the narrator's trip to Poland to revisit Nelly's childhood home in July 1971, and the narrator's writing of Nelly's story from November 1972 to 1975. What, Wolf would have us ask, can possibly bind together these periods of personal history? Memory? Narrative? Identity? The use of the first person? "We would suffer continuous estrangement from ourselves," she observes, "if it weren't for our memory of the things we have done, of the things that have happened to us. If it weren't for the memory of ourselves" (p. 4).

Does memory indeed provide a basis for continuous identity, uniting us to our acts, our experiences, our earlier selves? For Wolf's narrator, who cannot say "I" to herself, to remember is to fall into "a time shaft, at the bottom of which the child sits on a stone step, in all her innocence, saying 'I' to herself for the first time in her life" (p. 5). This initial probe into the past, into her earliest childhood memory, only deepens the narrator's sense of self-estrangement; time and the narrator's "unreliable memory" make Nelly, her earlier self, "inaccessible" to her. This sense of rupture, moreover, is compounded when she interprets the child's discovery of the first person as a rupture in its turn: when a child says "I," he "severs himself from the third person in which he has thought of himself up to that point" (p. 7). The use of the first person, then, provides no shield against self-estrangement, early and late. No wonder that the narrator proceeds warily, speaking of herself as an "intruding stranger" (p. 119) who approaches Nelly sometimes with diffidence, more often with aggression. She reminds us endlessly of the limits of her knowledge of Nelly, for Nelly in turn is another stranger.

The narrator's refusal of the first person, her "strange" (p. 3) choice of the second and third persons to portray her relation to her earlier self—these rhetorical moves mirror Nelly's psychological situation, the fissure in the fiction of continuous identity wrought by the trauma of the war. One of Wolf's great achievements in *Patterns* is her reconstruction of Nelly's progressive sense of dissociation, giving us the etiology of the narrator's view of her earlier self as a "third person." The early stages show us a child splitting in two, acting and observing at the same time and learning to fib (pp. 131–132). Sensitively attuned to how others see her, Nelly learns "to cheat herself out of her true feelings" (p. 160). By the time she embraces the heroic fantasies of her Hitler youth group, she has waded so far into denial, she has become so practiced in dissimulation and self-deception, that it takes the screams of a refugee mother at the death of her frozen baby to shock Nelly into the collapse of her illusions in the last days of the war; her brain shuts down, leaving a "memory gap" (p. 281).

Nelly becomes a refugee herself, fleeing with her family across a ravaged landscape, putting Germany's recent past and her own behind her, or so it would seem. The flight becomes a metaphor for the move-

ment of Nelly's consciousness from manifold fears and "inner alien-
ation" (p. 231) into a general "emotional numbness" (p. 297) and dis-
integration. Wolf interprets Nelly's subsequent recovery during the
occupation as a kind of "emergency maturity" whose premise is
"being quite unfamiliar with herself" (p. 350); Nelly, she believes, had
become a new person (pp. 368, 379).

As the narrator reconstructs it, then, Nelly's story opens and closes
with discontinuities of identity: the child sitting on the stone step saying "I" and the teenager at the end of the war are both dissociated
from the selves they had been. The curious result, however, is that the
narrator's dissociation from Nelly becomes one more link in a length-
ening chain of dissociations. Thus the rhetorical premise (the refusal
of "I") designed to represent the autobiographer's disidentification
with her early self is steadily controverted by parallel behaviors that
reveal the underlying continuities between identities early and late.[18]
What Nelly feared then, the narrator fears now: their participation in
the enormities of the Third Reich—Kristallnacht, the final solution,
the camps.

Amnesia, fueled by fear, binds them together. When the narrator
revisits the site where Nelly's Jungmädel unit held its rallies, she finds
that she cannot recall a single face.

> Where Nelly's participation was deepest, where she showed de-
> votion, where she gave of herself, all relevant details have been
> obliterated. Gradually, one might assume. And it isn't difficult to
> guess the reason: the forgetting must have gratified a deeply inse-
> cure awareness which, as we all know, can instruct our memory
> behind our own backs, such as: Stop thinking about it. Instruc-
> tions that are faithfully followed through the years. Avoid
> certain memories. Don't speak about them. Suppress words,
> sentences, whole chains of thought, that might give rise to re-
> membering. Don't ask your contemporaries certain questions.
> Because it is unbearable to think the tiny word "I" in connection
> with the word "Auschwitz." "I" in the past conditional: I would
> have. I might have. I could have. Done it. Obeyed orders.
> (pp. 229–230)

To speak in the first person is to assume the burden of history in the face of the collective repression of an entire generation determined not to wake up, to remember (pp. 149, 154). From this perspective, Wolf's seemingly unusual choice to write about her earlier self in the second and third persons seems if anything overdetermined. No wonder, too, that the act of composition was halting and protracted.[19]

The narrator's perseverance in the process of anamnesis and identity reconstruction despite her manifold ambivalences and fears recalls Nelly's courage at the end of the war in willing her battered identity into a form of "emergency maturity." In returning to the past, she confronts the identity costs of Nelly's premature, accelerated maturation, deferred and repressed; whether the costs can ever be repaid is a different question. Wolf's narrator, however, does not claim for the fiction of memory she has fashioned the therapeutic power to heal the wounds that experience and history visited upon her identity. She wisely concludes: "The child who was hidden in me—has she come forth? Or has she been scared into looking for a deeper, more inaccessible hiding place? . . . And the past, which can still split the first person into the second and the third—has its hegemony been broken? . . . I don't know" (p. 406).

In the light of the existential imperative driving our claims to continuous identity, it is hardly surprising that autobiographers should prove to be ambivalent with regard to memory, sometimes embracing both dynamic and invariant concepts. As makers themselves, autobiographers are primed to recognize the constructed nature of the past, yet they need at the same time to believe that in writing about the past they are performing an act of recovery: narrative teleology models the trajectory of continuous identity, reporting the supreme fiction of memory as fact.

References

Bruner, J. (1990). The invention of self: Autobiography and its forms. Conference on Autobiography and Self-Representation, March 3–4. University of California, Irvine.

Eakin, P. J. (1992). *Touching the world: Reference in autobiography.* Princeton: Princeton University Press.

Fivush, R. (1988). The functions of event memory: Some comments on Nelson and Barsalou. In U. Neisser and E. Winograd (Eds.), *Remembering reconsidered: Ecological and traditional approaches to the study of memory* (pp. 277–282). New York: Cambridge University Press.

Fivush, R., and Reese, E. (1992). The social construction of autobiographical memory. In M. A. Conway, D. C. Rubin, H. Spinnler, and W. A. Wagenaar (Eds.), *Theoretical perspectives on autobiographical memory* (pp. 115–132). Dordrecht, The Netherlands: Kluwer Academic Publishers.

Gergen, K. J. (1994). Mind, text, and society: Self-memory in social context. In U. Neisser and R. Fivush (Eds.), *The remembering self: Construction and accuracy in the self-narrative* (pp. 78–104). New York: Cambridge University Press.

Grosz, E. (1994). *Volatile bodies: Toward a corporeal feminism.* Bloomington: Indiana University Press.

Hirst, W. (1994). The remembered self in amnesics. In U. Neisser and R. Fivush (Eds.), *The remembering self: Construction and accuracy in the self-narrative* (pp. 252–277). New York: Cambridge University Press.

James, W. (1890/1981). *The principles of psychology,* 2 vols. Cambridge, MA: Harvard University Press.

Kerby, A. P. (1991). *Narrative and the self.* Bloomington: Indiana University Press.

Lejeune, P. (1989). The autobiographical pact. In P. J. Eakin (Ed.), *On autobiography* (K. Leary, Trans.) (pp. 3–30). Minneapolis: University of Minnesota Press. (Original work published 1973)

Lejeune, P. (1991). La mémoire et l'oblique: Georges Perec autobiographe. Paris: P. O. L.

Levy, S. (1994). Dr. Edelman's brain. *New Yorker,* May 2, pp. 62–73.

Malouf, D. (1986). 12 Edmondstone Street. In *12 Edmondstone Street* (pp. 1–66). Ringwood, Victoria, Australia: Penguin. (Original work published 1985)

Mandel, B. J. (1981). The past in autobiography. *Soundings, 64,* 75–92.

Miller, P. J. (1994). Narrative practices: Their role in socialization and self-construction. In U. Neisser and R. Fivush (Eds.), *The remembering self: Construction and accuracy in the self-narrative* (pp. 158–179). New York: Cambridge University Press.

Miller, P. J., Potts, R., Fung, H., Hoogstra, L., and Mintz, J. (1990). Narrative practices and the social construction of self in childhood. *American Ethnologist, 17,* 292–311.

Nabokov, V. (1966). *Speak, memory: An autobiography revisited.* New York: Putnam's.

Neisser, U. (1988). Five kinds of self-knowledge. *Philosophical Psychology,* *1,* 35–59.

Neisser, U. (1994). Self-narratives: True and false. In U. Neisser and R. Fivush (Eds.), *The remembering self: Construction and accuracy in the self-narrative* (pp. 1–18). New York: Cambridge University Press.

Nelson, K. (1988). The ontogeny of memory for real events. In U. Neisser and E. Winograd (Eds.), *Remembering reconsidered: Ecological and traditional approaches to the study of memory* (pp. 244–276). New York: Cambridge University Press.

Nelson, K. (Ed.). (1989). *Narratives from the crib.* Cambridge, MA: Harvard University Press.

Proust, M. (1934). *Remembrance of things past* (C. K. S. Moncrieff, Trans.), 2 vols. New York: Random House. (Original work published 1913–28)

Ricoeur, P. (1984–88). *Time and narrative* (K. McLaughlin and D. Pellauer, Trans.), 3 vols. Chicago: University of Chicago Press. (Original work published 1983–85)

Rosenfield, I. (1988). The invention of memory: A new view of the brain. New York: Basic Books.

Sacks, O. (1987). *The man who mistook his wife for a hat, and other clinical tales.* New York: Harper. (Original work published 1985)

Schacter, D. L. (1995). Memory distortion: History and current status. In D. L. Schacter (Ed.), *Memory distortion: How minds, brains, and societies reconstruct the past* (pp. 1–43). Cambridge, MA: Harvard University Press.

Schacter, D. L. (1996). *Searching for memory: The brain, the mind, and the past.* New York: Basic Books.

Searle, J. R. (1995). The mystery of consciousness: Part II. *New York Review of Books,* November 16, pp. 54–61.

Sheringham, M. (1993). The otherness of memory. In *French autobiography: Devices and desires* (pp. 288–326). Oxford: Clarendon Press.

Shotter, J. (1989). Social accountability and the social construction of "you." In J. Shotter and K. J. Gergen (Eds.), *Texts of identity* (pp. 133–151). London: Sage.

Snow, C. E. (1990). Building memories: The ontogeny of autobiography. In D. Cichetti and M. Beeghly (Eds.), *The self in transition: Infancy to childhood* (pp. 213–242). Chicago: University of Chicago Press.

Squire, L. R. (1995). Biological foundations of accuracy and inaccuracy in memory. In D. L. Schacter (Ed.), *Memory distortion: How minds, brains, and societies reconstruct the past* (pp. 197–225). Cambridge, MA: Harvard University Press.

Thernstrom, M. (1991). *The dead girl: A true story.* New York: Pocket Books. (Original work published 1990)

Wolf, C. (1980). *Patterns of childhood* (U. Molinaro and H. Rappolt, Trans.). New York: Farrar. (Original work published 1976)

Wolf, D. P. (1990). Being of several minds: Voices and versions of the self in early childhood. In D. Cichetti and M. Beeghly (Eds.), *The self in transition: Infancy to childhood* (pp. 183–212). Chicago: University of Chicago Press.

Young, K., and Saver, J. L. (1995). The neurology of narrative. Session on Autobiography and Neuroscience, Modern Language Association convention, December 29, New York.

Notes

1. In *Touching the World: Reference in Autobiography* (Eakin, 1992), I argue that autobiography is governed by a referential aesthetic, that the autobiographer signals to the reader in various ways "an intended fidelity of some kind to a world of biographical reference beyond the text" (p. 28).

2. The etymology given in the *American Heritage Dictionary of the English Language* reads as follows: "fiction [Middle English *ficcioun,* invention, from Old French *fiction,* from Latin *fictio,* a making, fashioning, from *fictus,* past participle of *fingere,* to touch, form, mold]" (p. 488).

3. Poststructuralist deconstructions of transcendental notions of selfhood are legion. The most promising newer approaches to study of the self repudiate Cartesian dualism in favor of the self as embodied. See, for example, Grosz (1994) and Kerby (1991).

4. Similarly, Gerald M. Edelman captures this constructivist view of the brain when he observes, "Your brain *constructs* . . . It doesn't mirror" (Levy, 1994, p. 62). Surveying memory research in the twentieth century, Daniel L. Schacter emphasizes the "constructivist" tendency of recent findings (1995, pp. 12–13).

5. For a brief discussion of this issue, see Lejeune (1991), pp. 74–77. He cites Stendhal, Mary McCarthy, Georges Perec, Nathalie Sarraute, and Guy Bechtel as rare examples of autobiographers who expose and explore the problems of memory.

6. Very little work has been done on the subject of memory in autobiography, perhaps because critics writing about autobiography themselves unwittingly subscribe to the "secular myth" of invariant memory. Sheringham's work (1993) gives the best overview (see his chapter 9, "The Otherness of Memory," pp. 288–326). For an important early study, see Mandel (1981). Adopting a phenomenological perspective, Mandel observes, "Since my past only truly exists in the present and since my present is always in motion, my past itself changes too—*actually changes*—while the illusion created is that it stays fixed" (p. 77; emphasis in original).

7. For the *petite madeleine* episode, see Proust (1934), Vol. 1, pp. 33–36. Sheringham (1993) wisely cautions, "Memory in Proust is by no means a

purely joyous affair," for it displays "a power to disrupt and problematize identity" (p. 292).

8. As Melanie Thernstrom (1991) puts it at the end of her memoir, *The Dead Girl*, "There is a place where everything is intact" (p. 428). Even so wary a student of memory's lures and deceptions as the French novelist Nathalie Sarraute is not immune to the siren call of belief in invariant memory. See Eakin (1992), pp. 31–39.

9. William Hirst (1994) has studied "the way in which the psychology of memory, narrative telling and self interact to effect changes in the self." He concludes that "people alter their concept of themselves as their life narratives shift" (pp. 252–253).

10. In a characteristic statement, the philosopher Anthony Kerby (1991) claims that "*self-narration*" is the defining act of the human subject, an act which is not only "descriptive of the self" but "*fundamental to the emergence and reality of that subject*" (p. 4; emphasis in original).

11. I am grateful to James Olney for prompting me to read this chapter of *The Principles of Psychology* in working out the connections among memory, narrative, and identity. In speaking of the "owning" of consciousness as central to an individual's sense of identity, I am using *own* in the sense of *acknowledge* rather than *possess*. It may well be that the former sense plays into the latter and is further implicated in the concept of "possessive individualism," but that is another matter. Edelman posits "the ability to discriminate the self from the nonself" (Searle, 1995, p. 54) as one of the fundamental attributes of primary consciousness.

12. See Ricoeur (1984–88) for a searching study of the relation between narrative and the human experience of temporality.

13. See, for instance, Kay Young and Jeffrey Saver (1995), who conclude that various brain injuries and lesions may impair the ability to construct narrative, thereby damaging identity: "Individuals who have lost the ability to construct narrative have lost their selves" (n.p.).

14. See also Neisser (1994), who comments: "Selves are not supported by narrative alone . . . amnesics have no current autobiographical memories and no on-going self-narratives . . . Nevertheless each of them has, and is aware of having, an obvious and distinct identity" (pp. 14–15).

15. In these adult-child exchanges about the past the child learns what is reportable: "such discussions mark for the child the incidents that should qualify as memorable and thus as narratable" (Snow, 1990, p. 225).

16. Nelson argues that "the distinctive thing about the autobiographical memory system is that the memories it contains do appear to be valued for themselves" (p. 266), and that they form "a personal history that has its own value independent of the general memory function of prediction and preparation for future events" (p. 267). Commenting on this view, Fivush (1988) notes that the same event memory may have a dual func-

tion, both predictive and autobiographical. If she is correct, this observation would link autobiographical memory to event memories with a more obviously identifiable adaptive purpose. As a student of self-narration, I like to think of its having an adaptive value of some kind in the perspective of human evolution.

17. Wolf's autobiography violates Lejeune's (1989) notion of the autobiographical pact and the related convention that author, narrator, and protagonist of an autobiographical text share the same name and identity. Contributing to this scrambling of autobiography's conventional generic signals, the back cover of the paperback edition identifies *Patterns of Childhood* as a novel.

18. We need to recognize an inevitable circularity in the evidence here, keeping in mind that everything that we know about Nelly is supplied by the autobiographical narrator performing an act of retrospect twenty-five years after the fact. Wolf's narrator projects a lively sense of the extent to which she may be manipulating the character Nelly for purposes of her own: "Aren't you fooling yourself by thinking that this child is moving on her own, according to her own inner laws? . . . The child is your vehicle" (p. 210).

19. For characteristic passages on the difficulties encountered in writing this narrative, see as examples Wolf's pages 164, 357–358.

Acknowledgments

This chapter appears in different form in my book *How Our Lives Become Stories: Making Selves* (Ithaca: Cornell University Press, 1999), and is used by permission of the publisher.

Autobiography as Moral Battleground

Sissela Bok

> The autobiographer has ex officio two qualifications of
> supreme importance in all literary work. He is writing
> about a topic in which he is keenly interested, and about
> a topic upon which he is the highest living authority. It
> may be reckoned, too, as a special felicity that an
> autobiography, alone of all books, may be more valuable
> in proportion to the amount of misrepresentation which it
> contains. We do not wonder when a man gives a false
> character to his neighbour, but it is always curious to see
> how a man contrives to give a false testimonial to himself.
>
> *Leslie Stephen*

When Sir Leslie Stephen wrote these magisterial and calmly
ironical lines, he was editor of the first twenty-six volumes of the
British *Dictionary of National Biography*. As a biographer, seeking to
dispel the myths woven by those writing about their own lives, he
could attest to the special pleasure in being "admitted behind the
scenes and [able to] trace the growth of that singular phantom which,
like the spectre of the Brocken [a mountain in Germany], is the man's
own shadow cast upon the coloured and distorting mists of memory"
(1881/1904, p. 185).

At the time, Stephen could hardly have predicted that his own
daughter Virginia Woolf, not yet born, would one day portray him
and other family members and intimates in her novel *To the Lighthouse* from perspectives so unfamiliar and diverging as to further
challenge any presumption of unique authority—either the biographer's or the autobiographer's. Nor could she, in turn, have predicted
the flood of memoirs, critiques, and biographies that would continue
to focus on the lives she evoked in that novel, much less the role that

autobiographical accounts would come to occupy over the course of our century in literary, therapeutic, and legal controversies.

It is against this contemporary backdrop of often bitterly contested memories explored in best-selling memoirs, therapy sessions, and courts of law, that I take up the role of the autobiographical account as moral battleground. I suggest that although some of the arenas in which such confrontations take place today may seem peculiar to our age and the attendant waves of publicity appear unprecedented, there is nothing new about such controversies in their own right—nor about the jarring perspectives of the *dramatis personae* in such accounts: the perspectives of the "I," the "you," and the "he, she, and they."

I begin by discussing the first-person perspective of the narrator; then turn to the second-person perspective of the reader or listener, often as skeptical as that of Leslie Stephen; and finally consider the third-person perspective of the author's relatives and other persons described in autobiographical accounts. This last perspective is rarely forgotten by the narrator, but often ignored by most of the rest of us as readers, listeners, and critics.

First-Person Perspective

Let us begin, then, with the first-person perspective of authors. For them, memory and belief are crucially at issue—not only their own memories and their own beliefs but their efforts to influence how they are to be remembered and the beliefs that will be entertained about them. Autobiographical accounts constitute, in part, empirical and moral claims that individuals stake out about their lives and, in the process, about the lives of others they have known. As authors attempt to recapture, relive, sometimes recreate their memories, they are led to praise and to question, to repent, ask forgiveness, accuse, and justify. They aim to shape belief not only about themselves but also about their relations to family members, colleagues, friends, lovers and enemies.

Such a process of writing about oneself offers temptations to rewrite one's life, even to write persons out of one's existence altogether. Saint Teresa's and John Stuart Mill's mothers are as conspicuously all but absent from their written lives as are the fathers of Saint

Augustine and Jean-Paul Sartre. Yet most parents or siblings in *Mommy Dearest*-type exposés would pay dearly for the privilege of being relegated to such obscurity. It is no wonder that in the back-ground of many a candid self-portrait hover bitter relatives, colleagues, friends, and enemies, some of whom are perplexed or resentful at having their personal lives exhibited, perhaps ridiculed or maligned; nor that writing about one's life involves intense moral confrontation, both with self and with those others, raising both aesthetic and moral questions of *treatment*. Authors show doubly how they treat individuals—themselves and others—in their texts and in the lives they trace out for readers.

For some who write about themselves, what matters most is being remembered at all: not confused with others or lost to posterity, but acknowledged in their own right and as the persons they take themselves to be. This is how Margaret Cavendish, Duchess of Newcastle, put it in *The True Relation of My Birth, Breeding, and Life*, in 1656:

> I hope my readers will not think me vain for writing my life, since there have been many that have done the like, as Caesar, Ovid, and many more, both men and women, and I know no reason I may not do it as well as they; but I verily believe that some censuring readers will scornfully say: why hath this Lady writ her own life? since none cares to know whose daughter she was, or whose wife she is, or how she was bred, or what fortunes she had, or how she lived, or what humour or disposition she was of. I answer that it is true, that 'tis to no purpose to the readers, but it is to the authoress, because I write it for my own sake, not for theirs. Neither did I intend this piece for to delight, but to divulge; not to please the fancy but to tell the truth.
> (pp. 317–318)

"Since none cares to know." It is this indifference that Cavendish, like so many autobiographers, writes above all to dispel. Whether she is describing her childhood, with its emphasis on "breeding" and compliance, or conveying her desire to write rather than do needlework, or recounting her marriage to her husband, William Cavendish (whose biography she has already written in glowing terms), or recalling the suffering and exile she shared with him during Britain's civil wars, or stressing her own efforts at contemplation, her prolific writing, and her extravagant ambitions for world fame, she is staking out a claim for her own life as one that is worthy of being long remembered. She ends by saying that she does not want to risk being confused with some other Duchess of Newcastle: "for my Lord having had two wives, I might easily have been mistaken, especially if I should die and my Lord marry again" (p. 315).

It is first and foremost against oblivion, against the confusing of their persons with others after death, against the wiping out of all traces of their lives, that many autobiographers write. Their ancestors, their families, all that went into shaping their existence matters, they insist. Their activities and efforts to change were not for naught. Even their suffering must have had meaning. For the brief duration of their lives, they had a unique perspective on the world that they knew. They saw, felt, heard, loved, and hated from their own vantage point. Why should it be, how *could* it be, that in the long run none should care to know?

Although oblivion may be the gravest peril in the minds of many who write about their lives, it does not threaten the most famous among them; not, for instance, Saint Augustine, Rousseau, or Tolstoy, all of whom were well known in their time, always controversial whether loved or hated, but certainly destined never to be forgotten, even as they sat down to write their *Confessions*. Far more troubling to these writers than the unlikely risk of not being remembered was that of being forever *mis*remembered—misunderstood, misinterpreted, cast in a false light. Their autobiographical works may be directed in part as defenses against adversaries and detractors, but authors like Saint Augustine and Tolstoy, who have undergone a religious conversion, also intend to contradict their own previous writings about their lives. These authors want to leave but chosen traces, erasing others, sometimes crossing and recrossing them like squirrels in the snow.

The religious overtones in these texts are often passionate both in the self-flagellation and in the repentance they express. To the extent that their authors have come to believe that they were culpable in misleading their public in the past, they may feel under a special obligation to render a truer account and to set matters straight. So for instance when Saint Augustine, after converting to Christianity, came to reject most of his early beliefs, he looked back at what he had written and taught as not only mistaken but as a tissue of lies. From his nineteenth to his twenty-eighth year, he writes in Book IV of the *Confessions,* he was led astray and led others astray in turn.

> We were alike deceivers and deceived in all our different aims and ambitions, both publicly when we expounded our so-called liberal ideas, and in private through our service to what we called religion. In public we were cocksure, in private superstitious, and everywhere void and empty / . . . . / Let the proud deride me, o God, and all whom you have not yet laid low and humiliated for the salvation of their souls; but let me still confess my sins to you for your honor and glory. Allow me, I beseech you, to trace in memory my past deviations and to offer you a sacrifice of joy. (397–398/1961, p. 71)

In the same manner, Tolstoy in *Confession* looks back with revulsion at his past life as having been hollow and false, and at his having written *War and Peace* and *Anna Karenina* as an intentional betrayal of the public: "In order to acquire the fame and the money I was writing for, it was necessary to conceal what was good and to flaunt what was bad" (p. 18).

Second-Person Perspective

The second-person perspective, that of the reader or listener to whom autobiographers address themselves and without whom all memory of them would perish, is more familiar to most of us than that of either the first or the third person. Most immediately, the readers the authors address are contemporaries: thus Saint Augustine addresses his *Confession* not only to God, but very much also to all those throughout the known world who, as he puts it in Book X, "have not their ear at my heart, where I am what I am, [yet want to] hear from my confession what I am inwardly" (p. 209).

As readers of such accounts, however, we have more to go on than the texts themselves. We can study what these authors wrote before and after, and what others have written in response. As a result, when we come across claims such as those of Saint Augustine or Tolstoy dismissing their past activities as deceitful or wrong-headed, we may balk. When authors aim as passionately as they did to be remembered in an entirely new way, they are driven to disparage their past perceptions and statements and to insist on special confidence in their current insights. Yet why should we, as readers, accept the latest versions as thus privileged? The reader's second-person perspective is of necessity more qualified and often considerably more skeptical than that of the author.

For readers of Tolstoy's great novels, the assertion that he wrote them purely for fame and money rings utterly false, the more so to the extent that we know from his diaries and other sources all that went into composing these works. This may be one reason why Tolstoy's biographers have been especially scathing in their treatment of his *Confession*. Thus A. N. Wilson views Tolstoy's rejection of his novels in that work as one of many elements that render it a "transparent piece of self-deception: transparent, that is, to everyone except the author" (1988, p. 312). This castigation blinds Wilson, I suggest, otherwise one of Tolstoy's most perceptive biographers, to the illuminating literary and philosophical qualities of the *Confession* and prevents him from examining it in the light of the long tradition of confessional works by Rousseau and others that Tolstoy had in mind when writing.

Biographers may be especially prone to such withering skepticism regarding the autobiographical works of the authors they study—prone, like Leslie Stephen, to dismissing these as efforts on the part of authors to give false testimonials to themselves, or like Wilson in holding that Tolstoy's *Confession* is nothing but blatant self-deception. Biography, after all, calls for the sharpest of eyes with respect to factual inconsistencies, exaggerations, inaccuracies, falsehoods, and self-deceit.

Such a professional focus intensifies and deepens the second-person perspective of the reader; but it risks allowing concern for accuracy to deflect fuller understanding of autobiographical texts. This risk mirrors and reverses the risk of claims to omniscience to which Stephen pointed for those assuming the first-person perspective. If I may coin a word or two, slipping into the posture of *panskepticism* or *omnidubience* is as dangerous for us as readers, and above all for biographers, as is slipping into that of *omniscience* for authors.

In Albert Camus' novel *The Fall,* Clamence, a compulsive reader of confessions, exemplifies this devouring skepticism. He warns readers against falling for the belief that authors who write about themselves, especially if they claim to be offering confessions, will truly reveal themselves as they are. They feign to confess, rather, in order to say nothing of what they know. "When they pretend to begin their avowals, it is the moment to be on your guard, they will be putting makcup on the corpse" (Camus, 1962, p. 141; Bok, 1989, p. 74). Yet Clamence himself is ceaselessly engaged in self-revelation even as he warns against its impossibility. Shifting between telling his story and listening to tales of others, he explores for us, the readers of Camus' novel, the allure of self-revelation for both speakers and listeners as well as its inevitable shortfalls from either perspective.

Authors vary in the awareness they show of the doubts that their claims may evoke, depending on the dissonances in their works between a past, discarded life and a new, fuller, supposedly more legitimate existence; between the evanescence of memories and the firmer reality of the present; and between the lived experience of both past and present and the prospect of oblivion, erasure, and death. But most authors recognize the skepticism with which at least some readers will view their accounts. To buttress the validity of their reports, they often insist on the very first page that they are going to be exceptionally truthful and remarkably open. Thus Montaigne declares, in introducing his *Essays,* that if only custom allowed he would "gladly have portrayed myself here entire and wholly naked" (p. 2). Queen Christina of Sweden, in her exceptionally insincere *Autobiography,* asks God to ensure that all she is going to say will bear witness to the truth, however damaging to herself (1681/1959, pp. 7–8). Edward Gibbon begins his *Autobiography* by saying that "truth, naked, unblushing truth, the first virtue of more serious history, must be the sole recommendation of this personal narrative." And Eleanor Roosevelt indicates in her *Autobiography* that her objective is "to give as truthful a picture as possible of a human being" (1961, p. xv).

The French critic Philippe Lejeune, in *Le Pacte autobiographique,* characterizes such declarations on the part of authors as efforts to establish a pact with readers, one underscoring the identity, in some sense at least, between author and subject; and as assurances that the accounts provided are as faithful as authors can make them. Autobiographies, memoirs, and all the writings Lejeune characterizes as "intimate" imply, he suggests, a pact quite unlike that in works of fiction. The pact signals that because one is both the author and the person whose life is conveyed through the text, one must be prepared to "honor one's signature" in a special way. In fiction, on the contrary, no such claim is made. The result is something of a paradox: the more autobiographers insist on their veracity, the more readers look for discrepancies between the written life and what they know of the author's life; whereas when confronted with autobiographical fiction, the effort of readers is, rather, to try to discern similarities between the author and the central character in the novel.

From the point of view of most readers, however, the full reliability of the claims made by authors of autobiographical works turns out to be secondary to the deep immediate interest aroused by the best of their works. Long before we discover that Montaigne and Rousseau are not as candid as they profess to be, we are drawn to their writings; long after, we read on. We come to recognize how much they reveal to us, even as they select and reinvent, at times misremember or misjudge, aspects of their lives.

Authors differ in their approach to the challenge and the peril of writing about themselves: the challenge of conveying a human life so as to make it memorable and alive to others long after they themselves die; and the peril of being nevertheless forgotten, misunderstood, disappointing to readers, false to those of whom one writes, and in the end false to one's own hopes—doubly lifeless. The greatest autobiographical works succeed in meeting that challenge and in transcending (without necessarily eliminating) that peril. In so doing, they come close to overcoming all barriers between author and reader. They show us the possibility of setting forth a human life with the precision, uniqueness, and depth that we sense but cannot put into words.

Even authors whose perspective seems especially lopsided, immature, or superficial, such as those engaged in what the late J. Anthony Lukas has called "the exploitation of personal dysfunction for private gain" (1997, p. 19), cannot help bearing witness to crucial issues of character and conduct. Whether they malign or sugarcoat family relations or disparage, ignore, or misrepresent former friends or spouses, their treatment of these others is as revealing of character in what they write as in how they live.

Third-Person Perspective

One category of readers, however, cannot afford the equanimity and distance with which we may now coolly weigh, for instance, Rousseau's attacks on former intimates or Tolstoy's revisionist view of his past activities as meaningless. These are persons occupying what I have called the third-person perspective, that of the author's relatives and others described in autobiographical accounts. The readers in this third category are more prone to skepticism than the sternest of biographers. For contemporaries of even the finest authors of memoirs and other autobiographical accounts, the question of the accuracy of the memories such works convey and of the validity of the beliefs that may be driving their authors matters far more personally and directly—and never more than if they find themselves included in such accounts. To them it may matter crucially who was right about, say, the breakup of a friendship, the question of whether or not sexual abuse took place, or the circumstances under which a father or mother died. It is here that the contesting of memories can be most bitter; and here that such accounts can most easily be visualized as moral battlegrounds.

Readers who have such a personal stake in what others convey about their lives have little patience with any confusion between what they perceive as fact and as fiction, regardless of how it is labeled by the author. All the distinctions stressed by literary scholars, such as that between autobiographical fiction and nonfiction, or between memoirs, confessions, and apologias, are as nothing to those relatives or other intimates who see themselves falsely portrayed in published works. And all the protestations by authors—that they were not aiming at absolute accuracy or intending harm to someone's reputation—do not assuage anyone who feels wounded by such works.

The confrontation between authors and third parties becomes public whenever some among the latter choose to offer their own first-person accounts of particular characters or incidents. It is rarely a more searing encounter than when former friends or once-close siblings take to the pen. To illustrate such diverging accounts among contemporaries, I shall briefly consider Rousseau's *Confessions* and Madame Louise d'Epinay's autobiographical novel, *Histoire de Madame de Montbrillant*; then turn to the memoirs of five of the six children of Sofya and Lev Tolstoy who lived on after the traumatic events of his death.

Louise d'Epinay and Jean-Jacques Rousseau were formidable opponents in a conflict that involved most of the figures in the French Enlightenment and lasted long after their own deaths (Bok, 1984). Each knew from the confidences they had exchanged during their years of friendship in the 1760s that the other was working on autobiographical materials; each was a master of psychological dissection and subtle blame; after they quarreled, each realized that the nature of their dispute might well form part of what the other was writing down and that intimate matters once told in confidence might then be revealed and most likely distorted; and each ached—and knew the other ached—to convey in writing a stronger consistency between living and professed beliefs than gossip and rumor and the distortions of the other might indicate. As with military adversaries imagining "worst-case scenarios," so Rousseau and Madame d'Epinay pondered the worst that the other might have to utter and prepared to respond in kind.

This is not to say that they did not have other, more important purposes in writing about themselves. But part of the story they would tell would be an effort to paint the other in "truer" colors than that other might provide without such correction. Rousseau in his *Confessions* depicted Madame d'Epinay as first having lured him into believing in their close, lasting friendship, then betraying that friendship in despicable ways. Among her offenses, he included her revealing to Voltaire the secret he had once confided to her: that he had abandoned at the public foundling-home one after the other of the children he had fathered with his caretaker and companion, Thérèse Levasseur, thus making possible a vicious and, in Rousseau's view, partly false attack by Voltaire.

In turn, Madame d'Epinay, in her epistolary novel about Madame de Montbrillant, provides a fascinating portrait of herself as the woman of letters that Rousseau claimed she could never become. She includes letters of his that give a decidedly less flattering view of his actions to precipitate the breach in their relations. The unpublished manuscript of her novel, which she willed at her death to the Baron Grimm, suffered many vicissitudes, including being packed up by guards during the French Revolution and labeled "worthless scribblings," then being published thirty years later in a truncated and altered version mislabeled *Memoirs and Correspondence of Madame d'Epinay*.

Rousseau's *Confessions* were also published after his death; but before then, the fact that he read aloud selected passages from that work in Paris salons proved so painful to Louise d'Epinay that she felt compelled to ask the police to issue an injunction against further readings on his part. From the moment of its publication, *Confessions* has been regarded as one of the world's great autobiographical works. As readers, we approach it on many levels quite apart from the question of factual accuracy. Madame d'Epinay's novel is at last coming to be read for its own worth, instead of being seen solely as part of some vendetta against Rousseau (Badinter, 1983; Weinreb, 1993).

For us, when we occupy the second-person perspective of readers, the chance to see the two works together provides a more illuminating portrait of the age and of the various protagonists in the struggles recounted in the two books. This helps us gain a deeper understanding of Rousseau, who is so elusive in his *Confessions* in spite of his declaration that in it he would show himself "in all the truth of nature" (1782/1964, p. 3). It helps us better to perceive his genius, his capacity for self-deception, his paranoia, but also the sense of broken bonds that both drew on that paranoia and intensified it. In the same way, we come to understand Madame d'Epinay too, and what she tried to do in her novel. Her spirit, her efforts at change and at standing on her own feet, what she took and what she rejected in her relations with Rousseau, her insights into human motives and her concern for those close to her, are cast in a deeper, more complex light once we consider both accounts.

If we try to put ourselves in *their* positions, however, I think we also understand better why neither one would be prepared to seek the distance to look at the work of the other as literature or social commentary alone. Once you are portrayed as one of the *dramatis per-*

sonae in such a work, no matter how splendid its literary merits, it is almost impossible to judge it without first asking about the justice or injustice of the characterizations it provides of yourself and of people you know well.

But such questioning carries its own risks of bias and distortion. Readers in this third-person perspective run *both* of the risks to which I have pointed in the first- and second-person perspectives. Someone whose character, and often also veracity, is at issue in the writings of another risks yielding to both a sense of *omniscience* about their own version of the disputed facts and a devouring *omnidubience* or panskepticism about anything their adversary recounts. "If they can be so wrong about what I know is the case about experiences we shared and about myself, then how can I trust what they say about anything else?"

This two-pronged risk of a skewed perspective is perhaps never greater than when the protagonists are members of the same family. Tolstoy's words, at the beginning of *Anna Karenina,* that happy families are all alike but unhappy families unhappy each in their own way, received a fitting commentary by the critic John Leonard: "*All* families are Russian novels!" And when a family, as Tolstoy's own or Virginia Woolf's, becomes the object of public debate, such a family "novel" can easily become a *roman fleuve,* with never-ending contributions from family members, friends, hangers-on, and critics—all attempting to explain "how it really was."

The Tolstoy family may be in a class of its own in the category of families in which both parents and children have published autobiographical accounts. Of the six Tolstoy children who survived Sofya and Lev Tolstoy, all but one wrote about how it was to grow up in that family. Their parents had kept passionately explicit diaries for many years that they had often shown to each other, at times to others in the house, sometimes day by day. A few years after Lev Tolstoy died in 1910, Sofya published her diaries, and later on also her memoirs. Over the ensuing decades, the children's books rang forth, in the course of many years—first in Russian, then in English, French, and German, depending on where each one settled after the Revolution. Among them are Sergei Tolstoy's *Tolstoy Remembered by His Son;*

Lev Tolstoy's *Truth about My Father;* Tatyana Tolstoy's *Friends and Guests at Yasnaya Polyana, The Tolstoy Home,* and *Tolstoy Remembered;* Ilya Tolstoy's *Tolstoy, My Father;* and Alexandra Tolstoy's *Léon Tolstoy, mon père, Tolstoys Flucht und Tod, The Tragedy of Tolstoy,* and *Out of the Past.*

Each of the Tolstoy siblings had, of necessity, an insider's perspective differing from that of the public, even on an illustrious confessional work such as their father's. They had witnessed many of the events he described. They knew his other writings and those of their mother, and the daily dramas in their home during the last decades of his life. They lived with the veneration and controversy and extraordinary worldwide publicity that he generated. As for their siblings' published views regarding what they might otherwise have taken to be their shared experience of family life, they were often startled to see sharp discrepancies from their own memories.

In their various memoirs, several among the Tolstoy siblings react to another's accounts, clearly troubled by incongruities that they come across and sometimes prepared to rethink their own earlier accounts as a result. As reasons for bringing out their own books, they often point to all the falsehoods written about their home and their family. Two of the six—Tatyana, the finest, most perceptive writer among the siblings, and Alexandra, or Sasha, born long after the others and rejected from the first by her mother—return again and again to the effort at sorting out their memories in print. And Lev, named for his father and aching to emulate his career as a writer, publishes his account first in French and then, somewhat altered, in English.

The siblings dwell especially often on the last, titanic battles between their parents before their father fled the family home in October 1910, at age eighty-two, became feverish, developed pneumonia, and died at the Astapovo railroad station, surrounded by reporters and photographers from the Russian and world press. Sofya Tolstoy had taken the train to join her husband when she learned his whereabouts from the newspapers; but Alexandra and Sergei, who were among those at his bedside, at first deceived him into believing their mother was still at home. Then, when she stood outside the station house, her face against the window of the room where he lay, they would not allow her to join him until he had become unconscious, near death, on the grounds that it would "excite him too much."

Reading these books together, one sees how the siblings are surprised at what they see in one another's books, how they try and try to think through what really must have happened, how they reread their own diaries, how they reevaluate their earlier reactions and ways of proceeding within the family (sometimes with genuine contrition), and how even those who stood implacably against one another for decades at last manage to seek contact with one another at the end of their lives.

Their conflicts and changing reactions are perhaps most thoroughly and humanely discussed in Ilya's *Tolstoy, My Father*. He looks back at the situation of his father and his mother and at how the siblings came to choose sides, most often against their mother, to the point of preventing her from approaching her husband as he lay dying. Now Ilya looks at this as a cruel mistake. And the reasons? They go far back in all their lives, but "have more to do with accusations than with guilt" (1971, p. 274).

Even for Alexandra, the unwelcome last child who became her father's secretary and ever-present helpmate during his last years and who had been most relentlessly hostile to her mother and those brothers who sided with her to the end—even for her, contempt and hatred have ebbed away by the time she writes *Out of the Past*, her last book: "Only now, when I near the end, can I remember my childhood without bitterness" (1981, p. 521). Her mother, she writes, before dying had asked her forgiveness for having never loved her. At last it was possible for Alexandra fully to forgive her mother, and to forgive herself in turn.

We as outside readers can approach the siblings' passionate, at times contradictory, family chronicles from a second-person perspective that also reaches for more complete understanding of the differing first- and third-person perspectives. It is my sense that this became possible for a number of the siblings as well. They could allow themselves to lay down their arms, helped in this regard by straining to view their lives from all three perspectives, not merely one or two. They could see the many-sidedness of the conflicts in which they had been enmeshed and struggle to understand each protagonist instead of choosing up sides as before. It was not that they would regard facts and fiction as indistinguishable, or that it was not possible to tell certain rights from certain wrongs. It was a fact, for example, that their father died at the Astapovo train station and that their distraught mother stood outside, looking in. For at least some of them, keeping her outside had come to seem no longer right but clearly wrong, however necessary it had seemed at the time.

Research concerning memory and belief can shed new light on the three perspectives on autobiographical writings discussed in this chapter, and thereby help to sort out some of the difficulties and conflicts they inevitably generate. Our growing understanding of how false memories and beliefs are generated, and of processes such as "source monitoring" and "perspective taking," is going to be indispensable to the literary and psychological study of such texts. In turn, scrutiny in this new light, perhaps especially of texts that sometimes support and sometimes contradict one another, can illuminate the conclusions derived from this research.

Both the scientific and the literary approaches have limitations, however, when it comes to fully understanding the complexity of human memory regarding oneself and one's world. These limitations are the more constricting to the extent that we do not fully take into account the experience of all three perspectives. One who knew that multiple experience especially well, and articulated it most subtly in all its shadings, was Virginia Woolf. She was as omnivorous a reader of autobiographies as her father, Sir Leslie Stephen, and as aware as he of how authors invariably cast their shadow "upon the coloured and distorting mists of memory" (p. 185). In addition, she knew from within the problems of those who attempt to write such accounts. A great many of them fail, she suggests, because the authors find it so difficult to describe themselves. "So they say: 'This is what happened'; but they do not say what the person was like to whom it happened" (Woolf, 1976, p. 65). Woolf goes on to use her own earliest memories to point to a second difficulty facing authors: that of comparing oneself to others, situating oneself in their midst, with anything like the necessary insight and accuracy.

Woolf's own writings about her childhood and her family, published posthumously, memorably convey her struggles to overcome these failures. She reflects there on the nature of memory itself as she tries to visualize and reexperience her childhood. In so doing, she endeavors to pinpoint experiences that neuroscientists and psychologists are still struggling to elucidate.

> In certain favourable moods, memories—what one has forgotten—come to the top. Now if this is so, is it not possible—I often wonder—that things we have felt with great intensity have an existence independent of our minds; are in fact still in existence? And if so, will it not be possible, in time, that some device will be invented by which we can tap them? I see it—the past—as an avenue lying behind; a long ribbon of scenes, emotions. There at the end of the avenue still, are the garden and the nursery. Instead of remembering here a scene and there a sound, I shall fit a plug into the wall; and listen in to the past. I shall turn up August 1890. I feel that strong emotion must leave its trace; and it is only a question of discovering how we can get ourselves attached to it, so that we shall be able to live our lives through from the start. (Woolf, 1976, p. 67)

It is perhaps in her novel *To the Lighthouse* that Woolf manages, in the most profound and humane way, to reflect a family life that was quite as many layered and complicated as Tolstoy's—one similarly fraught with conflict, but without the same external signs of domestic warfare. She succeeds in that novel in capturing and reexperiencing memories from her childhood and in entering with extraordinary acuity into the often narrow, at times brutal, perspectives of siblings and parents and family intimates. And she respects, precisely, the many-sidedness of perspectives, reflects each one so as to conjure forth individuals as whole persons rather than as stiff figures in her own drama. She has not put makeup on any cadavers, neither has she tried to dishonor them. With the clearest of eyes, she has borne witness to cruelty, tenderness, life at its most intense and ephemeral, and to the nearness throughout both of intensely felt memory and of death and oblivion.

References

Augustine, Saint. (397–398/1961). *Confessions*. New York: Penguin Books.

Badinter, E. (1983). *Emilie, Emilie: L'Ambition féminine au dixhuitième siècle*. Paris: Gallimard.

Bok, S. (1984). The contested portrait of Madame d'Epinay. *Ploughshares*, Nos. 2 and 3, pp. 166–178.

Bok, S. (1989). *Secrets: On the ethics of concealment and revelation*. New York: Vintage.

Camus, A. (1962). *La Chute*. Paris: Bibliothèque de la Pléiade.

Cavendish, M. (1656/1886). *The life of William Cavendish, Duke of Newcastle. The true relation of my birth, breeding, and life*. London: John C. Nimmo.

Christina, Queen. (1681/1959). *Självbiografi och aforismer*. Stockholm: Natur och Kultur.

Epinay, Louise, Marquise d'. (1818). *Mémoires et correspondance de Madame d'Epinay*. Paris: Brunet.

Epinay, Louise, Marquise d'. (1989). *Histoire de Madame de Montbrillant*. Paris: Mercure de France.

Gibbon, E. (1796/1978). *Autobiography*. Oxford: Oxford University Press.

Lejeune, P. (1975). *Le Pacte autobiographique*. Paris: Seuil.

Lukas, J. A. (1997). Symposium: The memoir revolution. *Authors Guild Bulletin*.

Montaigne, Michel de. (1588/1965). *Essays* (D. M. Frame, Trans.). Stanford: Stanford University Press.

Roosevelt, E. (1961). *Autobiography*. New York: Harper.

Rousseau, J. J. (1782/1964). *Les Confessions*. Paris: Garnier Frères.

Stephen, L. (1881/1904). *Autobiography: Hours in a library*. New York: Putnam.

Tolstoy, A. (1916). *Léon Tolstoy, mon père*. Paris: Amiot-Dumont.

Tolstoy, A. (1925). *Tolstoys Flucht und Tod*. Berlin: Bruno Cassirer.

Tolstoy, A. (1953). *The tragedy of Tolstoy*. London: Oxford University Press.

Tolstoy, A. (1981). *Out of the past* (K. Strelsky and C. Wolkonsky, Eds.). New York: Columbia University Press.

Tolstoy, I. (1971). *Tolstoy, my father: Reminiscences*. Chicago: Cowles.

Tolstoy, L. (1880/1983). *Confession*. New York: Norton.

Tolstoy, L. L. (1923/1979). *La Vérité sur mon père*. Paris: Bibliothèque cosmopolite, translated by himself and somewhat altered as *The truth about my father* (New York: D. Appleton, 1924).

Tolstoy, S. (1962). *Tolstoy remembered by his son*. New York: Atheneum.

Tolstoy, S. (1989). *Tolstoy et les Tolstoy*. Paris: Perrin.

Tolstoy, T. (1951). *The Tolstoy home: Diaries of Tatiana Sukhotin-Tolstoy.* New York: Columbia University Press.

Tolstoy, T. (1977). *Tolstoy remembered.* London: Michael Joseph.

Weinreb, R. (1993). *Eagle in a cage of gauze: Louise d'Epinay, femme de lettres.* New York: AMS Press.

Wilson, A. N. (1988). *Tolstoy.* New York: Fawcett Columbine.

Woolf, V. (1927). *To the lighthouse.* London: Hogarth Press.

Woolf, V. (1976). *Moments of being: Unpublished autobiographical writings* (J. Schulkind, Ed.). New York: Harcourt, Brace, Jovanovich.

Thinking about Belief:
Concluding Remarks

Antonio R. Damasio

The conference on memory and belief on which this volume is based gave support to the idea that understanding the nature of belief is essential for making sense of human behavior in a comprehensive manner. The conference brought together the disciplines and the approaches required to make progress in the investigation of this problem, and the discussions that ensued fully justified the decision to include both the traditional disciplines of the humanities and the less conventional and hybrid disciplines such as cognitive neuroscience. As a topic, belief is indeed that wide and that tall.

All things considered, the prospect of making inroads into the problem is good. This is a time of explosive developments in neuroscience and cognitive science. It is likely that such developments, along with the refined scholarship the humanities are offering, will permit new progress on the issues of belief and memory that confronted the participants.

A Working Definition of Belief

Although none of the participants asked to have his or her definition of the term "belief" endorsed by a vote, it became apparent, as the conference evolved, that a certain consensus was being reached. Perhaps I should begin by indicating my sense of that agreement by spelling out what the term means to me. In order to do so, I will make a distinction between *belief* and *knowledge*. I use the term "belief" when I refer to the attribution of truth value to a particular thought content, either perceived or recalled. It makes no difference whether the perception or recollection is that of an action, or an event, or an entity, or whether the perceived or recollected material is concrete or abstract. As I see it, to believe is to qualify a perception or recollection as true, false, or somewhere in between. Whereas the term "knowledge" refers to a datum in and of itself, the word "belief" refers to a datum qualified. The qualification is based on the use of a scale on which truth and falsity are at opposing poles, and on which, in between, is a greater or smaller probability of being close to one or the other pole. The believer is confident of the qualification. Belief belongs in the same family of meanings as conviction and certainty.

It also became apparent from the discussion that there is an advantage in circumscribing the domains over which one can hold a belief. In general, one does not use beliefs to qualify *any* datum from *every* domain of knowledge. One uses beliefs to qualify data from some domains of knowledge far more frequently than others. We can, of course, hold beliefs about the preferable shapes of doorknobs and broomsticks, but if one would see a character on stage talking about such beliefs, one would immediately realize that the character was comedic. The reason is that we tend to hold beliefs about certain kinds of matters—mostly, as it turns out, about matters of life and death. The proper subject matter is almost any topic that gravely affects our well-being, in both the physical and the spiritual senses. This range includes matters of moral behavior, matters of faith, matters of life—for instance, how to define life early in an organism's development or late in that development, in certain conditions of disease— matters that have to do with the constitution and organization of social groups, political systems, distribution of wealth, the running of the economic enterprise, and the state of the culture. Lastly, belief is about matters that have to do with the idea we hold of ourselves.

The Future of a Discussion

I would like to make a brief comment on the future, on some possible way of continuing the focused discussion on belief that began in this conference. I would think that one way of doing so is by engaging in a program to investigate the cognitive and neural underpinnings of belief. Let me give an idea of where I would start.

If belief pertains to the attribution of truth value to a particular mental content, then in order to understand the nature of belief we probably need to understand the mechanism of that attribution. We need to elucidate the means by which we qualify a certain datum in terms of its truth value. Let us consider some possible means of producing such an attribution and qualification.

I begin with the most transparent of those means, which I call openly cognitive, in the usual sense of the term. What I have in mind is the activation of some collection of explicit facts that are codisplayed around the central content of a given datum. Those coactivated facts help establish the provenance and interconnections of the content under scrutiny. They define the circumstances and conditions under which that content arose. The coactivated facts that we retrieve, declaratively—explicitly, in full consciousness—are available for manipulation using the strategies of logical reasoning, and the manipulation allows us to draw inferences about the truth or falsity of the datum, given the premises embodied in the coactivated facts.

There is probably no better way of building or expressing rational beliefs than using precisely this mechanism. Curiously, however, we do not often use this strategy. First, I venture that we come to hold beliefs by manipulating knowledge in a far less clear and declarative manner. Second, we tend to express beliefs using a different mechanism. We tend to "believe" even when we do not have many facts available for coactivation. In fact, even on occasions in which we have relevant facts potentially available, we nonetheless shortcut to the concluding belief without coactivating the facts, let alone operating logically on them. When we are in the process of articulating a belief, we often cite no facts at all. The foundational facts for the belief, correct or incorrect, remain hidden. Our neural and cognitive systems allow us to jump to a conclusion or even to an action without relying on intervening cognitive steps.

Seen in this perspective, belief is a result of intuition, the ability to make elliptic shortcuts from a situation stimulus to a response. We should note, however, that we can have intuitions about anything whatsoever—and those intuitions can pertain to any aspect of whatever content we are considering in our intuitive process—but that is not quite so with belief. As we have noted, the domain for belief is constrained. Further, the aspect of the content about which one intuits in belief pertains to its truth value rather than to its essential factual constitution.

There is one other trait to mark the difference between general intuition and the intuition of the qualification that constitutes belief. Intuition is one among many general tools of the creative mind, and the intuited content can be used, discarded, or modified fluidly in the ongoing thought process. But in the intuited qualification that constitutes belief, the subsequent intellectual analysis is often suspended or slowed down. The intuited qualification dominates the cognitive landscape, with a distinctive emotional force and vehemence. It is in the nature of belief to accept the qualification of a fact—its existence, for instance—without the need for immediate proof, or for any proof. There is a weakening of the process that Marcia Johnson has described as "source monitoring," that is, the checking of the facts surrounding the provenance of the belief or the consequences of the datum believed to be true (see Chapter 2).

Perhaps a recent example will clarify my meaning. Many of us would probably agree that, taken out of context, some of the facts adduced by the Unabomber in his manifesto may be true. When we read the document in its entirety, however, we realize that each fact and each argument depends on a very small pool of information, and that once the author has expressed a belief—for instance, that technology is evil—no further information is analyzed. When it comes to the "source monitoring framework," the Unabomber's reasoning is rather weak. He has an inordinate emotional investment in the narrow pool of information on which he concentrates, and he fails to consider countervailing information. When we are confronted with the same basic ideas, we are able to conjure up balancing facts that tell us that while technological advances can have an adverse effect on society, they can also bring numerous benefits. Following the presentation of the first negative content, our management of the problem would be quite different.

Having said this, I must confess that I worry about the dividing line between the beliefs of sane individuals and the irrational beliefs of neurological and psychiatric patients. I suspect it is not as wide as one might wish. Many beliefs are by nature "arational," and many are downright irrational. Belief makes me think of a thought unexamined that is not worth having.

The Nonconscious Processing of Belief

The above comments on a possible mechanism of belief and the alignment of belief with the process of intuition underscore the partly nonconscious nature of the processing underlying belief. Although we hold and express beliefs about contents that are in clear consciousness, it is likely that the mechanisms which allow us to develop the basis for beliefs, as well as the mechanisms by which we retrieve and express them, are operated in a largely covert manner. Beliefs are held in implicit memory and are retrieved from it (see Schacter, 1996, for appropriate background).

What could be the mechanism, neurally speaking, behind the elliptic shortcut I have just described? I suspect that the development of the rapid ellipsis depends on an implicit memory of a particular nature, the kind of memory that bonds certain categories of facts and certain categories of internal biological states, including those that can be expressed in the form of an emotion and perceived as a feeling. In other words, I propose that beliefs rely on particular kinds of composite memories that hold a link between categories of fact and categories of internal state. I have proposed the existence of such memories in order to explain certain aspects of personal and social decisionmaking and I suspect that the world of belief requires those memories as well (Damasio, 1994).

When such implicit composite memories are activated, the result is the deployment of a number of bioregulatory responses. These can operate in an entirely nonconscious manner and act as biasing signals in a variety of neural structures, thus covertly affecting the process of reasoning. The responses can also produce an overt emotional state, which can be perceived as feeling. In either instance, by dint of covert bias or overt emotional response, the positive or negative homeostatic value embodied in the covert signal or the overt emotion helps to establish the qualification of the content under scrutiny in terms of the truth scale mentioned earlier.

In conclusion, I suggest that either covert bioregulatory signals or overt emotions play the role of qualifiers in the ongoing mental formulation process. I also assume that certain kinds of internal biological states have a positive value that is aligned with consonance and truth, or a negative value that is aligned with dissonance and falsity (and every possible pairing in between). The sense of truth, the sense of falsity, and the confidence invested in that sense are related to bioregulatory operations including, of course, those we know as emotions and feelings.

It is becoming clear that the brain is equipped with all sorts of systems that can help produce the implicit memories I am considering here, and that help deploy them by activating bioregulatory signals. A large collection of neural structures in the brain stem, hypothalamus, limbic system, prefrontal cortices, and somatosensory cortices is engaged in the production of such memories and in the enactment of the ensuing signals.

Approaching the Neurobiology of Belief

There are a number of possibilities for studying belief from a neurobiological point of view. Human studies using both functional neuroimaging in normal subjects and the lesion method in neurological patients offer fruitful approaches. Consider, for instance, the process I will go through if I am asked to recognize my wife. Not only do I conjure up factual information to the effect that she is who she is and that we are married, but I also coactivate a number of affective states, some of which I become aware of but most of which I probably do not, facts that pertain to my prior emotional experience in interacting with her.

In specific conditions of disease, nature can alter this process in a variety of ways. For instance, we know that certain brain lesions will prevent recollection of the factual data just alluded to, and that, as a result, recognition is effectively blocked. The condition in which that strange manifestation occurs is known as prosopagnosia, or face agnosia. If I were to become prosopagnosic, I would no longer be able to recognize my wife, although I would be able to recognize her as a woman and describe her face. I would have no recognition of her identity and I also would not have any belief relative to the truth or falsity of her identity. Were I told that she was my wife, I would have to accept the fact without a truth evaluation, confessing in so doing that although she was my wife I did not know that directly (Damasio, Tranel, and Damasio, 1990).

In the strange condition known as Capgras syndrome, we can find a virtual inversion of the prosopagnosic problem and search for possible clues on the underpinnings of belief. If I were struck by Capgras, I would look at my wife and say: "This is very interesting; this person looks exactly like my wife, or almost exactly like my wife, but I sense that she is not my wife. In fact, in all likelihood, she is an impostor posing as my wife. She just *looks like* my wife."

The recognition mechanisms impaired in prosopagnosia are clearly operational in the Capgras condition. The stimulus situation does manage to evoke the facts necessary for the recognition of identity. Yet something else is missing. Perhaps because of that something, the Capgras patient is given logical latitude to make the inference that the subject under scrutiny is an impostor and to state the inference in the form of a vehement belief.

The Capgras condition is useful in a variety of respects. It provides yet another example that facts alone are not all that memory allows. In addition, it suggests that something is amiss with either the covert or overt emotional accompaniment that I described as necessary for normal beliefs to occur. Intriguingly, a bit of evidence in favor of that possibility comes from studies which reveal that patients with Capgras fail to generate skin conductance responses to the faces of people whom they almost recognize but consider impostors (see Chapter 3). The finding is notable, in that we have shown that patients with prosopagnosia who fail to recognize familiar persons but who have no evidence of abnormal belief do indeed generate normal skin conductance responses to the faces they fail to recognize (see Tranel and Damasio, 1985). Skin conductance responses, incidentally, are just one index of activity in the bioregulatory machinery that underlies emotions.

Tantalizing as the finding is, we need a word of caution here. We have also shown that patients with ventromedial frontal lobe damage, who recognize unique persons perfectly well but who do not confabulate them as aliens or impostors, fail to generate skin conductance responses to those same well-recognized persons (Tranel and Damasio, 1995). They truly do not have an emotional response to those individuals, yet they recognize them normally. What this discrepancy probably means is that some additional mechanism needs to be discovered to give a comprehensive and satisfactory account of the problem in Capgras. Perhaps the lack of an emotional signal is not sufficient to explain Capgras, or perhaps there are so many different kinds and levels of emotionally related signals that impairment in one does not predict an impaired consequence consistently. Another way of refining the account is by invoking something that Chris Frith has brought forth nicely in his work: humans often construct original interpretations to cope with the misinformation available to them. In patients with certain kinds of brain damage or certain psychoses, that natural tendency probably contributes to the generation of irrational beliefs (see Chapter 4). From this point of view, the mere lack of an emotional signal would not be likely to lead anyone to believe that others are impostors. However, such a lack, combined with a peculiar way of coping with the misinformation that an "emotional absence" would constitute, might lead to an irrational formulation. The same argument applies to the equally irrational beliefs that patients with anosognosia profess so easily and that are so blatantly at odds with reality.

I hope that our understanding of the cognitive neuroscience of belief will make considerable progress as we advance our understanding of the underpinnings of memory, of emotion and feeling, and of the biological nature of the self. I see the last as especially critical. After all, the constrained domain in which we hold and express beliefs and the attribution that constitutes belief, is closely related to the notion of an *individual organism* and to the neural and mental representation of that individual organism, that is, to the *self*. We hold beliefs about things that matter to the self, and beliefs pertain to truth or falsity, attributions that are correlated with states of emotional concordance or discordance experienced by the self. Curiously, many patients who exhibit abnormalities of belief suffer from impairment of the representation of self, their self-representation being unstable or incomplete, as is patently the case in the condition known as anosognosia (Damasio, 1999).

References

Damasio, A. (1994). *Descartes' error: Emotion, reason, and the human brain,* New York: Putnam.

Damasio, A. (1999). *The feeling of what happens: Body and emotion in the making of consciousness.* New York: Harcourt Brace.

Damasio, A., Tranel, D., and Damasio, H. (1990). Face agnosia and the neural substrates of memory, *Annual Review of Neuroscience, 13,* 89–109.

Schacter, D. 1996. *Searching for memory.* New York: Basic Books.

Tranel, D., and Damasio, A. (1985). Knowledge without awareness: An autonomic index of facial recognition by prosopagnosics. *Science, 228* (21), 1452–54.

Tranel, D., and Damasio, A. (1995). Double dissociation between overt and covert face recognition. *Journal of Cognitive Neuroscience, 7,* 425–432.

Contributors

Mahzarin R. Banaji, Yale University, Department of Psychology, New Haven, Conn.

R. Bhaskar, Yale University, School of Management, New Haven, Conn., and Federal Trade Commission, Washington, D.C.

J. Alexander Bodkin, McLean Hospital, Belmont, Mass.

Sissela Bok, Harvard University, Harvard Center for Population and Development Studies, Cambridge, Mass.

Antonio R. Damasio, Department of Neurology, College of Medicine, University of Iowa, Ames, Iowa

Daniel C. Dennett, Center for Cognitive Studies, Tufts University, Medford, Mass.

Raymond J. Dolan, Institute of Neurology, University College, London, England

Paul John Eakin, Professor of English, Indiana University, Bloomington, Ind.

Howard Eichenbaum, Department of Psychology, Boston University, Boston, Mass.

Chris Frith, Institute of Neurology, University College, London, England

Marcia K. Johnson, Department of Psychology, Princeton University, Princeton, N.J.

Martin Lepage, Rotman Research Institute of Baycrest Centre, University of Toronto, Toronto, Canada

Katherine Nelson, Department of Developmental Psychology, Graduate School, City University of New York, New York, N.Y.

335

V. S. Ramachandran, Center for Brain and Cognition, University of California, San Diego, Calif.

Carol L. Raye, Department of Psychology, Princeton University, Princeton, N.J.

Michael Ross, Department of Psychology, University of Waterloo, Waterloo, Canada

Elaine Scarry, Department of English and American Literature and Language, Harvard University, Cambridge, Mass.

Daniel L. Schacter, Department of Psychology, Harvard University, Cambridge, Mass.

Endel Tulving, Rotman Research Institute of Baycrest Centre, University of Toronto, Toronto, Canada

Chris Westbury, Department of Psychology, University of Alberta, Alberta, Canada

Anne E. Wilson, Department of Psychology, University of Waterloo, Waterloo, Canada

Index